THE FIRST WHOLE REHAB CATALOG
A COMPREHENSIVE GUIDE TO PRODUCTS AND SERVICES
FOR THE PHYSICALLY DISADVANTAGED

THE FIRST WHOLE REHAB CATALOG

A COMPREHENSIVE GUIDE TO PRODUCTS AND SERVICES FOR THE PHYSICALLY DISADVANTAGED

A. Jay Abrams & Margaret Ann Abrams

BETTERWAY PUBLICATIONS, INC.
WHITE HALL, VIRGINIA

Published by Betterway Publications, Inc.
P.O. Box 219
Crozet, VA 22932
(804) 823-5661

Cover design by David Wagner
Typography by Park Lane Associates

Cover photos courtesy of: (Clockwise from left) Iron Horse Productions; "Un-Skru," Multi Marketing & Manufacturing, Inc.; "Recreation Belt," The Freehanderson Company; "Retaining Reacher," CME Medical Equipment Corporation; Touch Turner; "Stair-Tree," Garaventa (Canada) Ltd.

Library of Congress Cataloging-in-Publication Data

Abrams. A. Jay.
    The first whole rehab catalog : a comprehensive guide to products and services for the physically disadvantaged / A. Jay Abrams and Margaret Ann Abrams.
        p. cm.
        Includes bibliographical references.
        ISBN 1-55870-131-1 : $16.95
        1. Physically handicapped--United States--Equipment and supplies--Catalogs. 2. Physically handicapped--Services for--United States--Directories. I. Abrams, Margaret Ann. II. Title.
HD9995.H563U5422   1990
362.4'0483--dc20   89-29934
                                                                CIP

Printed in the United States of America
0 9 8 7 6 5 4 3 2 1

To Adam Abrams . . . a constant inspiration.

Acknowledgments

We take great pleasure in expressing our appreciation of those individuals who in many ways have supported the efforts that enabled us to produce *The First Whole Rehab Catalog*. Specific acknowledgment is made to Ruth Houska and Gloria Greenhill for their generous assistance in the preparation of this manuscript, and to our editor Hilary W. Swinson for her suggestions, constructive criticism, and encouraging interest. We would also like to express our gratitude to the many businesses and other organizations that are included in this work, for their courteous and helpful cooperation.

CONTENTS

Introduction

According to the "Digest of Data on Persons with Disabilities" provided by the National Institute of Handicapped Research, it is estimated that there are as many as 36 million non-institutionalized physically, intellectually, and/or perceptually challenged people living in the United States. And about 350,000 are added each year as a result of disease, and automotive and industrial accidents. This book was compiled as a basic tool for getting information about independent living aids and services to these consumers.

The First Whole Rehab Catalog can help you find out what commercial products are available, where and how to get them and, in many instances, what you can expect to pay for them. With the *Catalog*, you won't be tied to a few local sources and the hit-or-miss kind of information that is too often provided by caregivers. And you can actually comparison shop to find the products that most appropriately match your requirements.

We've divided the product listings into sections to make it easier to find what you're looking for and to expose you to related items that may not be familiar. The major categories include Home Management, Personal Care, Access, Communication, Mobility, Transportation, Health and Fitness, Recreation, Education and Vocation, Catalogs, and Books. The section on catalogs refers to commercial catalogs that contain a variety of products and are most often published by product distributors.

A surprisingly large number of the items described in this book were developed by consumers. Over the past several years, many enterprising people have created products and services to meet their own needs and alleviate their frustrations. These products and services are helping to reshape our perceptions of what is possible. On another front, technological advances in the field of rehabilitation engineering are rapidly changing both the capabilities and aesthetic characteristics of rehab products.

In certain respects, this *Catalog* is an "idea book." In addition to providing information about things you can buy, we hope that it stimulates your creativity. With access to the right materials and proper information, you might well find yourself thinking about finding new approaches to familiar problems.

The Appendix of the book offers an abundance of resources that can help you to keep informed and connected with others. We've included information about support groups, independent living centers, magazines and newsletters, accessible travel, protection and advocacy, legal resources, sports and recreation, and databases, as well as organizations of general interest.

Although we've made every effort to ensure that the information furnished in this book is accurate, up-to-date, and as complete as possible, the reality is that with a project of this kind omissions and changes are a fact of life. Should you have difficulty contacting any organization or business listed in this book, or if you haven't found the specific information you're looking for, or if you've used one or more of the aids or services that we've described and would like to share your impressions, please let us know. Our mailing address is: S.R. 12479 - Box 209, Phoenicia, NY 12464.

When it comes to ordering, keep in mind that every company has its own policies and procedures. We've tried our best to include only those firms that are willing and able to sell directly to consumers ("end users"). In many instances we've excluded prices, either due to the complexity of pricing a particular item, or the probability that the price will have changed by the time the book is in print. Prices given are expressed as ranges or approximate prices. We recommend that you contact companies directly for the most up-to-date cost information. Also, please realize that the information in this book is advisory in nature and is not offered as an endorsement, approval, or a certification of the products described.

To the companies and organizations that are represented in this work: should addresses, phone numbers, or other information prove to be incomplete or inaccurate, please let us know so that we can make the necessary changes in our files. With regard to those that have not been included, please accept our sincerest apology and our invitation to submit any information that you would like us to consider for inclusion in the next edition.

CHAPTER ONE

HOME MANAGEMENT

CLOTHING AND DRESSING

WHEELMATES

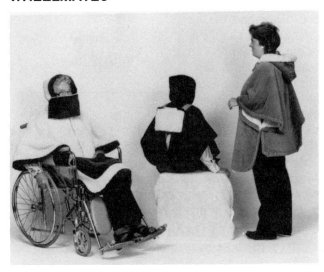

Wheelmates "Special Needs Ponchos" were designed to make life easier for wheelchair users. Styled for convenience, they may be put on before or after seating, and will not drag or catch on wheels. A practical inside front lap pocket is provided, and Velcro type fasteners ensure that "buttoning up" is fast and simple. The attached hood includes a single-string that makes retieing unnecessary once properly adjusted. Nose and face covers are optional, as are front corner loops —handy for securing poncho to wheelchair on windy days.

Special Needs Ponchos are also available for use with shoulder support straps and lap-boards, and for infants and young children "Cuddle Bug" Ponchos are offered.

Prices range from about $85.00 up.

VICKI WADE
611 E. Washington
Pittsfield, IL 62363
(217) 285-6520

****

COMFORT CLOTHING

The stylish Comfort Clothing line includes dresses, separates, lingerie, underwear, hosiery, night and loungewear. Four options in back design are offered: the "back wrap," for those who require a back-open garment but are ambulatory; the "center back-open," for the difficult to dress and for the incontinent, non-ambulatory individual; the "shoulder closure," for the individual requiring a completely open back; and the "yoke back," for the non-ambulatory incontinent individual who does not want Velcro. All Comfort Clothing garments are produced in easy care washable fabrics.

Yoke Back Dress

Great styling with contrast collar and tie, elastic belt. 100% polyester knit prints.

Sizes XXS, XS, S, M, L. Priced well under $100.00.

Open Back Separates

Open back T-shirt in poly/cotton blend, prints and solids. Closes at center back with Velcro tabs.

Sizes: XS, S, M, L, XL. Priced under $50.00.

Elastic back pants feature drop panel to facilitate toileting. Button and Velcro closures. 100% polyester knits. Sizes: XS, S, M, L, XL, XXL. Priced around $50.00.

COMFORT CLOTHING KINGSTON INC.
21 Harvey Street
Kingston, Ontario K7K 5C1
(613) 546-7716

****

IRWIN/TAYLOR

Irwin/Taylor is a company that designs career clothing, leisure wear, evening clothes, and undergarments for women with arthritis and other physical challenges.

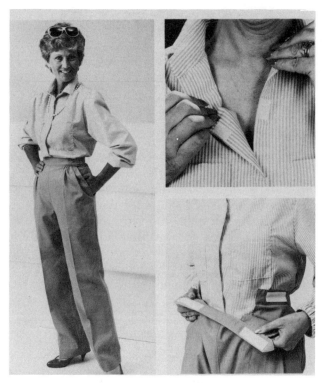

The idea grew out of a conversation Taylor had with Irwin at a dinner party. Taylor asked Irwin, a fashion designer, to design "easy-on" dresses for a friend. The dresses were so successful that Irwin and Taylor created a line of back opening apparel for women who use wheelchairs. Fourteen months into their business, Irwin and Taylor expanded their clothing line to include the more than 24 million active women with arthritis in the "dressing" joints of the body (fingers, wrists, shoulders, hips, and knees).

Dresses, jumpsuits, blouses, pants, skirts, lingerie, and accessories are all made with easy closures. With fashions by Irwin/Taylor there is never a need for pulling, hooking, tying, snapping, or buttoning!

Irwin/Taylor fashions enable physically challenged women to dress with ease. Difficult pulling, buttoning, and fastening are eliminated. Hidden Velcro closures, innovative design make fashions accessible.

IRWIN/TAYLOR
P.O. Box 10510
Rochester, NY 14610
(716) 381-4304

＊＊＊＊

"Flex-O-Lace"

Lace your shoes just once! At one end of the lacing is a flat, round piece of metal that holds the lacing intact in the bottom eyelet. The lacing goes through the remaining eyelets. At the other end of the lacing is the usual tip, behind which is an adjustable slide fastener that permanently secures the lacing

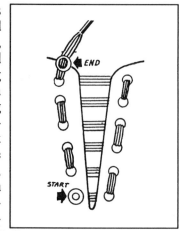

at the top eyelet. Thus the lacings can be adjusted to the wearer's comfort and the security of the shoe. The shoe can be removed or put on without untying or tying the laces, as the lacings are elastic. Moreover, because the lacings are stretchable they adjust comfortably with each step.

Laces come in black, brown, or white.

CECIL CORPORATION
P.O. Box 654
Evanston, IL 60204

＊＊＊＊

E-Z Shoe-On (U.S. Patent No. 4709839 and 3527492)

This convenience product lets you pick up, put on, or remove shoes, whether sitting (20") or standing (30"), without putting your feet on the floor. The 20" or 30" inch length helps you retrieve shoes from high shelves and under beds. The E-Z SHOE-ON is built to provide a lifetime of service. A combination of shoe horn, gripper and reacher, the trigger-action makes it fun and useful for people of all ages.

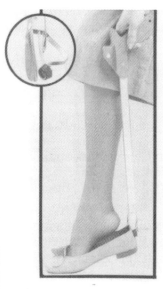

Weight 8 oz. Stem length 20 inches. About $25.00.

Weight 9 oz. Stem length 30 inches. Between $25.00 and $30.00.

ARCOA INDUSTRIES
888 Rancheros Drive
San Marcos, CA 92069
(800) 621-0852 Ext. 165

See CATALOGS for other Arcoa products.

****

ADAPTIVE FASHIONS

Adaptive Fashions designs custom garments for men and women that are fashionable as well as functional, using comfortable and attractive fabrics. Adaptive features include back openings, side openings, back cut-outs, catheter openings, Velcro front openings, and other special designs to help solve dressing problems.

Men's Slacks

Their front-flap slacks with a false fly are designed for the man with a catheter, or for easy urinal use while seated. The adjustable elastic back gives a good, secure fit, and simplifies dressing for the independent man. Priced well under $50.00.

ADAPTIVE FASHIONS, INC.
5641 Bartlett Blvd.
Mound, MN 55364

****

Sasa Sock and Shoe Aid

The Sasa sock and shoe aid can be used with just one hand since there are no clips or tapes to pull. A half-funnel shaped sleeve is inserted into the sock or stocking and the lock slid into place. After the foot has been inserted the lock holds the hosiery until it has been pulled entirely into place on foot and leg. The lock is then released and the aid removed. A shoehorn-type tip helps getting in or out of shoes or boots, and the tong-like gripper can be used as an aid in putting on clothing. The surfaces are smooth enough to handle fine hosiery and the gripper strong enough to hold a 10 lb. object. The gripper can even be used as a reacher to pick up small items. An added advantage is a polyester sponge mitt that fits over the end for use in bathing. The aid is molded out of strong ABS plastic and permanently snapped together. Weight is only 8 oz. Dimensions are 5" x 5 1/2" x 20 1/2" long. Shipping weight 1 lb.

Panty Hose Aid

The Panty Hose Aid consists of a double shaped plastic sheet rigid enough to keep panty hose legs open, but flexible enough to curl to form a channel for the foot. Three cloth tapes are attached to the plastic sheet by grommets, and also to elastic mounted garter clips. In use, the plastic forms are withdrawn from the panty hose legs after the foot is in place; the panty hose is then pulled up by the garter clips. The upper ends of the three tapes are attached to a plastic strap which keeps them in position and provides equal tension at three points.

MADDAK INC.
Pequannock, NJ 07440
(800) 443-4926

See CATALOGS for other Maddak products.

****

Clawson Rocker

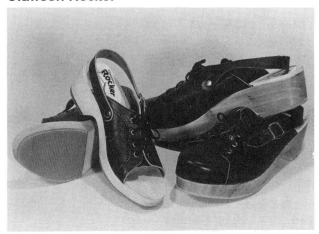

The Clawson Rocker is a therapeutic aid to ambulation. Thanks to a chance discovery by a person with multiple sclerosis, Mrs. Carolyn Clawson, the Clawson Rocker can act as a substitute for lost ankle/knee movement. This is done by means of a rigid sole with a special inner contour and bottom sole dimension which acts as a fulcrum point over which the body weight is distributed. Thus, for those with ankle or knee restriction, this unique shoe gives back a lost freedom in walking.

The Clawson Rocker shoe is not a panacea for all walking problems. Persons who have sensory loss, severe muscle weakness, or constant equilibrium imbalance will not benefit from this product. Also, this is not offered as a corrective shoe for foot problems.

To obtain the fullest benefit of the Clawson Rocker shoe, proper fitting is a must. Your local Clawson Rocker dealer is trained to correctly fit your shoe and to instruct you in proper use.

For further information, and/or to locate the Clawson Rocker dealer nearest you, contact:

NEW FREEDOM, INC.
P.O. Box 472
Rexburg, ID 83440
(208) 356-0061

∗∗∗∗

"SAY WHAT" Apparel Identification Marker

Specially designed for the visually impaired—to identify clothes on hangers. The reusable identifier fits wood, slack, and regular wire hangers. The sturdy plastic has a circular looped end and a 7/8" diameter opening. Tags are 1 1/2" wide by 5 3/4" long. "Say What" includes enough plastic strip to make 23 labels 1/2" wide by 3" long. Each kit has 10 tags and a roll of tape for brailling. Under $10.00.

Placket Sweatshirt

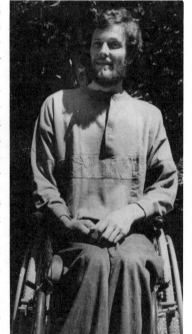

The placket sweatshirt features a Velcro neck closure and a wonderfully generous cut. Made of soft, comfortable 50% polyester, 50% cotton fleece, it sports a cotton woven inset on the front and a patch pocket with a Velcro closure. The cuffs and hipband have a knit rib trim. This sweatshirt comes in white, blue, or melon.

Adult sizes S, M, L, XL. Priced well under $50.00.

LAUREL DESIGNS
5 Laurel Ave., #9
Belvedere, CA 94920
(415) 435-1891

See CATALOGS for other Laurel products.

∗∗∗∗

Money Organizer Wallet

This practical organizer for the visually impaired has four separate compartments for one, five, ten, and twenty dollar bills so that folding of paper money is unnecessary. There are also four separate change purses for pennies, nickels, dimes, and quarters, and five slots for credit cards. An extra compartment is provided to hold slate, checkbook, signature guide, or charge slips. And there is a large toss-all purse for unsorted change, keys, etc. As an extra benefit, there is an expandable loop that's perfect for holding either pen or pencil-shaped stylus. Compact ... not much bigger than a small folding checkbook; wheat colored fabric with brown binding and Velcro closures. Under $25.00.

LS&S GROUP, INC.
P.O. Box 673
Northbrook, IL 60065
(800) 468-4789
(312) 498-9777 in Illinois

See CATALOGS for other LS&S Group products.

∗∗∗∗

DANMAR PRODUCTS

Danmar Products provides a wide range of proven equipment including headgear, swim aids, positioning aids, and custom products as requested.

Soft Shoe

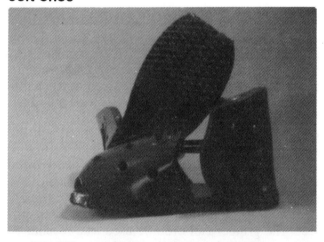

Combine cushiony comfort, easy access, and hand washability with a lightweight, ventilated shoe and you have Danmar's popular Soft Shoe.

1/2" thick, shock absorbent foam is vinyl coated and given a tread sole for easy maintenance and long life. So welcome to the foot that is sensitive or requires uniquely shaped footwear. Available in custom sizes and colors. We recommend wearing them with cotton socks. Shoelaces included.

Sizes S, M, L, XL. Priced well under $100.00.

DANMAR PRODUCTS, INC.
221 Jackson Industrial Drive
Ann Arbor, MI 48103
(313) 761-1990

See CATALOGS for other Danmar products.

✳✳✳✳

"Touch-Time"

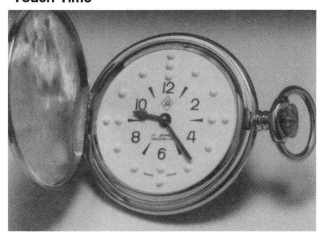

The men's "Touch-Time" quartz pocket watch is battery operated, very accurate, and because there are few internal parts it's less likely to need repair than a wind-up watch. Handsome brushed gold finish, with gold face, black numerals and hands, and raised dots so you can read it without looking at it. No winding needed. Over $50.00.

Timex Easy-reader—Women's Quartz Watch

An easy to read large face watch that's water resistant. Specifically styled for a woman. Quartz accuracy with a genuine Quinn band imported from England. Three year battery included. One year limited warranty. Well under $50.00.

Talking Wristwatch

LCD printout supplemented by a talking function. This handsome watch not only tells the time, but can also be used as a timer and can be set as an alarm to wake you, remind you of an appointment, etc. Batteries included. Under $50.00.

INDEPENDENT LIVING AIDS, INC.
27 East Mall
Plainview, NY 11803
(516) 752-8080

See CATALOGS for other products offered by Independent Living Aids.

✳✳✳✳

THE COMFORT COLLECTION

The Comfort Collection by Salk is a complete line of quality home care apparel, designed exclusively for the person convalescing at home. All Comfort Collection clothing and accessories offer superior comfort and convenience combined with an exceptional range of choice in style, color, and fabric.

The Winter Warm Laprobe—With Leg Pouch and Hand Pocket

This multi-function Laprobe with leg pouch is designed to provide extra warmth and convenience for the person confined to a wheelchair or an ordinary chair for most of the day. Made of insulated Vellux (by West Point Pepperell) it provides maximum warmth during travel or while sitting outdoors for a breath of fresh air. The ample leg pouch (a Salk exclusive) completely encloses the wearer's legs for warmth and comfort. The Laprobe may be self-tied around the waist or tied to chair arms to prevent slippage. The outdoor Laprobe comes with the added benefit of a special pocket with side openings for the patient's hands. An absolute must for mobile persons, the Laprobe is a great traveler and washes beautifully. Priced under $25.00.

THE SALK COMPANY, INC.
119 Braintree Street, P.O. Box 452
Boston, MA 02134
(800) 343-4497
(617) 782-4030

✳✳✳✳

Hemiplegia Shoe Horn

Swiveling enables the Hemiplegia Shoe Horn to be easily inserted into the back of a shoe. When handles are aligned, a holding disc moves under the outside back of the heel forming a clamp that holds the shoe in place. The user is then able to put on the shoe without it moving away. Shipping weight 2 lbs.

CLEO, INC.
3957 Mayfield Road
Cleveland, OH 44121
(800) 321-0595

See CATALOGS for other things by Cleo, Inc.

****

Apron Hoop

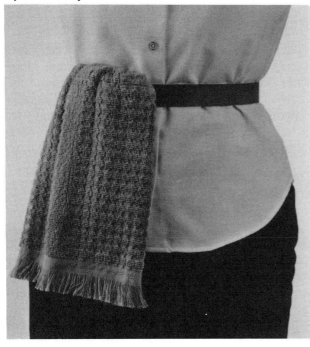

The Swedish Rehab Apron Hoop is a convenience with a number of practical applications. After the plastic hoop has been opened and placed around the waist it springs back to hold pants, apron, or skirt snugly in place.

LUMEX/SWEDISH REHAB
100 Spence Street
Bay Shore, NY 11706
(800) 645-5272

See CATALOGS for other Lumex/Swedish Rehab products.

****

AMERICAN FOUNDATION FOR THE BLIND

The American Foundation for the Blind makes a wide variety of tactual watches available. The covers open and time is determined by the location of the sturdy hands in relation to raised dots at each hour. All dials have three raised dots at 12:00, two raised dots at 3:00, 6:00, and 9:00, and a single raised dot at each other hour. The majority of watches that open at the 6:00 position are thumb operated. Button opened watches have spring-loaded hinges located at 3:00 unless otherwise specified.

All watches are made in Switzerland, and come with expansion bands or leather straps. There is a good selection of quartz, manually wound, and self-winding models.

Before a watch is shipped, it is thoroughly checked and tested for accuracy. All parts are guaranteed against defects in materials and workmanship for a period providing the watch has received normal use and been given adequate care.

Aluminum Clothing Tags

Brailled multi-colored identification tags, with holes at each end for sewing into garments, are distributed by the American Foundation for the Blind through the generosity of the Telephone Pioneers of America.

They are offered at no charge when ordered along with other items from the Foundation's catalog. The price to order them separately is $2.00.

AMERICAN FOUNDATION FOR THE BLIND
Consumer Products
15 West 16th Street
New York, NY 10011
(212) 620-2000

****

Jumpsuit

This all-purpose jumpsuit has been designed for versatility and comfort. It can be worn at any hour, in any season, alone or paired with other garments. It has a long front zipper and comfortable knit rib at the wrist and ankle. A double layer of fabric reinforces the knee area at the front and back. Priced well under $50.00 with additional charges for options.

Options:
• Move zipper to back
• Add gastrostomy tube access
• Add adjustable elastic waist
• Add full snap crotch
• Add 4 buttons to fasten bib
• Attach foot covers

Culotte Dress

This loose fitting Culotte Dress has a dropped waist, and can be worn alone or paired with a shirt or bodysuit. Try it for winter wear over a long sleeved jumpsuit, or button an appliqued bib to the front for a completely different look. Double buttons at the shoulder allow for size adjustment. The left side opens the full length of the garment and fastens with snaps for ease in dressing. Full snap crotch. Priced under $25.00.

Options:
• Replace snaps w/ Velcro
• Add gastrostomy tube access

Overalls

These roomy overalls are very comfortable and practical. The front panel opens to hip level and fastens at the waistband with Velcro. Soft pleats and a false fly front add to the appeal. Double buttons at the shoulder make it possible for this garment to "grow" with your child. The knee and seat areas are reinforced with a double layer of fabric for extra wear, and deep hems make an attractive finished cuff if the bottoms are turned up. Priced well under $50.00 with additional charges for some options.

Options:
• Add wrist loops
• Replace Velcro w/ buttons
• Add full snap crotch

For these items as well as the many other beau-tiful, functional garments that can be found in the Special Clothes line, you can use your imagination as you select fabric and style options to customize your choice. They also offer outerwear, swimwear, underwear, bibs, and accessories.

SPECIAL CLOTHES
P.O. Box 4220
Alexandria, VA 22303
(703) 683-7343

✳✳✳✳

OTHER SOURCES OF CLOTHING AND DRESSING AIDS:

ABBEY MEDICAL
ALIMED INC.
CONSUMER CARE PRODUCTS
J.A. PRESTON CORPORATION
KAYE'S KIDS
ST. LOUIS OSTOMY AND MEDICAL SUPPLY
THERAFIN CORPORATION

For additional information, including addresses and phone numbers, see CATALOGS.

FOOD PREPARATION

Un-Skru Jar & Bottle Opener

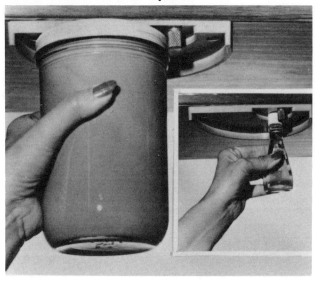

The Un-Skru is not a gadget, but a top-quality, lifetime kitchen tool. Molded of ABS plastic, with a case-hardened serrated steel gripper, this rugged jar opener comes with a 5-year guarantee. It offers the advantage of eliminating the strain to finger and wrist joints that typically accompanies the twisting motion of jar opening and is of particular benefit to older people who may no longer have the strength in their hands to hold a jar firmly with one hand while operating an opener with the other.

The Un-Skru is out of the way, out of sight, yet always ready when needed. It can be attached permanently to the underside of any table, counter, cabinet, shelf, or bar. And it can open any size screw lid from 1/2" to 5"—from a toothpaste tube to a gallon jar—with no adjustments. It has no moving parts to jam, and nothing to take apart, wash, or lose. Priced under $10.00.

MULTI MARKETING & MFG., INC.
P.O. Box 896
Cedaredge, CO 81413
(303) 856-3170

✳✳✳✳

Honeywell Lo-Vision Thermostat

Enlarged raised numbers indicate temperature range for easy recognition by touch or sight. A "click" is heard and indent is felt for every two degrees of dial movement. Enlarged temperature dial and indicator arrow. Replaces virtually all 24 volt thermostats. Comes with complete installation instructions, large print Users Hang Tag, and Braille card. Priced well under $50.00.

"Say When" Liquid Level Indicator

"Say When" is a compact electronic device that hangs over the lip of a cup, glass, or other container. It buzzes and vibrates when liquid nears the top. Useful for blind and deaf-blind persons at home, restaurants, vending stand operations, and in other applications. Comes ready to use with long-life, standard replaceable 9 volt battery. "Say When" is a blind-made product. Priced around $15.00.

AMERICAN FOUNDATION FOR THE BLIND
Consumer Products
15 West 16th Street
New York, NY 10011
(212) 620-2000

See CATALOGS for other aids offered by the American Foundation for the Blind.

✳✳✳✳

Cutting and Slicing Knife

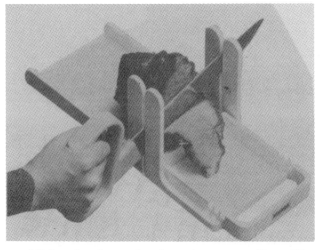

Make simple work of cutting even slices. The cutting aid is molded of smooth, strong, ABS plastic. Frame guides assure straight, even slices from 1/16" to 1" thick. The slicing knife features a molded polypropylene saw-type handle for comfort and better use of hand strength. The 9" long Swedish steel blade is tapered from 1 3/8" wide to a pointed end and is serrated along its length for improved cutting. Cutting aid and knife are sold separately and priced between $15.00 and $25.00 each.

Braille Kitchen Scale

Ideal for household weighing of all kinds. Excellent quality, with double post construction for accuracy and durability. 6 1/4" inch dial is slanted to make the large numbers easier to read. Raised dots at each 1/4 pound, double raised dots at each whole pound, and triple raised dots at each 5 pounds. Weighs up to 25 pounds by ounces; platform is 6" square. Base size 8 1/2" x 6 3/4". White and gray steel dial with baked enamel finish. One year warranty. Under $25.00.

LS&S GROUP, INC.
P.O. Box 673
Northbrook, IL 60065
(800) 468-4789
(312) 498-9777 in Illinois

See CATALOGS for other aids offered by LS&S.

****

Milk Carton Holder

Allows you to hold a standard square milk carton easily with one hand. Slips over the top of the carton for a secure grip. The handle snaps on or off to conserve space in the refrigerator. Durable dishwasher proof plastic. Under $5.00.

Box Topper

Don't struggle with cereal boxes, detergent boxes, any sealed box. This molded plastic blade quickly slices through any box, and the sponge rubber grip makes it easy to use. Under $5.00.

Slit-A-Bag

Now that so many foods are packaged in tough plastic bags to retain freshness, the "Slit-A-Bag" is as much a necessity as a can opener. Its sharp prong is easily pushed into the bag, and then pulled, opening the bag as it moves. Very inexpensive.

CAN-DO PRODUCTS
Independent Living Aids, Inc.
27 East Mall
Plainview, NY 11803
(800) 537-2118

See CATALOGS for other aids offered by Can-Do Products.

****

Contour Tap Turner

The Contour Tap Turner is a multi-purpose tool for turning taps, knobs, keys, etc. When pressed against an object the spring-loaded metal pins help provide an improved grip for a person with weak hands. Handle length 4". Priced around $15.00.

Cheese Slicer

The Cheese Slicer has a solid angled handle which makes cutting work easier for people with energy and/or movement impairment of the hand and arm. The thickness of the slices can be adjusted by changing the angle of the cutting tool. The handle is made of plastic and the cutting tool of stainless steel. Dishwasher safe. Priced under $20.00.

Suction Grater

The Suction Grater was designed to be held securely in place by suction feet. Perfect for the one-handed user, it comes with one reversible plastic grating plate. A bin holds grated food for easy use and convenient cleanup. Priced under $15.00.

CLEO INC.
3957 Mayfield Road
Cleveland, OH 44121
(800) 321-0595

See CATALOGS for other aids offered by Cleo.

****

Hemi Can Opener

This useful can opener was designed with the one-handed operator in mind. A lever snaps the cutting blade into position; turning the handle easily removes the lid. Made of lightweight durable plastic with a cutting blade that will stay sharp for cutting can after can.

Wash Up Brush

A simple household convenience, this brush features a tube clamp that readily attaches it to faucets, making scouring and cleaning utensils far less troublesome.

Tongs

Available in four variations, these practical tools have seemingly endless applications. All feature soft spring-loaded, self-opening handles with non-breakable, reversible nylon spring bands.

Item:

100400 (Kitchen Tongs with straight handles)

100330 (Kitchen Tongs with loop handles)

100340 (Spatula Tongs, featuring a spatula on one side)

100630 (Turner Tongs, featuring two spatulas instead of tongs)

LUMEX

Division of Lumex, Inc.

100 Spence Street

Bay Shore, NY 11706

(800) 645-5272

See CATALOGS for additional aids offered by Lumex.

****

Electronic Kitchen Timer

This pocket-size, battery operated unit times from 99 minutes down to one second. Conveniently equipped with a handy clip, magnet, stand, and hanging hole, it has an LCD display, and a loud electronic tone that signals when time is up. Perfect for the visually impaired individual, the timer can be easily set with buttons arranged in three rows. A 1 1/2 volt G 13 button battery and casette instructions are included. Priced around $15.00.

Pot Watcher

This device, shaped like a drink coaster, will prevent liquids from boiling over in a pot. Made of heat resistant glass, it is about 3" in diameter. Simply place it in the bottom of a pot and it will keep watch, making a rattling sound when liquid is boiling. Very inexpensive.

OPTION CENTRAL

1604 Carroll Avenue

Green Bay, WI 54304

(414) 498-9699

See CATALOGS for other aids offered by Option Central.

****

Maddatap

The Maddatap permits the intermittent use of water from a standard tap without shutting off or turning on the valves each time. The Maddatap screws onto the end of the faucet (where a filter is normally attached). The water is then turned on but will not run out of the faucet until the slim plastic rod hanging down from the spout is pushed. The rod can be gently pushed with a cup, bottle, or by hand to obtain water flow from the faucet. As soon as the container is removed, the water stops. The Maddatap has the advantage of being operated with one hand in a simple motion. It also saves water because the stream stops immediately when the pressure against the plastic rod is released. The Maddatap is adaptable to faucet ends having internal or external threads. The plastic rod hangs down only 3 3/4".

Kettle Tilter

The Maddak Kettle Tilter is adjustable and adaptable to any water or tea kettle from 6 1/4" to 8" in diameter. This household convenience is ideal for use by the geriatric population and individuals with weak wrists or tremors who find an unaided kettle difficult to handle. The tilter takes the pressure off the user's hand, arms, and shoulders when pouring hot liquids. It is simply operated by applying gentle pressure to the kettle's handle or to the wooden post at the rear of the platform. The tilting platform moves easily but is restrained by tension coil springs that control its movement and return it to the back-tilt rest position. The base is supported on four skid-proof rubber pads. The base and the platform are both epoxy coated steel. Posts, made of wood, are adjustable for the size of the kettle.

Double Claw Peeling Machine

This hand operated peeling machine grips potatoes, oranges, lemons, apples, pears, etc. between two plastic claws that rotate. A crank handle at one side turns the gripping claw and rotates the item being peeled against a U-shaped blade that follows the contour of the item, peeling it evenly. The peeling blade is adjustable for peel thickness. The cast metal frame must be clamped to a table or board using the screw clamp supplied. Open space between grips is adjustable from zero to 3 5/8". Center to frame gap radius is 2 1/4". Overall length is 10 1/2", shipping weight 2 1/4 pounds.

MADDAK INC.

Pequannock, NJ 07440-1993

(800) 443-4926

(201) 694-0500

See CATALOGS for additional aids offered by Maddak.

****

Fold Away Cart

The Fold Away Cart is particularly useful for transporting objects safely while walking. Unhampered movement is facilitated by easy glide casters. The cart folds flat for storage. Carrying surfaces measure 25 1/2" by 16 1/2". Height 29". Priced under $50.00.

ALIMED INC.
297 High Street
Dedham, MA 02026-2839
(800) 225-2610
(617) 329-2900

See CATALOGS for other aids offered by AliMed.

✳✳✳✳

OTHER SOURCES OF FOOD PREPARATION AIDS:

J.A. PRESTON CORPORATION
THERAFIN CORPORATION

For additional information, including addresses and phone numbers, see CATALOGS.

SLEEPING

Daniel Ortho Bed Lift

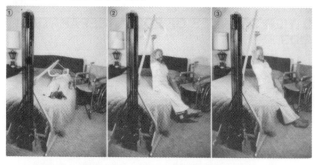

The Daniel Ortho Bed Lift is efficient and easy to use. A slight squeeze on a hand-held or clip-on remote button smoothly lowers a handlebar to the right height for your grasp. Then, holding the bar and with a touch on the handle-mounted remote button, you are gently lifted forward and upward to a sitting position.

The caster-mounted lift can be moved and positioned with ease and can be adjusted quickly to individual requirements without using tools. Its clean simple design allows it to fit conveniently under the foot of the bed. The room's wall socket is the economical power source. A remote control permits a variety of ortho tasks such as position-holding. An automatic light with a 4 1/2 minute delay provides safe, convenient middle-of-the night use.

RADCO
9859 N. 110th Avenue
Sun City, AZ 85351
(602) 933-7337

****

Airmate Deluxe Air Support Bed Pad

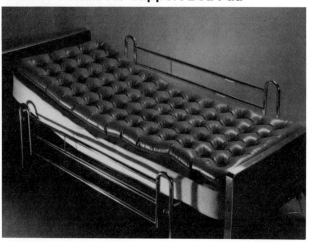

The AirMate is an inexpensive, reuseable, washable, fire retardant air mattress that needs no continuously operating air pump and comes with a six month warranty. It provides support on a cushioned network of over 100 air-filled convoluted cells that redistribute your weight and reduce pressure.

AirMate is easy to inflate with the free valve adapter and your own inflator or canister-type vacuum cleaner. An optional AirMate Air Inflator is also available. Under $50.00.

Multi-Part Decubitus Care Flotation Mattress

This Spinal Tech flotation system includes a patented water or gel flotation mattress proven effective against decubitus ulcers in two published hospital studies. Unlike one-piece type flotation mattresses, it is made up of seven separate components which together make it easy to fill or drain and use on a daily basis.

The system consists of an air frame-safety liner, three separate baffled water chambers in addition to its own special insulation pad, incontinence cover, and buoyancy pad. They form a sophisticated, yet very economical, lightweight flotation mattress which, if placed on top of an adjustable hospital bed mattress, can be elevated to any angle or position without the water pooling. Priced around $150.00.

SPINAL TECHNOLOGIES
859 Route 130
East Windsor, NJ 08520
(800) 257-5145
(609) 443-8083

****

Stop-Leak Gel Flotation Mattress

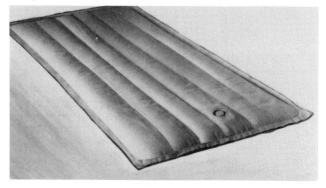

The Stop-Leak Gel Flotation Mattress provides the benefits of flotation support and pressure distribution without the risk of messy leaks. Made from a formulation of vinyl and nylon that was developed to prevent small repairable punctures from becoming large holes, the mattress is light enough so that it can be easily installed on top of any hospital bed mattress. Should it ever be accidentally punctured, a permanent repair can be made instantly with the repair kit provided. Priced under $75.00.

Econo-Float II—Water Flotation Mattress

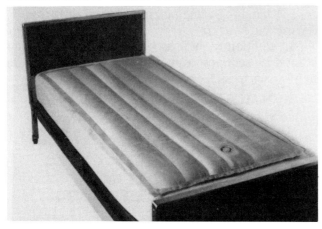

By utilizing the principles of flotation and displacement, the Econo-Float II reduces and distributes pressure. It offers full body flotation support while its internal baffles reduce water motion. It is simple and lightweight and can be ready to use in as little as ten minutes. A built-in fill level indicator is provided, and there is only one wide-mouth, screw-on-type valve to fill. The Econo-Float II is rugged and comes with a twelve month warranty. Under $50.00.

JEFFERSON INDUSTRIES
205 Nassau Street
Princeton, NJ 08540
(800) 257-5145
(609) 924-2040

✳✳✳✳

Wal-Pil-O Cervical Pillow

The Wal-Pil-O "4-in-1" cervical pillow relaxes muscles while correctly aligning the head and neck. Its applications include: headaches, neck and shoulder pains, whiplash injuries, arthritis related disorders, strains and sprains, pinched nerves, TMJ Syndrome, and tight muscles. The firm narrow/wide borders plus soft and medium center sections provide four combinations of comfortable head and neck support. With the pillow, the natural weight of the head serves as gentle traction to stretch, and

thereby relax, irritated muscles and ligaments whether the user sleeps on his or her side or back. Four models are available to accommodate children and adults, whether at home or traveling.

Good 'N Bed™ Support Products

Good 'n Bed™ support products offer a complete line of Hi-Tech Marsh-Mello Plus™ Foam including an adjustable wedge, a roll, a body pillow, and a neck pillow. The non-allergenic lavender foam is sculptured into rows of puffs to distribute the body's weight effectively. The "hills and valleys" increase air circulation, while reducing pressure, heat, and moisture build-up.

ROLOKE CO.
5760 Hannum Avenue
Culver City, CA 90230
(213) 649-1807

✳✳✳✳

Para-Quad™ Bed

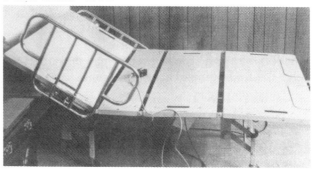

The Para-Quad™ Bed includes many features which previously were not available in combination from a single manufacturer. Its steel deck provides even weight distribution and firm support for the orthopedic multi-density foam mattress (approved by V.A.). Deluxe hand controls facilitate full electric operation (dual controls for king and queen size units). The height range of the deck is from 13 3/4" to 22 1/4". Half length safety side rails are provided. The bed is available in standard and custom sizes. Prices range from approximately $2500.00 to $5000.00.

CHERRY HILL MEDICAL, INC.
815 Hylton Road, Suite 9
Pennsauken, NJ 08110
(800) 238-8181
(609) 663-5677

✳✳✳✳

Jobst™ Hydro-Float™ Flotation Pad

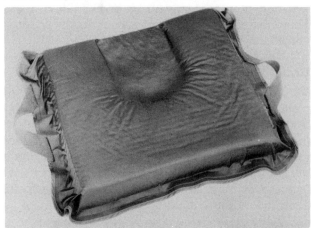

The Jobst™ Hydro-Float™ Flotation Pad reduces pressure on tissue over ischium and coccyx, yet permits easy transfer to and from a wheelchair. Both hydrostatic and mechanical buoyancy principles are combined in the pad, a permanently sealed unit covered with heavy-duty, thin nylon fabric.

Under normal care and use the pad will not crack, split, or develop pin holes. The pad also finds efficient application in the bed when used in conjunction with a 2" foam leveling pad cutout to receive the flotation pad at critical points.

JOBST™ INSTITUTE, INC.
Box 653
Toledo, OH 43694
(419) 698-1611

****

"Bye Bye Decubiti" Air Mattress OverLays

"Bye Bye Decubiti" Air Mattress Overlays convert any bed into a flotation unit when used between the conventional mattress and pad. Fabricated from heavy-gauge rubber, five separate inflatable sections are held together in a strong pocketed cover of soft fleece and velour material. Made in two sizes to fit either of the standard hospital beds, the unit will conform to any head or leg positioning. It may be folded zig-zag or rolled up for ease in handling while making the bed or for transferring and storage.

In addition to their use in the mattress unit, the inflatable sections may be used individually as pelvic pads in bed, or on easy chair, sofa, etc.

KEN MCRIGHT SUPPLIES, INC.
7456 South Oswego
Tulsa, OK 74136

****

OTHER SOURCES OF SLEEPING AIDS:

ALIMED INC.
CLEO INC.
DANMAR PRODUCTS
J.A. PRESTON CORPORATION
LUMEX
MADDAK, INC.
ST. LOUIS OSTOMY AND MEDICAL SUPPLY

For additional information, including addresses and phone numbers, see CATALOGS.

HOUSEKEEPING

Retaining Reacher

CME offers a number of lightweight, versatile reachers. The Retaining Reacher measures 32 1/2" in overall length and weighs only 8 ounces. It offers a modified trigger mechanism for people with limited hand dexterity that will delicately but firmly hold objects. It enables the use of either one or both hands for lifting. Folding and clip-on models are also available.

CME MEDICAL EQUIPMENT
CORPORATION
1130 Donamy Glen
Scotch Plains, NJ 07076
(201) 561-0906

✳✳✳✳

The Mailhawk

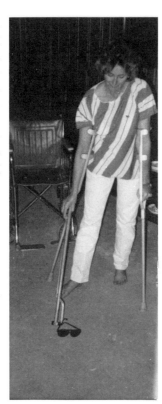

The Mailhawk tool features a good feeling wooden handle and spring operated aluminum jaws. Sensitive tapered plastic jaws facilitate picking up small objects. Three convenient lengths are available, measuring 20", 28", and 42". Ruggedly contructed, the Mailhawk was designed for daily use by rural mail carriers. Priced under $15.00.

MAILHAWK
MFG. COMPANY
P.O. Box 445
Warm Springs, GA
31830
(404) 655-3849

✳✳✳✳

Environmental Controls

A versatile environmental control unit which can serve as a simple five function scanner and controller or can be set up to control many additional functions. It has a built-in ultrasonic receiver for remote operation from a wheelchair or bed, and can be used with a variety of accessories, for: placing and receiving phone calls, unlocking doors, controlling TVs, operating call bells, and more. Priced around $1500.00.

JAMES (from FST, Switzerland) is a trainable infrared transmitter capable of replacing most infrared remote control units. By placing James in front of the remote control unit you wish to copy and executing a few manipulations, the new functions are instantly registered. James can be used to operate the Encoscan 4010 and other Tash products that have built-in receivers. Priced around $800.00.

TASH, INC.
Technical Aids & Systems for the Handicapped
70 Gibson Drive, Unit 12
Markham, Ontario L3R 4C2
(416) 475-2212

See CATALOGS for other products offered by Tash, Inc.

✳✳✳✳

Deuce

Du-It makes an impressively powerful, fully mobile distributed ECU system called MECCA. It controls telephone, ECU accessories like page turners, and the X10 remote control system which allows you to control lamps and appliances all around your home, and all this from your powered wheelchair by radio remote control. But let's face it, some people don't want that much environmental control. And some can't afford it.

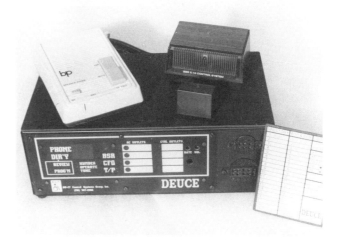

For under $1000, DEUCE controls a standard or speaker phone, up to eight ECU accessories, and an X10 remote control system. A full-scale system costs under $1500.

SRC Scanning Remote Control

The SRC is an infrared remote control unit designed to take the place of hand held, finger-operated controls. It can function as one giant remote control or two smaller ones and can be custom programmed by Du-It to control your equipment, from either a single or double switch. Priced around $400.00.

DU-IT CONTROL SYSTEMS GROUP
8765 TR 513
Shreve, OH 44676
(216) 567-2906

See CATALOGS for other products offered by Du-It Control Systems.

****

OTHER SOURCES OF HOUSEKEEPING AIDS:

ACCESS TO RECREATION, INC.
ADAPTIVE PRODUCTS INCORPORATED
ALIMED INC.
AMERICAN FOUNDATION FOR THE BLIND
ARCOA INDUSTRIES
CLEO INC.
J.A. PRESTON CORPORATION
J.T. POSEY CO., INC.
LAUREL DESIGNS
LS&S GROUP, INC.
LUMEX
MADDAK, INC.
RADIO SHACK
ST. LOUIS OSTOMY AND MEDICAL SUPPLY

For additional information, including addresses and phone numbers, see CATALOGS.

HOUSEHOLD FURNISHINGS

Upright Standing Frame

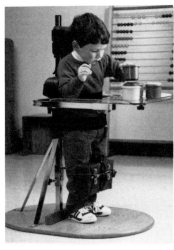

The Ortho-Kinetics Upright Standing Frame is designed for children up to 50" in height (minimum height 23") with mild to moderate levels of neuromuscular involvement. This fully adjustable standing system is ideal for home or educational settings, providing a secure upright standing posture and putting the child at peer level.

All framework and adjusting hardware is conveniently located to the rear for easier placement, handling, and assessment. Adjustments can be made quickly, without tools. (Not recommended for user under one year of age.)

Dynamic Posture Chair

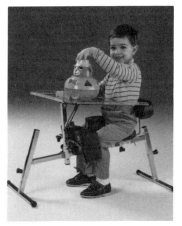

The Dynamic Posture Chair has been designed to provide optimum posture and control of the trunk and lower extremities for children with mild to moderate motor involvement due to conditions such as Cerebral Palsy. This sturdy yet portable chair is easily adjustable from child to child. Features include an adjustable angled seat to allow for proper positioning of the pelvis and lumbar spine; a pommel to minimize sliding forward; adjustable lumbar/pelvic ring to provide support and prevent excessive lateral or posterior movement; and removable knee pads. An optional upper extremity support tray is also available.

Other Ortho-Kinetics products include: adaptive commode/shower chair, PONY II, battery-powered three-wheeler; and care and travel chairs.

ORTHO-KINETICS, INC.
W220 N507 Springdale Road
P.O. Box 1647
Waukesha, WI 53187
(800) 558-7786
(800) 522-0992 in Wisconsin

＊＊＊＊

Assist-A-Lift

The Assist-A-Lift is a moderately priced chair offering a variety of features. Operated by a single switch that's always in easy reach, the entire chair raises slowly and steadily to bring the user to a standing position. The back can be removed without tools for transporting or cleaning.

Assist-A-Lift chairs are available in 12 designer colors and three fabrics, are Medicare approved, and are covered by a one-year limited warranty.

ACTION ENGINEERING, INC.
1689 N. Topping Avenue
Kansas City, MO 64120
(800) 247-7344
(816) 241-7344

＊＊＊＊

Easy Kneeler Stool

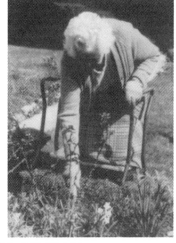

A practical aid for kneeling or sitting, the Easy Kneeler Stool can make many gardening tasks far more comfortable. The frame is constructed of steel with a stove enamel finish. The kneeler board is made of wood. Cartoned for easy home assembly.

CORRIE OF PETERSFIELD
J.B. CORRIE & CO. LIMITED
Petersfield, Hants GU32 3AP, England

＊＊＊＊

Bean Bag

Now becoming more and more widely used in schools and day centers, Bean Bags are also very useful in the home. Filled with tiny polystyrene beads, which shape to the body making it extremely comfortable, it is an acceptable form of seating for most members of the household. The PVC cover is easily wiped clean.

> NEWTON WHEELCHAIRS U.S.A.
> 21209 Lago Circle, 12 E
> Boca Raton, FL 33433
> (407) 483-7184

✳✳✳✳

OTHER SOURCES OF HOUSEHOLD FURNISHINGS:

ABBEY MEDICAL
ACCESS TO RECREATION, INC.
ADAPTIVE PRODUCTS
ALIMED INC.
ARCOA INDUSTRIES
CLEO INC.
CONSUMER CARE PRODUCTS
FLAGHOUSE, INC.
J.A. PRESTON CORPORATION
KAYE PRODUCTS INC.
KAYE'S KIDS
LS&S GROUP, INC.
LUMEX
MADDAK, INC.
RIFTON
WINCO INCORPORATED

For additional information, including addresses and phone numbers, see CATALOGS.

PERSONAL CARE

EATING, FEEDING, AND DRINKING

ALTERNATE STONEWARE

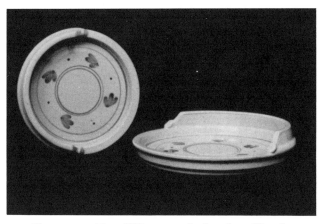

Georzetta Ratcliffe was admitted to Charleston General Hospital in West Virginia with a broken neck, a damaged spinal cord, several dislocated vertebrae, collapsed lungs, and a massive head injury.

In the summer of 1976 at the age of eighteen, she began a new life.

A quadriplegic for twelve years, today she is President of Alternate Stoneware, a company that designs and markets a unique line of stoneware plates.

An alternative to institutional-looking dinnerware, Alternate Stoneware adds a fresh, new look to the dinner table. Each piece is beautifully handcrafted and glazed. And because stoneware is fired at very high temperatures, it is more durable. Made of the finest natural clays, Alternate Stoneware is both aesthetically appealing and functional. The plates are designed to enhance the whole eating experience. A partially raised outer edge enables you to scoop food onto a fork or spoon with only a slight upper limb motion. Alternate Stoneware is stackable, chip resistant, ovenproof, microwaveable, refrigerator safe, and retains both heat and cold. Available in four designs, it can be purchased by the piece or in complete forty-two piece settings.

Additional matching stoneware pieces can be purchased for handicapped and non-handicapped family members. Brochures are available in both color and black and white. There is a $2.00 charge for the full color brochure.

Plates are priced well under $50.00 each.

ALTERNATE STONEWARE
P.O. Box 2071
Charleston, WV 25327-2071
(304) 346-4440

✱✱✱✱

The Winsford Feeder

The Winsford Feeder is designed for those who are able to sit in an upright position and have reasonable control of their head motion. While most food can be eaten with the feeder some, such as meat, spaghetti, or salad, must be cut to fit on the teaspoon.

The feeder's attractive appearance, its use of a normal dish and spoon, and its several means of control combine to provide ease of operation and personal dignity. It includes: dish, spoon, pusher, glass holder, chin switch rod, hand/foot switch, battery, and charger.

The Winsford Feeder has been in use since 1980. It is sold through medical equipment dealers in the United States and Canada. It is priced under $1500.00.

Headrest Switch

This is a two function rocker switch that is supported from the handles of a wheelchair. Turning the head to the left closes one switch and to the right closes the other. An adapter cable is required to connect it to the feeder.

WINSFORD PRODUCTS, INC.
179 Pennington-Harbourton Road
Pennington, NJ 08534
(609) 737-3297

✱✱✱✱

OTHER SOURCES OF EATING, FEEDING, AND DRINKING AIDS:

ABBEY MEDICAL
ALIMED INC.
CLEO INC.
DANMAR PRODUCTS
FLAGHOUSE, INC.
HOYLE PRODUCTS, INC.
J.A. PRESTON CORPORATION

KAYE'S KIDS
LS&S GROUP, INC.
LUMEX
MADDAK, INC.
MARSHALL MEDICAL
ST. LOUIS OSTOMY AND MEDICAL SUPPLY
THERAFIN CORPORATION

For additional information, including addresses and phone numbers, see CATALOGS.

BATHING

Eaton E-Z Bath

"I only wish to note that the bath lift is a marvel of simplicity and ingenuity and has afforded me the opportunity to take more baths with comfort and without fear of accident . . ."—H.H., Garden City, Kansas

The Eaton E-Z Bath was invented by J. W. "Willie" Eaton, a polio victim. Made of sturdy, non-corrosive aluminum, it is simple to install and easy to use. A support arm extends to the outside edge of the tub at wheelchair height for convenience in getting the bather onto the seat. Raising and lowering is accomplished with a crank. No plumbing or electrical work is required. Attach the support arm to whichever side fits your tub, and the E-Z Bath is ready for use. Priced around $600.00.

EATON E-Z BATH CO.
P.O. Box 712
Garden City, KS 67846

✳✳✳✳

EZ-Bathe™

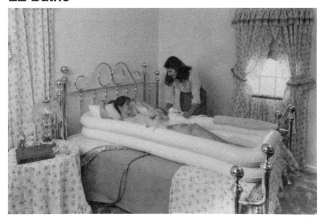

The EZ-Bathe™ inflatable tub can be a convenient alternative to conventional bathing methods. It provides an opportunity to experience the relaxing luxury of a real bath without getting out of bed. Its durable wet and dry vacuum inflates, deflates, and dries the tub. Priced around $350.00.

EZ-Shampoo™: Inflatable Shampoo Basin

When inflated by mouth or air pump the EZ-Shampoo™ becomes a form-fitting basin that comfortably cushions the neck and shoulders. A convenient drain hose efficiently removes soap suds and water. For cleanup, towel dry, deflate, and fold for storage in a space as small as a folded towel. Under $30.00.

EZ-Shower™

The perfect companion for the EZ-Shampoo™ Inflatable Basin, the EZ-Shower™ hangs on a bed post or I.V. pole, holds 2 1/2 gallons of warm tap water, and sports a flexible four foot hose for directing a gentle spray where it's needed. Under $20.00.

HOMECARE PRODUCTS
P.O. Box 88694
Seattle, WA 98188
(206) 251-9183

✳✳✳✳

One Piece Shower and Tub/Shower Modules

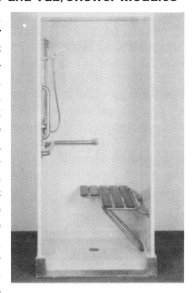

Fiat Products, Inc. offers a number of one piece acrylic shower and tub/shower modules. Each thermoformed from a continuous cast acrylic sheet to provide a seamless, non-invasive bathing environment. The smooth acrylic surface is warm to the touch, and grab bars are located in the proper supportive positions. Many of the units are designed with integrally molded seats; others can be supplied with a fold-up teakwood seat which facilitates accessibility without barriers. Convenient soap shelves are strategically located for shower or bath positions.

All Fiat units have anti-skid floor treatment, and are in compliance with the minimum guidelines issued by the U.S. Architectural and Transportation Barriers Compliance Board (A&TBCB), and with most city, state, and national standards for barrier free, accessible showering facilities. The Fiat acrylic modules come with a fifteen year limited warranty.

FIAT PRODUCTS
1 Michael Court
Plainview, NY 11803
(516) 349-7000

✳✳✳✳

TLC™ Bath Chair

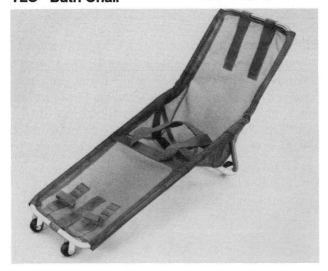

With the TLC™ Bath Chair from Ortho-Kinetics, a child can be bathed in a standard bathtub with a minimum of effort. It uses the edge of the tub to form a natural lever. This enables a transfer that doesn't require lifting the child's full weight. Once in the tub, washing of "hard-to-get-to" areas is made easier through the use of open mesh polyester fabric and a back that can be lowered to provide a neckrest during hairwashing. For versatility the TLC can be used for a variety of other activities, both indoors and out. It folds easily for taking on trips, to the beach, or on picnics.

6701—48"
6741—52"
6781—72"

> ORTHO-KINETICS
> W220 N507 Springdale Road
> P.O. Box 1647
> Waukesha, WI 53187
> (800) 558-7786
> (414) 542-6060 in Wisconsin

NOTE: See the Ortho-Kinetics Adaptive Commode/Shower Chair described with aids for Personal Hygiene.

✳✳✳✳

Minor-Aquatec Bath Lift

The Minor-Aquatec Bath Lift weighs just 25 pounds in the carrying case included with each lift. Hydraulically operated, it is quickly and easily installed in any standard bathtub.

With a lifting capacity of over 300 pounds, the Minor-Aquatec acts as a transfer bench, and gently lowers into the water with a simple finger pull. The user can remove the seatback for a fully immersed bath. Lowered, it is within three inches of the tub bottom. The covermat can be removed for washing in a standard washing machine. The lift is made of high impact plastic and stainless steel, and is completely non-corrosive. It has a two year parts and labor warranty (excluding covermat and carrying case).

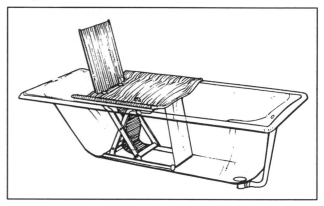

The Minor-Aquatec is an eye-pleasing aid to independence and privacy. Because of its compactness in the lowered position, there is no need to remove it when other household members wish to bathe.

A larger model covering the entire top of the tub is also available for those requiring more assistance in the bath.

> AQUATEC
> Health Care Products, Incorporated
> Allegheny Station P.O. Box 7066
> Pittsburgh, PA 15212
> (412) 322-7800

✳✳✳✳

Tri-Grip Rail

A security rail gives safety, comfort, and convenience while getting in and out of the bathtub. Frohock-Stewart's Tri-Grip offers three gripping heights, to aid in every bathing function. The adjustable clamps fits all modern style 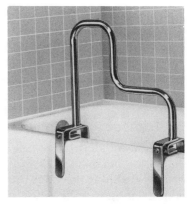 bathtubs. Special flexible strength steel allows them to conform to the tub walls when being tightened. The company also offers many other security rails, for a broad variety of applications.

Adjustable Height Bath Bench

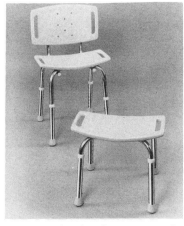

The seat and backrest of Frohock Stewart's Adjustable Height Bench, Model 85, are made of blow molded polyethylene plastic —air cushioned for comfort. Bright dipped anodized aluminum is used for the legs and back supports. The seat and back both measure 19" wide by 12" deep. The back rest can be adjusted to either of two positions, from 12 1/2" to 14" deep. A backless version, Model 75, is also available.

FROHOCK-STEWART, INC.
Bath Patient Aid Products and Bath Accessories
455 Whitney Avenue
P.O. Box 330
Northboro, MA 01532-0330
(800) 343-6059
(617) 393-2543 in Massachusetts

NOTE: See the Frohock-Stewart Adjustable Raised Toilet Seat and Toilet Guard Rails described with aids for Personal Hygiene.

✳✳✳✳

Just Add Water

The Silcraft Corporation offers a complete line of bathing and transfer systems.

The "Bather 2001" features comfortable sit down bathing and showering, hydrotherapeutic whirlpool massage, and sitz spray. The "Hi-Lo Supine Bath" provides easy entry in the lowered position and a convenient work height in the raised position, with full accessibility for bathing and whirlpool. The "Traverse" is a mobile power lift that can smoothly and quietly raise or lower a person weighing up to 350 pounds at the touch of a hand control.

Silcraft "Easy Access Shower Systems" are designed with "no threshold," and provide gentle entry for shower chairs. They are equipped with a pressure equalizing mixing valve to maintain a constant temperature of mixed water, and are supplied with a pulsating shower/massage wand, an acrylic bottle holder, and a flexible vinyl decorative bumper guard to protect the shower surface from damage.

"Special Care Acrylic Showers" offer one piece seam-free construction for ease of cleaning. Typical features include stainless steel grab bars, integral shelves, hand held shower/massage wand, and single lever water control valve. Silcraft "Bathmates" include a number of different products including a shower chair, transfer chair, bathside storage, and linen hamper. All are lightweight, durable, stain resistant, and constructed of high impact, unitized, tubular plastic. The lightweight covers are made of plastic coated polyester that can be laundered and disinfected easily. Cushions are filled with resin coated polyester padding. All casters swivel and are hooded, on bathing related products, to prevent hair and dirt buildup.

THE SILCRAFT CORPORATION
528 Hughes Drive
Traverse City, MI 49684
(800) 678-7100
(616) 946-4221

✳✳✳✳

Bath-O-Matic

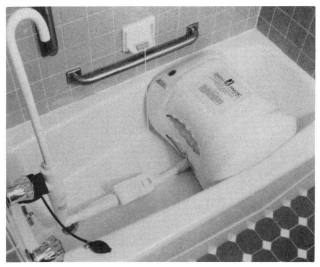

The Bath-O-Matic is a waterpowered bath lift. It can be used with either the tub faucet or shower-head, and requires no tools for installation. It permits full reclining and freedom in the tub, with an optional backrest that lifts and lowers with the bather. The unit fits inside any regular bathtub and is completely portable, weighing only 13 pounds. "It enables me to easily take a simple bath without assistance ... and is especially good for me when I travel."—M. S., Chicago, Illinois

Bath-O-Matic is priced under $500.00; the backrest is under $100.00.

INTERNATIONAL HEALTHCARE
PRODUCTS, INC.
State Route 83
Box 4180, Suite 104
Long Grove, IL 60047
(800) 423-7886
(312) 634-2626

✳✳✳✳

OTHER SOURCES OF BATHING AIDS:

ABBEY MEDICAL
ADAPTIVE PRODUCTS INCORPORATED
ALIMED INC.
ARCOA INDUSTRIES
ARJO HOSPITAL EQUIPMENT, INC.
CLEO INC.
INDEPENDENT LIVING AIDS, INC.
J.A. PRESTON CORPORATION
LAUREL DESIGNS
LS&S GROUP, INC.
LUMEX
MADDAK, INC.
RAYMO PRODUCTS, INC.
ST. LOUIS OSTOMY AND MEDICAL SUPPLY
WINCO INCORPORATED

For additional information, including addresses and phone numbers, see CATALOGS.

GROOMING

Sunbeam Dental Care System

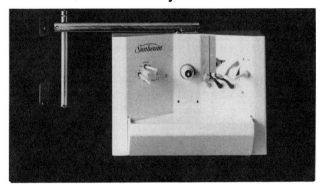

The Sunbeam Dental Care System allows hands-free toothbrushing for those who would otherwise be dependent on personal assistance to manage their dental hygiene. The unit mounts permanently to the wall with a swing-away bracket. Supplies of water, mouthwash, and toothpaste are stored inside and are replenished after 3-5 days' use. Toothpaste, in standard tubes, is attached to a mouthpiece via an adapter. Brushing action is activated by a toggle switch with a touch by the mouth, chin, or hand. Three toothbrushes, designed in several configurations, are stored in a convenient position to the right of the power head. By holding a toothbrush between the teeth, it can be moved from the storage pin to the electric toothbrush. A mirror mounted above and behind the brush storage area permits inspection of the entire face. With the Sunbeam Automatic Toothbrush the user is able to dispense toothpaste into his mouth, turn on the brush, rotate the brush angulation with respect to the teeth and gums, rinse the mouth with water, rinse the brush, and return it to the storage position by using only his lips, tongue, or teeth.

> NORTHERN ELECTRIC COMPANY
> P.O. Box 70
> Hattiesburg, MS 39401
> (601) 268-2880

✳✳✳✳

OTHER SOURCES OF GROOMING AIDS:

ALIMED INC.
CLEO INC.
INDEPENDENT LIVING AIDS, INC.
LS&S GROUP, INC.
LUMEX
MADDAK, INC.
MARSHALL MEDICAL
RAYMO PRODUCTS, INC.
SCIENCE PRODUCTS
ST LOUIS OSTOMY AND MEDICAL SUPPLY
THERAFIN CORPORATION

For additional information, including addresses and phone numbers see CATALOGS.

PERSONAL HYGIENE

Adaptive Commode/Shower Chair

The Ortho-Kinetics Adaptive Commode/ Shower Chair was designed to solve a difficult problem: how to provide children with adequate support and effective seating while toileting or showering.

It offers overall head and trunk support as well as a chest harness for proper positioning. Completely adjustable, it allows for use over toilets of different heights and can adapt to a child's growth over the years. Functional in three ways, it can be used independently with a commode pan, over a toilet, and in the shower.

6901 — Adaptive Commode
6902 — Shower Chair

ORTHO-KINETICS, INC.
P.O. Box 1647
Waukesha, WI 53187
(800) 558-7786
(800) 522-0992 in Wisconsin

****

SALK PRODUCTS

Salk products include briefs, panties, disposable and reusable pads and diapers, waterproof sheeting, plastic ware, and patient gowns.

Prefer Incontinence Briefs

The reusable Prefer brief and panty feature the convenience of a zippered fly-front sleeve for holding an absorbent disposable pad.

The pad can be changed quickly and easily without lowering the garment and without handling the soiled portion of the pad. The brief is made of 100% cotton rib with a 3/4" waistband. The panty is made of form fitting 100% cotton jersey, with a picot elastic trim at the waist and leg.

Disposable Absorbent Pads

Salk disposable pads are designed for a wide range of incontinence care needs. Salk pads adhere neatly to the garment by means of secure adhesive strips, eliminating shifting and offering freedom of movement.

Salk pads are made from soft, non-woven disposable paper, absorbent cellulose fluff, and a strong lightweight polyethylene backing. They are completely disposable, eliminating laundry and associated storage problems. Together with the appropriate Salk brief, they deliver protection and comfort.

Ostomate

Ostomate is intended for use by ostomates to replace their regular underwear. This multi-purpose garment conceals the plastic collection pouch to make it completely undetectable under clothing. It provides comfort to the wearer by holding the pouch in place, eliminating discomfort and skin irritation. Clips arc kept away from the abdomen, no belts are required.

For the male wearer, the garment allows the person to urinate through the front fly opening. This opening also enables the male wearer to have more normal sexual experiences while wearing the garment by reducing the stigma of seeing or touching the collection pouch.

The Salk line of Plastic Ware is made of rigid, non-autoclavable reusable plastic.

Sitz Bath

This sitz bath fits all toilet bowl sizes and can be used without assistance. Water flows from front to back so the user doesn't have to turn around in order to control cleansing. It includes convenient 60" tubing with a shut-off clamp.

Carefor Disposable Wipes

CareFor disposable wipes are premoistened and lanolized for softness. Large enough to accommodate an adult's needs, they are made from a non-woven paper material. The pop-up dispenser is great for home, office, or travel use.

THE SALK COMPANY, INC.
119 Braintree Street
P.O. Box 452
Boston, MA 02134
(800) 343-4497
(617) 782-4030

****

Safe and Dry

The Safe and Dry liner/pant incontinence system contains urine leakage so clothing and bed linen stay protected day and night. The all cotton pant is front opening, designed with easy-to-use Velcro tabs. The waistband is soft and stretchable. Absorbent, disposable polymer liners provide protection from leakage without bulkiness.

HYGIENICS INDUSTRIES,
INCORPORATED
3111 W. Allegheny Avenue
Philadelphia, PA 19132
(215) 229-3377

****

Showerlet

Showerlet is designed to comfortably clean and dry people who either cannot take care of themselves effectively, cannot use toilet tissue, or require a higher level of sanitation and hygiene than toilet tissue provides. It consists of a toilet seat and cover, water spray nozzle, blow dryer, push button controls, and pump. It is designed to clean and dry quickly, comfortably, and completely. A heated seat with adjustable temperature control is optional.

Showerlet can be installed in just a few minutes on "tank" type commodes; no additional plumbing is required. A bedside portable commode is also available with the Showerlet. The Showerlet is priced under $500.00 and the Portable Showerlet is under $600.00.

SANLEX INTERNATIONAL, INC.
P.O. Box 14717
Dayton, OH 45414
(513) 297-3011
(800) 424-1224

****

Leg Bag Emptier

"I am a quadriplegic and have been for thirteen years. I developed the Electric Leg Bag Emptier for my own use and found it has increased my independence as well as improved my health. I am convinced it will do the same for others."–Richard J. Dagostino

The Emptier enables the user to drain his or her leg bag at their convenience, with no outside help. Because of this, users increase their fluid intake which, in turn, reduces the frequency of urinary tract infections.

It is a small, lightweight valve connected to the bottom of the leg bag. Its size makes it very easy to conceal under a pant leg. The operating switch can be located anywhere on a wheelchair, depending on individual needs.

The Electric Leg Bag Emptier with Standard Switch is under $200.00; the Electric Leg Bag Emptier with Standard Switch, Battery, and Charger is under $400.00.

R.D. EQUIPMENT, INC.
12 Herring Run Road
Harwich, MA 02645
(508) 432-3948

****

CONVATEC PRODUCTS

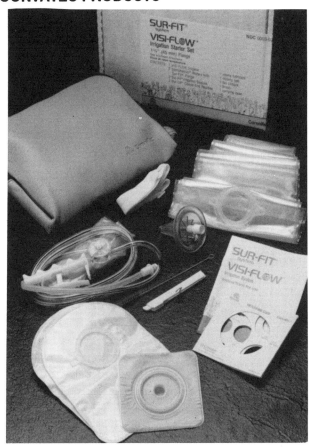

Convatec offers a wide range of ostomy and incontinence products. As an example, their "Visi-Flow" Irrigation Starter Set contains: (1) Irrigator with Stoma Cone, (2) "Stomahesive" Wafers with Flange, (2) Irrigation Sleeves, (2) Closed-End Pouches, (1) stoma lubricant, (1) ostomy belt, (1) tail closure, (1) brush, and (1) carrying case. The Starter Set is priced around $50.00.

E. R. SQUIBB & SONS, INC.
P.O. Box 4000
Princeton, NJ 08543-4000
(201) 359-9224

Consumers are invited to call collect with inquiries between 8:30 a.m. and 4:30 p.m., Eastern Time.

****

Adjustable Raised Toilet Seat

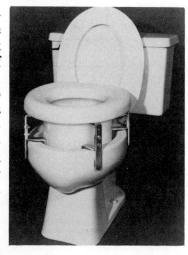

Frohock - Stewart's Adjustable Raised Toilet Seat adds up to 6 1/2" of height adjustment, in 1" increments, to a standard toilet. Its lightweight reinforced molded construction makes it easy to remove or replace. The mounting brackets, made of non-corrosive anodized aluminum, are slotted for adjustability. Swiveling them 360 degrees will lock the seat securely, to prevent slipping or tipping.

Adjustable Toilet Gard−Rails

Bright chrome plating and comfort-grip arm rests make this unit both attractive and useful. The height can be adjusted from 26" to 30", with legs that are rubber tipped to prevent marking floors. For maximum sturdiness, it bolts securely to the toilet.

FROHOCK-STEWART, INC.
455 Whitney Avenue
P.O. Box 330
Northboro, MA 01532-0330
(800) 343-6059
(617) 393-2543 in Massachusetts

****

Restop Relief System

"My husband is in a wheelchair, and when we are out and away from home, Restop really comes in handy. I used to hunt for special restrooms, or else have him use a portable urinal, but it was really smelly and I hated to have to wash it out. Restop is easy for him to use, and all I have to do is just drop it in a trash can."

Star Pioneer Products, Inc. offers a personal relief system called Restop. It contains a chemical polymer absorbent packet that solidifies urine and eliminates odor. Designed for easy use and compact storage, Restop's "funnel bag" easily adapts to women, men, and children. It can be used while standing or sitting, without spilling or leakage. Disposal is simple: twist the neck of the bag, place it in the provided "zippered disposal bag," and drop it in the nearest trash can.

Information about companies that distribute the Restop system can be obtained from:

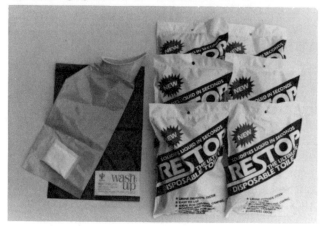

STAR PIONEER PRODUCTS, INC.
1395 Manassero Street
Anaheim, CA 92807
(714) 779-8833

****

Freshette

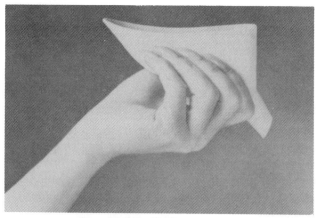

Freshette is a three-way modular urinary care system designed specifically for women. It can be used while sitting, standing, or lying down. The basic components−"collector bags," "extension," and "director"−fit into a convenient pouch that's small enough to be slipped discreetly into purse, pocket, pack, or glove box. Freshette provides an instant restroom wherever and whenever nature calls. Priced under $10.00.

SANI-FEM/FRESHETTE
7415 Stewart & Gray Road
Downey, CA 90241
(213) 928-3435

Uro-Safe Leg Bag

The Uro-Safe Leg Bag has a patented silicone inlet valve that's interference free, self-cleaning, and prevents back flow, thereby reducing the potential for bladder distention and possible infections. Made of soft transparent vinyl, or opaque white vinyl back with transparent vinyl front, the Uro-Safe Bag comes with a choice of "easy twist" drain valve or thumb operated tube clamp. The bag is packaged individually with two latex leg straps having reinforced eyelets.

Many other urinary incontinence products are also available from Urocare. These include: Leg Straps, Catheters, Bedside Drainage Systems, Extension Tubes, Connectors, Clamps, Foam Strips, and Discs.

UROCARE PRODUCTS, INC.
2419 Merced Avenue
South El Monte, CA 91733
(800) 423-4441
(818) 442-3477

∗∗∗∗

OTHER SOURCES OF PERSONAL HYGIENE AIDS:

ABBEY MEDICAL
ALIMED INC.
CLEO INC.
COLUMBIA MEDICAL MANUFACTURING
FLAGHOUSE, INC.
INDEPENDENT LIVING AIDS, INC.
J.A. PRESTON CORPORATION
KAYE PRODUCTS
KAYE'S KIDS
LS&S GROUP, INC.
LUMEX
MADDAK, INC.
RIFTON
ST. LOUIS OSTOMY AND MEDICAL SUPPLY
THERAFIN CORPORATION
WINCO INCORPORATED

For additional information, including addresses and phone numbers, see CATALOGS.

SEXUALITY

ErecAid System

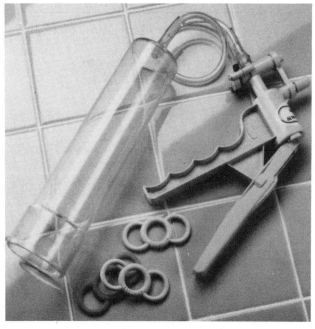

The ErecAid System is a nonsurgical product approved by the Food & Drug Administration for impotence management. Through the utilization of the Osbon Technique of vacuum therapy, the system mimics the natural process of erection causing rapid influx of arterial blood into the corporal tissues of the penis when adequate negative pressure is utilized. Engorgement and rigidity are created while the erection can be maintained for an ex tended period using a tension prosthesis to reduce venous outflow, allowing for intercourse.

Dr. Roy Witherington, M.D., Professor of Surgery and Chief of Urology, Medical College of Georgia, School of Medicine, Augusta, Georgia, supports ErecAid System in a chapter of *Urologic Clinics of North America*. It is his premise that the "acid test" of any impotence management procedure is the benefit (real or perceived) to the patient.

"The marked improvement of self-image noted by more than two-thirds of individuals using Erec-Aid System indicates that this particular device allows them to achieve penile tumescence of sufficient quality for sexual intercourse . . . Contraindications to the use of (ErecAid System) are few." (Witherington, R.: "Suction Device Therapy in the Management of Erectile Impotence." *Urologic Clinics of North America*, Vol. 15, No. 1, 123-128, 1988. Reprinted by permission of W. B. Saunders Company.)

ErecAid is an inexpensive alternative to abstinence, pharmacological injections, or prosthetic surgery. While it is easily adapted to by most users, some may require initial support. Each system is packaged with a comprehensive manual and training video. A toll-free telephone number is available for technical assistance.

OSBON MEDICAL SYSTEMS
P.O. Box 1478
Augusta, GA 30903-9990
(800) 438-8592

✳✳✳✳

ACCESS

TRANSFER DEVICES

EasyPivot

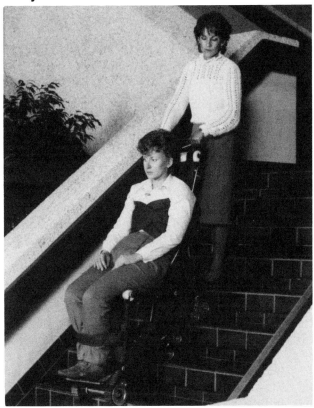

The EasyPivot is a machine suitable to many quadriplegics or others who have difficulty transferring themselves from wheelchair to bed or commode.

Transfers take less than a minute. A platform holds your feet, while a padded support steadies your knees. As your helper rotates the padded chest support, your torso lifts from chair or bed. In this semi-standing position you can be moved easily about the room. Straps support your knees during lift and transport.

There are no slings to slide under the buttocks.

Pants, dresses, and undergarments can be moved and repositioned while you're on the machine. This allows direct wheelchair to commode chair transfers without bedstops for clothing removal and sling repositioning. The motions when using the Easy-Pivot are similar to the "standing-pivot transfer" used when a helper bodily lifts and rotates you from place to place.

Designed to be unobtrusive in the home, the machine features a baked enamel finish and durable vinyl-covered, padded surfaces. The standard EasyPivot is adjustable to fit most persons. Prices range from $1200.00 to $2000.00.

This company also publishes a magazine entitled *Mobility Ltd*.

RAND-SCOT INCORPORATED
1418 West Oak Street
Fort Collins, CO 80521
(303) 484-7967

✳✳✳✳

Garaventa Evacu-Trac™

Getting out of a multi-story building during an emergency can present a serious problem for disabled or injured persons. Garaventa Evacu-Trac™ provides a solution to the problem of emergency egress. The Evacu-Trac™ is an evacuation chair that provides a fast, simple, and safe means of egress when elevators cannot be used. The chair moves on steel-belted rubber tracks with slip-resistant treads, allowing even petite attendants to safely move heavy individuals down stairways. It is ideal for any location where disabled persons live, work, or stay. Priced at about $1400.00; $1700.00 in Canada.

Garaventa Stair Lift

Garaventa Stair-Lift is an inclined wheelchair lift which provides access to many types of buildings. Stair-Lift Model GSL-1 can travel along turning stairways, stopping like an elevator at each floor to offer total building access. Model GSL-2 is designed for straight stairways without intermediate landings. Disabled users benefit from easy, independent operation as well as safety and security features.

Currently, Garaventa Stair-Lifts offer daily access at more than 1600 installations across North America.

Stair-Lift Price: Prices vary with size and complexity of installation.

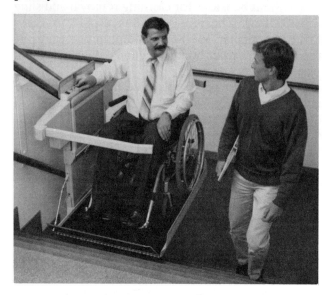

Garaventa Stair-Trac™

The Garaventa Stair-Trac allows an attendant to transport a person in a wheelchair up and down virtually any stairway. Stair-Trac is quickly and easily operated. Adding to its versatility is the fact that is powered by a chargeable battery, and that it folds in seconds for storage or transportation. (Stair-Trac fits easily into most car trunks!) The convenient Stair-Trac requires no installation, permits, or stairway modifications. And it is economical compared to elevators or fixed lifts. Priced under $5000.00.

For information write:

GARAVENTA (CANADA) LTD.
P.O. Box L-1
Blaine, WA 98230

GARAVENTA (CANADA) LTD.
7505 - 134A Street
Surrey, B.C. V3W 7B3
(800) 663-6556
(604) 594-0422

✱✱✱✱

HANDI-LIFT, INC.

Handi-Lift specializes in lifting aids, and offers a full range of products for elevating wheelchairs. Residential elevators, porch lifts, and inclined wheelchair lifts for straight or curved stairs are available. Prices for these items vary widely according to the requirements for each application. A stairway elevator for a straight stair of thirteen risers or less could be under $2700, depending upon added accessories and location. Curved stair units begin at $7000.

Offerings by Handi-Lift include products by Cheney, Garaventa, Waupaca, and D.A. Matot.

HANDI-LIFT, INC.
436 West Main Street
Wyckoff, NJ 07481
(800) 432-LIFT
(201) 891-8097

✱✱✱✱

CHENEY COMPANY

Cheney offers a full range of stairway elevators and wheelchair lifts for use in private or public buildings.

The Handi-Lift® Vertical Wheelchair Lift

The Cheney Handi-Lift® provides easy stairway access. It's adaptable to both indoor and outdoor applications in private homes, churches, schools, office buildings, and industrial plants.

The Handi-Lift® has an overall cabinet width of 48", allowing installation in very confined areas. Yet, a full twelve square foot platform is maintained. The loading rate is 500 pounds (with an optional 750 pound rating). Its design is aesthetically pleasing, and it comes in a variety of colors.

The Handi-Lift® is available in five lifting heights, ranging from 4 feet to 12 feet. The forward ramp/guard plate operates automatically, providing easy wheelchair access. A "3-Stop Package" that allows the passenger to exit or enter at 3 different levels is optional. The unit is operated by a passenger activated switch, causing the platform to raise and lower.

Handi-Enclosure®

If state or local requirements necessitate the use of a hoistway or restrictive access, the Handi-Enclosure® is available. It's adaptable to indoor applications and built so that the Handi-Lift® becomes a part of the structure. An "Outdoor Dome" is optional.

Victory Wheel'n Chair Lift

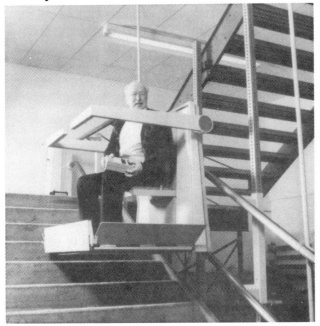

Cheney's Victory Wheel'n Chair Lift is a variable inclined stairway lift designed for carrying a person in a wheelchair or a seated passenger from one floor to another. It can traverse almost any stairway configuration up to three flights. It's sleek "space-age" design, steel rails, and hi-tech styling make it as attractive as it is functional. It contains three basic sub-systems: the rail system, the platform, and the main drive unit.

Parallel steel tubes provide the platform support and encase the drive system. The vertical platform housing is fabricated from formed sheet steel and includes padded security arms as standard equipment. Platforms are of lightweight construction and include load capacity sensing devices. Directional obstruction sensors are at the upper and lower ends of the platform. The empty platform will respond to a call/send signal only after folding. The carriage is provided with an over-speed sensor and brake to prevent uncontrolled descent. The unit features a special hydraulic power folding system that allows it to fold up flat for normal stair use.

The Lift has an infrared position sensing system that automatically slows it to a comfortable 12 feet per minute on turns and when it approaches each station. The passenger control panel can be easily removed form the control box for handheld convenience when riding on the built in auxiliary passenger seat. Or it can be left in place on the control box for convenient wheelchair user operation.

Code Key Card access limits operation to authorized passengers or attendants only. Victory's battery is automatically recharged at each exit or entrance landing.

Liberty Stair Lifts

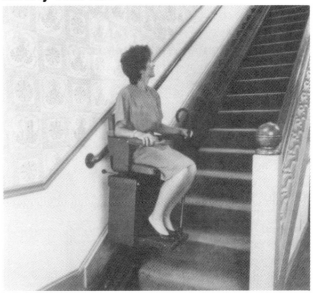

"As a retired engineer, I was greatly impressed with the excellent workmanship ... I was also impressed with the efficiency and expertise of the installer."—L.T., Washington, DC

The Liberty SP lets you ride comfortably facing sideways with a full 180 degree view. It has a large, cushioned 18" seat, padded armrest, and large footrest, all of which fold up to within 15" of the stairway wall. A "Feather Touch" constant pressure switch lets you start, stop, and reverse the chair any time. At the top landing, the seat swivels and locks at both 60 and 90 degrees, making it easier to get on and off. Power cutoff prevents the chair from moving unless the seat is in the riding position.

The Liberty LT is especially designed to make wheelchair transfers easier than with ordinary stairway lifts. The LT provides special features like the high backrest, special chest strap, and locking arm rests, and can accommodate virtually any stairway configuration.

The Liberty LX is the top-of-the-line. Designed for straight, curved, or even spiral stairways, this unit offers an array of special features. From decorator fabrics to contoured seats, from arms that gently surround you to lights that illuminate the stairs.

All Liberty models feature a 4" I-beam rail and cog drive.

CHENEY
2445 South Calhoun Road
P.O. Box 188
New Berlin, WI 53151
(800) 782-1222
(414) 782-1100

✳✳✳✳

Florlift—Residential Wheelchair Lift With Trapdoor

Florlifts are manufactured in various models for residential, commercial, and industrial applications. They are custom built to fit individual requirements, designed to carry up to 1000 pounds, delivered completely assembled, and installed in as little as six hours.

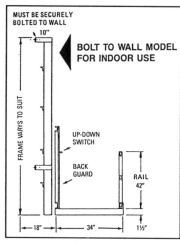

The Florlift travels vertically, either between the basement and first floor or the first and second floor. As it rises, it opens a trap door at the upper level, and when lowered the trap door closes automatically. In fact, the only time floor space is lost on the upper level is while the lift is traveling. Once the trap door is fully closed, it can be walked over.

Florlifts have been installed in over 1000 homes throughout the United States and have been approved by insurance carriers.

Totally Enclosed and Short Rise Lifts are also available from this company.

FLORLIFT OF NEW JERSEY, INC.
41 Lawrence Street
East Orange, NJ 07017
(201) 429-2200

✳✳✳✳

LIVING RAMPS

Well suited for entrances to churches and community buildings, these ramps feature an exclusive serrated sawtooth deck surface which provides safe and secure traction for indoor and outdoor use. Constructed of high strength aluminum, ramps are made in sections which join together with leg supports at all connecting points.

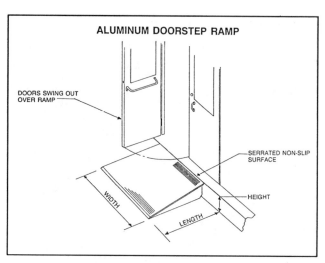

Ramps have full length raised safety curbs on both sides and are available with 32" high handrails on one or both sides. Level platform sections are available in a variety of sizes to enter doorways, extend from a porch, or make right angle or U-turns.

Standard ramp widths are 36" and 48" between safety curbs. Ramp lengths are based on local conditions, but usually follow the rule of thumb of 8" to 12" long for every 1" of rise. These lengths are based on the American National Standards Institute (ANSI) standard specification A117.1-1980, but the 1:12 rule is usually only required for new construction.

Purchase and leasing options are both available.

JH INDUSTRIES
8901 E. Pleasant Valley Road
Independence, OH 44131
(800) 321-4968
(216) 524-7520

✳✳✳✳

INDEPENDENT TRANSPORT

I✳TEC offers an independent transport system which allows such freedom and self-sufficiency that dressing, bathing, rising from bed, and transferring to a wheelchair can be accomplished without any assistance.

Ceiling-mounted or free-standing tracks guide the system to any location, and a push-button control box gives the operator a simple means of vertical and horizontal movement.

The SE 400 Automatic provides powered movement horizontally and vertically. It can be used unassisted by C 5/6 quadraplegics and also people with M.D., M.S., C.P., or spinal injury. The

SE 400 Semi-Automatic provides vertical power lift with manual horizontal movement. There is also a choice of monorail systems.

The ceiling mounted system affixes to joists in the ceiling and allows transfers from bed to wheelchair or bath areas. Special ordered curved track enables the system to go around corners.

The free standing system is designed for use where ceiling mounting is not practical, for example in apartments or in rooms where the bed position is temporary. The free standing system is available in straight track only. Lengths up to 20 feet may be special ordered allowing the supports to be against the walls.

I*TEC units have a low voltage control box and adjustable up/down limit switches.

I*TEC
Independence Technologies
5482 Business Drive, #C
Huntington Beach, CA 92649
(800) 622-ITEC
(714) 898-9005

✳✳✳✳

Wheel-O-Vator

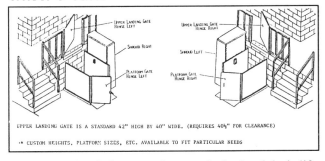

UPPER LANDING GATE IS A STANDARD 42" HIGH BY 40" WIDE. (REQUIRES 40½" FOR CLEARANCE)

** CUSTOM HEIGHTS, PLATFORM SIZES, ETC. AVAILABLE TO FIT PARTICULAR NEEDS

The Wheel-O-Vator is a vertical wheelchair lift. It can be installed at the side of a porch landing or at the end of a stairway (with the aid of a Wheel-O-Bridge). Each unit has key operated controls within easy reach of the rider. The lift has sturdy steel construction, weatherproof enamel finish suitable for interior or exterior use, and operates on standard 110 volt current.

Among standard features of the BC-model: a platform safety ramp, a skidproof ramp and platform, adjustable upper and lower limit switches, emergency manual operation, 24 volt control system, removable handrail and carriage to accommodate interior applications.

The Wheel-O-Vator is available in two models, the BC with lifting heights up to 12 feet, and the CDE, primarily used for commercial applications where an enclosure in required.

A most recent addition to the NWC line is the Stair Master Stair Lift.

Both the Wheel-O-Vator and the Stair Master are marketed and sold through a national network of selected health care dealers. Installation and service are normally handled by these factory-trained dealers.

NWC
The National Wheel-O-Vator Company, Inc.
P.O. Box 1308
Patterson, LA 70392
(800) 551-9095

✳✳✳✳

Patient Handling Sling

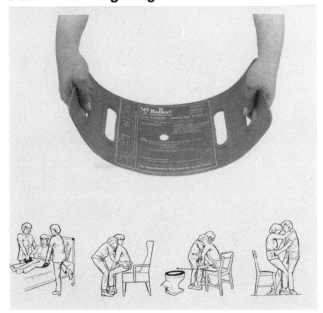

"St. Luke's Nursing Home initially purchased one sling on a trial basis. Because there was an overwhelmingly positive response from the staff, four more were purchased. One sling was placed on each of our four wings and one in the central bathing area. As usage and staff acceptance grew, ten more were purchased and placed in specific resident rooms. The ultimate goal is to have one sling in each room."—Assistant Director of Nursing

The Patient Handling Sling was originally conceived and designed by Dr. J.D.G. Troup, an internationally acknowledged consultant in the fields of orthopaedics and occupational health. His aim was to reduce the load on nurses' backs when handling patients. The Sling works by making the arms effectively longer, so that it becomes unnecessary to bend as far forward. The base polymer has exceptional physical properties which combine high tensile strength and low stretch with extremely good flexibility and durability. The Patient Handling Sling is one of the product range of MEDesign Ltd. Priced under $25.00.

BALLERT INTERNATIONAL, INC.
3677 Woodhead Drive #17
Northbrook, IL 60062
(800) 345-3456

****

OTHER SOURCES OF TRANSFER AIDS:

ABBEY MEDICAL

ACCESS TO RECREATION, INC.
ADAPTIVE PRODUCTS
ALIMED INC.
ARJO HOSPITAL EQUIPMENT, INC.
CLEO INC.
GUARDIAN
J.A. PRESTON CORPORATION
LUMEX
MADDAK, INC.
ST. LOUIS OSTOMY AND MEDICAL SUPPLY
SUNRISE MEDICAL

For additional information, including addresses and phone numbers, see CATALOGS.

HOUSEHOLD ACCOMMODATIONS

LEVERON®

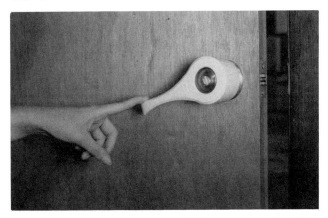

"A recent survey we carried out revealed that opening doors is one of the most difficult problems for people with arthritis of the hands."—Frederic C. McDuffie, M.D., Senior Vice President Medical Affairs, Arthritis Foundation

Utilizing a special thermoplastic material and a unique fastening principle, Leveron® is installed over any doorknob within two minutes by anyone with minimal mechanical ability. Considered a breakthrough in lever handle design, Leveron® requires less than one-third the force of metal lever hardware to operate.

Leveron® meets all safety and endurance requirements for home, public schools and universities, hospitals, industrial facilities, and public buildings. After three years of extensive field testing, Leveron® has V.A. approval, as well as endorsements by private and public agencies.

Leveron's® solid colors are almond, three metallics, and "Hi-Glow," the newest addition which remains visible in total darkness for several hours after the lights are turned off or electric power fails. Priced under $15.00.

LINDUSTRIES, INC.
21 Shady Hill Road
Weston, MA 02193
(617) 237-8177, 235-5452

✳✳✳✳

X-10® Powerhouse™

The X-10 Powerhouse™ Home Control system offers a variety of Controllers and Modules to aid in daily living.

The Wireless System RC5000 lets you control up to eight X-10 Modules from inside or outside your home. It can also dim and brighten lights connected to Lamp and Wall Switch Modules. The Transceiver is an Appliance Module and also sends signals to eight standard X-10 Modules over your house wiring. The system includes both the Remote Control and the Transceiver/Appliance Module. Priced around $50.00.

For your bedside, the Maxi Controller SC503 lets you control up to sixteen X-10 Modules at the touch of a button from anywhere in the house. Priced around $25.00.

Other components of the X-10 Powerhouse system include: Telephone Responder Set, Telephone Transmitter, Thermostat Set-Back Controller, Wall Switch and Receptacle Modules, Radio Home Control System, Timer/Controller/Alarm Clock, Home Control Interfaces with Software and Cable for IBM PC and Compatibles, Macintosh, Apple IIe & IIc, and Commodore 64 & 128.

X-10 (USA) INC.
185A LeGrand Avenue 1200
Northvale, NJ 07647
(800) 526-0027
(201) 784-9700

X-10 HOME CONTROLS INC.
Aerowood Drive, Unit 20
Mississauga, Ontario L4W2S7
(800) 387-3346
(416) 624-4446

✳✳✳✳

Power Access Automatic Door Opener

The Power Access automatic door operator has important built-in safety features—both mechanical and electrical.

The operator arm is not attached to the door. Instead, a wheel at the end of the operator arm rolls against the face of the door, pushing the door open. This feature ensures that the door can always be opened manually.

If the door meets an obstruction during the opening cycle, a built-in load sensing circuit automatically stops the operator and the arm returns to the at-rest, or closed position. The drive motor is thermally protected. Door hold-open time can be set for as long as thirty seconds, longer if necessary. A range of door sizes and opening forces can be accommodated. Left and right hand units are available as well as inverted, deep reveal, and door mounted units for special applications. Control options include: Push Button, Push Plate, Key, Touch, and Radio Transmitter. Installation is easy. No modification of the door or jambs is required and the unit plugs into a standard 110 volt A.C. wall outlet.

POWER ACCESS CORPORATION
Bridge Street
P.O. Box 235
Collinsville, CT 06022
(800) 344-0088
(203) 693-0751

****

The Ezra System

"Ezra has changed my life. Before Ezra, my only visitors were people who had a key to my house. Now I can unlock my front door for a variety of guests. Without Ezra I just sat in my chair in front of the TV like a robot and watched the same station all day long. Now I have my choice of programs and I don't feel so isolated."—M.B.

With the Ezra System a list of items appears on the TV screen and an arrow constantly moves down the list at the speed you select by adjusting a knob on the back. When the arrow points to the item you want, you push or puff your switch. If you select Bed Control, for instance, another list will appear allowing you to move the head, foot, or entire bed up or down. To make another selection return to the original list, the Main Menu. If you don't change the menus for a few minutes, the screen goes blank. When you need the menus again, push your switch and they'll reappear.

The switch is wireless and can be mounted on a bed or wheelchair. It's a half dollar-sized button requiring very little pressure to push. (The puff/sip switch is optional).

Ezra's base unit, with built-in radio, costs under $1000. In addition you need to provide a television to display Ezra's menus. If you want Ezra to control a TV, the TV must be a remote control model and the remote control must be modified by KY Enterprises. If you want to control the TV through your VCR, your VCR controller can be modified too. The price for modification of the remote controls is included in the base price.

Options include: Telephone, Electric Bed Control, Puff/Sip Switch, Flexible Stand, Remote Speaker Amplifier for phone, Speech Synthesizer—50-word list.

KY ENTERPRISES
Custom Computer Solutions
3039 East 2nd Street
Long Beach, CA 90803
(213) 433-5244

****

Access Real Estate

Access Real Estate specializes in the marketing of specially designed wheelchair accessible homes. They have established a national referral center through which buyers and sellers of homes may list their requirements. The service is available at no charge and any actual transactions that result are handled through licensed brokers at standard fees.

SEA REALTY
22 Sunset Avenue
Westhampton Beach, NY 11978
(516) 288-6244

****

Horton Automatic Sliding Door Operator

New energy saving regulations require the use of dual and triple glazed sliding glass doors in colder climates. These doors are built and weatherstripped to prevent air infiltration. Unfortunately, this requirement makes them heavy, tight, and more difficult for many people to open and close. But, with the Horton Automatic Sliding Door Operator, just push a button and the sliding glass door opens and closes automatically. The operator uses regular household current (115 volts, 2 amps) and is attached to the top of the fixed and moving panels of the door. It can be activated by one of three optional switches, a radio control remote, keyless entry or simple doorbell switch. The Horton Door Operator can be installed on an existing door as well as new construction. It is easily adjusted to operate doors of various sizes and weights. The door can be opened or closed manually if there is a power failure.

Series: 8700

Easy Access™

Horton also produces Easy Access™, a manual/automatic swing door operator for barrier free openings that may be installed on an existing swing door. It is low powered and slow-opening with an adjustable time delay to hold the door in the open position (it meets the requirements of ANSI standard A156.19 when adjusted in accordance with the standard). Two methods of activating the door are available: 1) manual when pushed and automatic when activated by a push-button; 2) automatic operation by either pushing the door or by pushing the button ("Push and Go").

Series: 7000

HORTON AUTOMATICS
A Division of the Dallas Corporation
4242 Baldwin Blvd.
Corpus Christi, TX 78405
(800) 531-3111
(512) 888-5591

✳✳✳✳

ABLENET

The Ablenet catalog offers a variety of useful switches, a universal switch mounting system and other practical aids.

Switch 100

Switch 100 is a single push switch 5" in diameter. It comes with a 6-foot cord for connection to control units, adapted battery-operated devices, and computers.

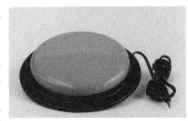

Control Unit

The control unit allows the operation of any two electrical devices up to a 1700 watt capacity. When the switch is activated the devices turn on. If the timer is used the attached device will remain on from 2 to 90 seconds.

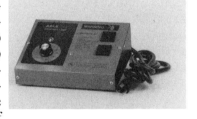

String Switch

The string switch is activated with less than 1/2 ounce of tension on the pull cord connected to it. To use the switch attach a string or piece of yarn to the pull cord. Then wrap it around the user's hand or other body part. The small base can be easily secured to any surface with Velcro or tape.

Plate Switch

The Plate Switch by Don Johnston Developmental Equipment, Inc. is a small versatile switch that can be easily mounted to accommodate a variety of hand and head movements. The Plate Switch is under $50.00.

Other switches include the L.T. Switch, a light touch version of the plate switch; the Computer Switch Interface, allowing single switch access to an Apple Computer.

Universal Switch Mounting System

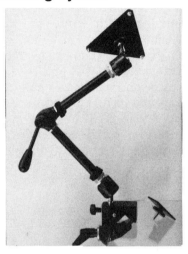

The Universal Switch Mounting System allows for switch placement in any position. It consists of an adjustable arm attached to a one-piece clamp that tightens onto a table or wheelchair. The length of the arm from the clamp to the switch is 20 1/2". Two switch mounting plates are included, along with two pieces of Poly-Lock™ to attach the switches. Priced under $150.00.

ABLENET
AccessAbility, Inc.
360 Hoover Street, N.E.
Minneapolis, MN 55413
(612) 331-5958

✳✳✳✳

Scanning X-10 Powerhouse

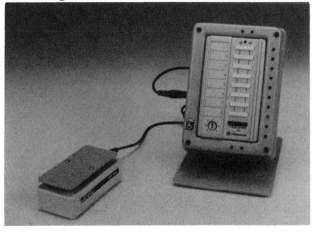

The Scanning X-10 Powerhouse permits control of up to 16 (see note) appliances and/or lights. Access is by either a single or dual control interface (switch), or the input controller for the Arrow powered wheelchair using the Switch Control Interface (Model 1551) made by Invacare Corporation. The user of an Arrow powered wheelchair simply activates the single switch to independently select between wheelchair drive and environmental control mode.

This compact environmental control unit is made up of a portable, battery-operated visual display transmitter and a receiver/control module with antenna. Both visual and auditory feedback are available.

Note: You can change the transmitter back and forth between 1-8 and 9-16 quite easily. The receiver, on the other hand, is not as easy to change back and forth. For this reason, if you plan on using more than eight lamp or appliance modules, you need to purchase an additional receiver so that you can set one receiver to 1-8 and the other to 9-16.

Control 1

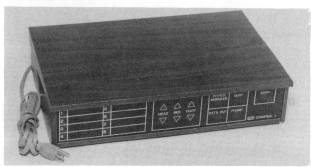

Control 1 represents a new approach to environmental control. While it can be used quite independent of a computer, Control 1 is designed to respond to computer type commands. Those commands could come from a computer or from an input display operated by a dual control switch or from a communication aid. The user need not have knowledge of, or interest in computers, but if so, may wish to write a program for his own computer to operate Control 1. When Control 1 recognizes a particular sequence of ASCII characters, it performs a particular task.

The Control 1 user can operate up to 256 AC power devices using BSR power control modules. These modules plug into standard power outlets and have receptacles into which the device to be controlled is plugged. Control 1 has eight control receptacles that can be used for the operation of accessories and other devices. Since the Control 1 user may also want to use a computer, a data output is provided.

Standard components:

- Control 1 unit
- BSR Appliance Module
- BSR Lamp Module

- Telephone cord, 25 feet
- Duplex phone jack
- Operator Manual

A variety of specialized devices are available for use with the PRC Control 1 (and older PRC environmental control systems). In many cases the accessory may be used as a self contained unit, apart from the main environmental control system. Control interfaces and adapter cables must be ordered separately and should be selected based upon the physical capabilities of the user.

PRENTKE ROMICH COMPANY
1022 Heyl Road
Wooster, OH 44691
(800) 642-8255
(216) 262-1984

✳✳✳✳

Telecaption 3000™

TeleCaption 3000™ displays closed captions as text on the lower portion of your TV screen, when viewing a Closed Captioned television program. Its small size and light weight (only four pounds) makes it truly portable—easy to carry between TVs in the bedroom or living room, or to take traveling. TeleCaption 3000™ gives access to full screen text channels such as TEXT News Service, PLUS (Program Selection Listings) and HINT (Hearing Impaired Specific News Text). Priced around $200.00.

AT&T
National Special Needs Center
Suite 310
2001 Route 46
Parsippany, NJ 07054-1315
(800) 233-1222
(800) 833-3232/TDD

(TeleCaption 3000™ is a trademark of the National Captioning Institute.)

✳✳✳✳

NATIONWIDE FLASHING SIGNAL SYSTEMS

Nationwide Flashing Signal Systems, Inc. (NFSS) is a nationwide-concentrated company whose primary business transactions are conducted through mail order, walk-in, and convention business. Formed in 1976, NFSS was the first company in the United States to overcome the barriers hearing-impaired persons had with smoke detector systems.

"As a deaf-owned and deaf-operated company, we manufacture and distribute products that we use ourselves." The NFSS product line ranges from doorbell, telephone, and baby cry signalers to alarm clocks, bed vibrators, pagers, smoke detectors, TDDs, answering machines, printers, TV decoders, and other everyday living accessories, including security alarm systems. Most of the products are approved by Underwriters Laboratories, Inc. "In our desire to produce high-quality and reliable devices, we maintain intense working relationships with our electronic engineers and we are continuously seeking ways to upgrade and/or modify our products to meet the needs of our customers. In addition, we are authorized repair agents and take pride in our large service center."

NFSS, INC.
8120 Fenton Street
Silver Spring, MD 20910
(301) 589-6670/TDD
(301) 589-6671/Voice

✳✳✳✳

Tactile Communicator, TC1001

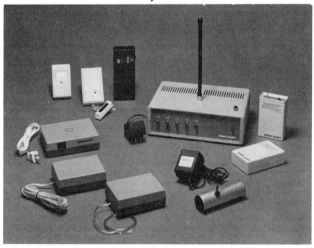

The Sonic Alert Tactile Communicator, TC1001 is a wireless radio and paging system designed specifically for deaf-blind com-munications. Its pocket-size receiver alerts the wearer to a signal being received by vibrating the receiver case. This allows users to have a com-munication link to their door-bell, telephone, fire alarm, or any other devices they select. (The right combination of signalers and remote receivers depends upon individual needs.)

The system was designed by the Research De-partment of the Helen Keller National Center to utilize the new handicap frequency 43.64 megahertz.

SONIC ALERT
1750 West Hamlin Road
Rochester Hills, MI 48309
(313) 656-3110/Voice or TTY

✳✳✳✳

Speak-A-Lock

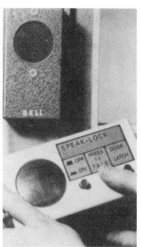

Speak-A-Lock lets you answer the door without moving from your bed or chair. When the doorbell rings a buzzer also sounds in the handset. After switching on, press the "Talk" to identify the person at the door. If you want to admit the caller, press the "Door Latch" button, releasing the lock on the door. Otherwise the door remains securely locked.

Speak-A-Lock can be operated with any "Yale" type lock, and does not interfere with normal operation of the door. Existing keys and locks can still be used. Speak-A-Lock runs on low voltage (12 volt) and is completely safe to use.

NEWTON WHEELCHAIRS U.S.A.
21209 Lago Circle, 12 E
Boca Raton, FL 33433
(407) 483-7184

✳✳✳✳

OTHER SOURCES OF HOUSEHOLD ACCOMMODATIONS:

ABBEY MEDICAL
ALIMED INC.
CLEO INC.
INDEPENDENT LIVING AIDS, INC.
J.A. PRESTON CORPORATION
MADDAK, INC.

For additional information, including addresses and phone numbers, see CATALOGS.

CHAPTER FOUR

COMMUNICATION

READING

VTEK Voyager

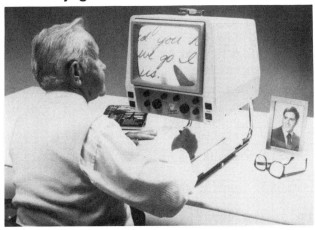

Voyager and Voyager Plus are easy to operate closed circuit television systems that magnify reading, writing, and other materials 3 to 45 times. They provide the independence to view books, photographs, or small print on medicine bottles, and to write letters, balance a checkbook, pursue hobbies, or accomplish work with ease. For individuals with impaired dexterity, they can be equipped with automatic focusing.

For maximum comfort and ease the Voyager and Voyager Plus display screen, video camera, and viewing table are designed to be used in one vertical configuration known as "in-line" viewing. Controls are conveniently accessible, easily distinguished, and clearly labeled on the front panel.

In addition to all the features of the Voyager, Voyager Plus offers spring legs, choice of screen, and split-screen capability.

Voyager XL

The Voyager XL and XL-Plus feature a 19 inch screen that allows magnification of up to 60 times the original size. The camera module is separate from the monitor so it can be detached and carried to and from home or work.

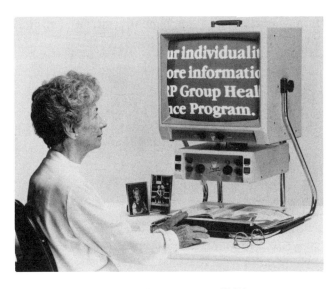

Large Print Display Processor (DP)

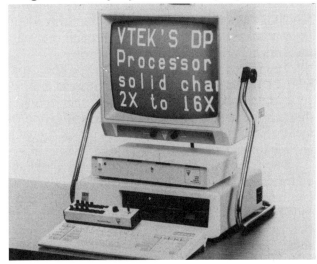

Large Print Display Processors enlarge normal dot-matrix computer display into solid, proportional characters up to 5 1/2" high in one of eight magnifications—up to 16 times. VTEK's software-transparent DP operates with the most popular word processing, database, and spreadsheet programs. DP-11 and DP-11 Plus support the IBM PC, XT, AT, and PS/2 Models 25 and 30, as well as most compatibles. DP-10 supports the Apple II, II+, IIe, and II GS.

The DP consists of three components—an interface board, processing box, and User Control Panel. The Control Panel features a four-directional joystick that conveniently moves a display window around the full screen.

VTEK
1625 Olympic Blvd.
Santa Monica, CA 90404
(800) 345-2256 Continental U.S. and Hawaii
(800) 338-4898 Canada
(213) 452-5966 Alaska and Puerto Rico

✶✶✶✶

TOUCH TURNER

The Touch Turner story began twenty years ago when a prominent Seattle professional engineer and inventor was told about polio patients at the area's respirator center, who did not have the capability of turning the pages of books and magazines.

The resulting invention was awarded the Gold Medal for Function and Design at the Switzerland International Polio Convention. Through the years the Touch Turner has continued to evolve.

Today, the Model CR brings to you the capability of turning pages both in the forward and reverse direction. The sensitive switch that actuates the turning action can be operated with a movement of the chin, a puffing of the cheek, or with any minimum movement.

The Touch Turner can operate on flashlight batteries for months without replacement. It can be used anywhere, and there is no danger of electrical shock. One simple adjustment enables the user to change from one book to another, or to a magazine. The angle is easily modified for reading in bed, wheelchair, or at a table. Special switches and adapters are available. Touch Turner is priced at around $600.00.

TOUCH TURNER
443 View Ridge Drive
Everett, WA 98203
(206) 252-1541

✶✶✶✶

Circline Magnifier

Dazor offers a full range of lighting and magnification aids. The Circline Magnifier has a built-in handle that allows you to maneuver the lamp more

easily. The 5" double-convex 3-diopter lens made of crown optical glass provides magnification of (+75%) at a focal length of 13". With the addition of the easy-to-attach Add-A-Lens accessory, the magnification can be increased to (+275%) at a focal length of 3 3/4". The fluorescent tube sheds even, shadow-free light from all sides, for optimum brightness without harshness. A 5-diopter lens is also an option, providing magnification of (+125%) at a focal length of 8".

Dazor's "floating arm" glides with the touch of a finger, and stays where you put it. There are no exposed springs to wear out, squeak, or distract from its sleek appearance.

DAZOR MANUFACTURING CORP.
4483 Duncan Avenue
St. Louis, MO 63110
(800) 345-9103
(314) 652-2400

✶✶✶✶

Viewscan®

Viewscan® is a portable large print reading device. Compact and attractively styled, it is small enough to fit into a briefcase.

The Viewscan® contains a flat display unit linked by a light cable to a miniature pocket-sized camera. By scanning this camera across the page the reader can see a bright magnified image of the text on the large Viewscan® display screen. At the touch of a switch magnification from 4x to 64x can be selected and either positive or negative image characters are shown on the high contrast, anti-reflective amber display. The carrying handle doubles as an adjustable stand which allows the display to be angled back to suit the viewing position. Automatic Threshold Control enables the unit to adapt instantly to different reading materials and changes in print quality. As the user's needs change Viewscan® can be upgraded to facilitate typing, calculating, word processing, computers, and access to electronic information. The whole unit measures only 15 1/2" wide, 8 1/2" high, and 2" thick. The Viewscan® with carrying case, manual, and scanning aid is priced at under $4500.00

Ransley Braille Interface™

The Ransley Braille Interface™ (RBI) is simply a box that connects between any standard computer or computerized source and any standard braille embosser. What this means is that a sighted secretary, teacher, co-worker, or anyone who knows nothing at all about braille will be able to produce automatically formatted Grade II braille in essentially the same way they would use a standard printer. An important feature is that RBI works with any computer, not just Apple II's or IBM PC compatibles. Price: around $900.00.

HUMANWARE, INC.
6140 Horseshoe Bar Road, Suite P
Loomis, CA 95650
(916) 652-7253

****

Pagemate™

The Pagemate™ is a well-designed easel that requires minimum space yet maximizes reading efficiency. It allows quick and easy page turning in either direction, and can accommodate all types of data. Because it's portable, it can be used wherever needed. A patented feature provides a sliding T-bar with foam pads to hold publications open and eliminate "flipping pages." The unit can be adjusted to the desired viewing angle to eliminate light glare. It folds flat to store or carry. Price: about $20.00.

Line-A-Timers®

Line-A-Timers® are moveable hi-liters that can adhere to a page and be moved as desired. They are available in yellow and blue in packets of four of varying lengths to accommodate different size pages or other source material.

EAGLE MARKETING
5321 S. Sheridan, Suite 34
Tulsa, OK 74145
(918) 663-4477

****

Large-Display Options

The National Institute for Rehabilitation Engineering (NIRE) offers a variety of large-display options for IBM-PC/XT/AT and PS/2 compatible computers. They also provide technical support for PC/XT/AT and compatible computers.

The National Institute for Rehabilitation
Engineering
P.O. Box T
Hewitt, NJ 07421
(201) 853-6585

****

Optacon II

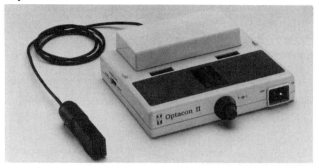

The Optacon II is a portable print reading aid that was jointly developed over four years by Canon, Inc. of Tokyo and Telesensory Systems, Inc. of Mountain View, California. The Optacon II is a dramatic redesign of the original Optacon of which 11,000 are in use in over seventy countries.

To read, the user scans text with the miniature camera and reads the vibrating image with his index finger. The device weighs only two pounds and measures 6" x 5.5" x 1.1".

Advantage™

Telesensory Systems also offers a large 19-inch screen magnification system called AdVantage™. With it, reading materials or other objects can be magnified from 4 to 60 times their original size. It can be used as the monitor for Vista™, the company's image enlarging system for IBM PCs and compatibles.

TELESENSORY SYSTEMS, INC.
455 North Bernardo Avenue
P.O. Box 7455
Mountain View, CA 94039-7455
(800) 227-8418
(415) 960-0920 International

OTHER SOURCES OF READING AIDS:

ALIMED INC.
AMERICAN FOUNDATION FOR THE BLIND
CLEO INC.
HOYLE PRODUCTS, INC.
INDEPENDENT LIVING AIDS, INC.
J.A. PRESTON CORPORATION
LS&S GROUP, INC.
MADDAK, INC.
RAYMO PRODUCTS, INC.
SCIENCE PRODUCTS
THERAFIN CORPORATION

For additional information, including addresses and phone numbers, see CATALOGS.

SPEAKING

Passy-Muir Tracheostomy Speaking Valve

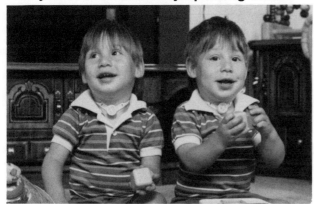

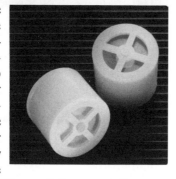

"The first time we heard our boys cry, we laughed; it was so wonderful. We feel it is important for children to get the Passy-Muir Tracheostomy Speaking Valve at the same time they get their trach tube so they don't lose valuable speech development." (Pierre & Jeremy Adler, two year old twins with Central Hypoventilation Syndrome)

The Passy-Muir Tracheostomy Speaking Valve is designed to eliminate the necessity of finger occlusion for the patient with a tracheostomy while allowing the user full-power uninterrupted speech. David Muir, a quadriplegic with a tracheostomy, has developed and used his tracheostomy speaking valve and makes it available for others. The Passy-Muir Tracheostomy Speaking Valve is a one-way valve made of lightweight plastic that attaches to the universal hub of all tracheosotmy tubes including pediatric sizes. This valve allows air to enter the pulmonary tree, easily inflating the lungs upon inspiration. On expiration the valve is closed directing the air into the trachea and up through the vocal cords creating speech as the sound passes through the oral and nasal cavities.

"The doctors and nurses started asking questions in the recovery room. It is very frustrating not to be able to answer normally. The Passy-Muir Tracheostomy Speaking Valve makes communication normal and gives me a feeling of independence. I don't feel helpless anymore."—Judith L. Rosendahl

Caution: U.S. federal law restricts this device to sale by or on the order of a physician.

PASSY & PASSY, INC.
4521 Campus Drive, Suite 273
Irvine, CA 92715
(800) 634-5397
(714) 856-2634

✳✳✳✳

Park Electronic Artificial Larynx

The Park Electronic Artificial Larynx offers the user an on/off switch and both volume and tone controls. Rotate the head of the unit and it will give softer or more strident sound. It is supplied with a battery charger, two rechargeable nickel cadmium batteries, oral adaptor, and carrying case. The larynx is 5" long and 1 1/2" in diameter. Price: under $500.00.

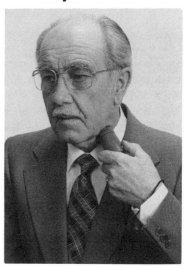

PARK SURGICAL CO., INC.
5001 New Utrecht Avenue
Brooklyn, NY 11219
(800) 633-7878
(718) 436-9200

✳✳✳✳

PRC Intro Talker

Intro Talker is a simple portable battery-powered speech output communication device for non-speaking people. It is a limited function device, offering only speech output with a limited vocabulary, and is intended for users who will not be held back by its limitations.

Intro Talker employs digitized processing, resulting in natural sounding speech. The standard unit includes memory for two minutes of extended speech or one minute of standard speech. Additional memory can be added to extend the capacity to eight minutes of extended speech. (One minute is enough time for more than 120 words or thirty short phrases.)

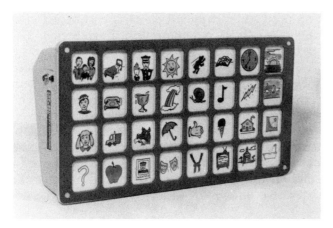

Intro Talker uses semantic vocabulary organization (Minspeak™) in a limited way. It allows vocabulary items to be retrieved using a sequence of up to three multi-meaning icons. The keyboard has thirty-two keys on 1 1/2" centers, requiring four ounces of force. An eight-location key guard is available.

Intro Talker is easily programmed in any language by a speaking person using the built-in microphone or an optional external microphone. Intro Talker users can benefit from much of the research and application support now available to users of the Minspeak system. Price: about $600.00.

Touch Talker™ & Light Talker

Touch Talker™ and Light Talker use computer technology to enable the user to store information and recall it at will. However, no computer knowledge is necessary to use these devices. Messages are stored by means of pictures and recalled when these pictures are activated by touch, a light sensor, or a control switch. The messages are then translated into synthesized speech. The number of pictures in the message and its complexity varies with the needs of the user.

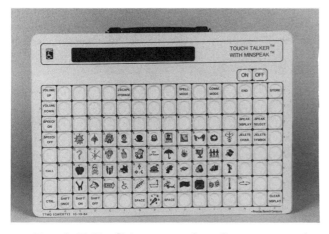

Touch Talker™ is appropriate for persons who

can use a keyboard with their fingers, a mouthstick, or a headpointer. Light Talker uses a light sensor to activate the keyboard. It is designed for persons without touch capabilities who have a single body movement that can be utilized, i.e., head movement, brow wrinkle, puff-sip, or the raising of a finger or a knee.

When you choose a Touch Talker™ or Light Talker, you choose one of two software packages, Express or Minspeak™, which enable the devices to grow and change with the needs of the user. Express software has been available since the 1970's. It permits communication vocabulary to be organized using levels and locations, pages or abbreviations. It is still used effectively by many non-speaking people and the professionals who serve them. Minspeak™, introduced in 1982, represents the very latest in communications software design.

Options:
TT-ME Touch Talker™ w/Minspeak™ and Echo™ Speech Price: under $3000.00
TT-MS Touch Talker™ w/Minspeak™ and SmoothTalker™ Speech Price: well under $4000.00
LT-ME Light Talker w/Minspeak™ and Echo™ Speech Price: about $3500.00
LT-MS Light Talker w/Minspeak™ and SmoothTalker™ Speech Price: under $4500.00

Memory Transfer Interface

The possibility of memory loss in a Touch Talker™ or Light Talker may cause apprehension in users and professionals. With the use of the Memory Transfer Interface, this apprehension can be minimized; the stored memory is transferred to a floppy disk.

The Memory Transfer Interface is useful for private users as well as professionals as a tool for cataloging stored memory. It also enables a professional to utilize one device for evaluating several clients without losing each client's stored text. Each client's text is transferred to a disk and is then transferred back to the machine when appropriate.

The Memory Transfer Interface contains the memory transfer interface unit, the transfer program (floppy disk), and a step-by-step operator manual. The only other components needed for use are an Apple (IIe, II+, or IIgs) computer with disk drive and a super serial card, available from your local Apple dealer. Price: about $100.00.

Note: Interfaces also available for use with Macintosh Plus, SE, and Macintosh 512.

Wheelchair Mounting Kits

Wheelchair Mounting Kits are hardware kits designed to facilitate the mounting of various items on a wheelchair. They contain the following components:

- Set of cast aluminum blocks for clamping to the standard 7/8" wheel+chair frame;
- Stainless steel tube which holds a mounting platform in front of the person;
- Wrench for attaching the system and making adjustments to it—included and stored below the mounting platform.

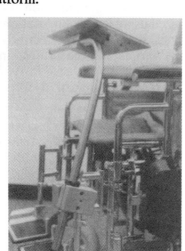

Position and angle of the wheelchair mounting kits is adjustable. In addition, the entire assembly swings away or can be removed easily for transferring into and out of the wheelchair. The kits can be attached to either the left or the right side.

WCMK-5 is used for the Introtalker.

WCMK-4 is used for the Light Talker.

WCMK-3 is used for the Touch Talker™.

WCMK-2 is used for Versascan.

In addition to PRC aids, the Wheelchair Mounting Kits can be used to mount other items such as manual communication boards or book and paper holders. The Wheelchair Mounting Kits are priced at around $250.00.

PRENTKE ROMICH CO.
1022 Heyl Road
Wooster, OH 44691
(800) 642-8255
(216) 262-1984

****

SonomaVoice

The SonomaVoice (SV) is a communication aid and teaching tool featuring low-cost, custom vocabulary speech synthesis. It was designed at Sonoma Developmental Center (SDC), Eldridge, California, to meet the needs of clients of that facility and of the Department of Developmental Services of the State of California. The SV is now produced and distributed on an at-cost basis to the public by the Communication Engineering Department at SDC.

The SV is currently used by people whose speech is impaired by various developmental, neuromuscular, and/or neurological problems. The youngest known user is three years old, and the eldest is eighty. During the research and development cycle, input from those familiar with the needs of persons with hearing impairments and/or cerebral palsy, and of those persons with poststroke expressive difficulties was used in refining the design.

A computer is used to store phrases for an individual user in a computer memory chip. This chip, when inserted in the SV, gives the machine its vocabulary. The maximum number of phrases which may be stored in the SV ranges from 64 (16 phrase keys with four levels) to 256 (16 phrase keys with 16 levels using the mode key option). The SV speaks a phrase when one of its 16 phrase keys is pressed. To increase the capacity beyond 16 phrases, a process called level selection is used. This arrangement provides four levels having 16 phrases each for a total of 64 phrases. If more than 64 phrases are desired, then the mode key option is needed; it increases the SV's capacity to 16 levels.

The voice in the SV is electronically synthesized. It is artificial sounding and in the "male" range. While this type of speech synthesis can provide fairly good quality speech, it does have its shortcomings. For this reason, each phrase is carefully programmed by the Communication Engineering staff and then the pronunciation is stored in a data base along with a code number referred to as the Phrase Code. Lists of the phrases and phrase codes in this data base are available on request. They can give you good ideas about what phrases other people have used on SV's and can save money. If the phrase codes are included with those phrases chosen from the data base, those phrases are free. Custom programming of new phrases is done on a fee-per-phrase basis. It is important to keep in mind, however, that it is the ability to customize the vocabulary of the SV for the particular needs of each user which makes it effective.

The SV runs on rechargeable batteries which will power it for an entire day. The battery charger included will recharge the batteries in about four hours. Typical battery life is about 14 to 18 months. Replacement batteries must be of the same type and can be obtained from Communication Engineering.

The SV keyguard is a formed piece of plastic

with rows and columns of 1 1/2" diameter holes. It is easily removeable, being attached to the unit by hook and loop fastener. User-supplied graphics may be affixed to the inner surface of the keyguard. A variety of options allow customization of the SV to meet individual needs.

The SV is available on loan for client evaluation purposes to licensed professionals and agencies. As with all of the activities of the Sonoma Developmental Center, lending is done on an at-cost basis.

COMMUNICATION ENGINEERING
Sonoma Developmental Center
P.O. Box 1493
15000 Arnold Drive
Eldridge, CA 95431
(707) 938-6306

✱✱✱✱

OTHER SOURCES OF SPEAKING AIDS:

ABBEY MEDICAL
CLEO INC.
FLAGHOUSE, INC.
INDEPENDENT LIVING AIDS, INC.
J.A. PRESTON CORPORATION
LS&S GROUP, INC.
MADDAK, INC.
TASH, INC.

For additional information, including addresses and phone numbers, see CATALOGS.

WRITING

Speakwriter 2000

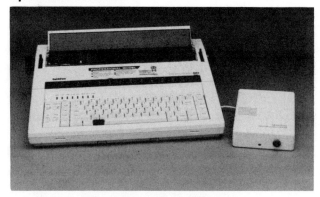

The Speakwriter 2000 (SW2000) is a talking typewriter designed for blind and visually impaired people who need to produce letter perfect documents, but who are not interested in working with computers and word processors. It plugs directly into a Brother CX-90 Typewriter and converts it into a talking typewriter using synthetic speech output.

The SW2000 is also ideal for use in centers where a variety of people need access to a typewriter. (The Brother CX-90 Typewriter can be used by both blind and sighted typists by simply plugging-in or unplugging an SW2000.) In order to become proficient with the SW2000 one only needs to know basic keyboard skills. With very little guidance a user can function autonomously.

Although word processing programs are clearly more powerful, sometimes a standard typewriter is still the more appropriate choice.

SW 2000 only Price: around $900.00
SW 2000 and Brother CX-90 Price: under $1400.00

HUMANWARE, INC.
6140 Horseshoe Bar Road, Suite P
Loomis, CA 95650
(916) 652-7253

✳✳✳✳

End-O-Line Lite

End-O-Line Lite has been designed for the typist who has a hearing impairment and finds it difficult to hear the bell which indicates the end of the typing line. As the carriage approaches the end of the typing line, a light comes on at the same time as the typewriter bell. The light remains activated for approximately six seconds, allowing the typist to ob-

serve the need to return the carriage. You may also plug End-O-Line Lite into your desk lamp which then can serve as your signaling device. End-O-Line Lite automatically adjusts to the right hand margin setting and is equipped with a cord which allows the typist to locate the unit wherever it is most convenient. Price: about $400.00.

Type Typewriter

Large-type typewriters with the standard keyboard for two hand typists are available for immediate delivery. They are office sized model D's which are fully electric and have been re-conditioned. The typewriters feature an easy to read large-type style having six spaces to the inch horizontally (as compared to the ten and twelve spaces of pica and elite). This is the largest type available on an electric typewriter having both upper and lower case letters. The typewriters are equipped with a ribbon which minimizes the strain of reading and produces a bold bulletin size print. The large-type typewriter is priced around $800.00.

A single case, five-pitch "E-Z Reader" is also available. Price: approximately $850.00.

Dvorak One-Handed Keyboard

At first glance these keyboards look like conventional machines. The keys are four banks high, just as they are on a standard keyboard, except that they have been rearranged. All of the frequently used letters are concentrated in the center, the basic advantage being the elimination of muscular contortions and strenuous reaches. Keyboards are available in right and left hand models.

On an ordinary standard keyboard, the left-hand typist does 40% of his typing with the weak little finger. The Dvorak assigns only 15.3% of the typing load to the little finger, 18.3% to the ring finger, 29.7% to the strong middle finger, and 36.7% to the index finger, providing a typewriting load to each finger in proportion to its strength and flexibility. The right-hand keyboard provides an almost identical distribution of the finger load.

The Typewriting Institute for the Handicapped has one-handed keyboards available for use with IBM PC and XT computers. For Apple IIe users, a keyboard converter is available. The Institute also offers left and right hand adapted IBM Correcting Selectric III's. A training manual is included with all Dvorak one-hand keyboards.

IBM Selectric III (with Dvorak keyboard) Price: around $1500.00
Keyboard for IBM PC & XT Price: around $750.00

Converter for Apple IIe Price: around $750.00

TYPEWRITING INSTITUTE FOR THE HANDICAPPED
3102 West Augusta Avenue
Phoenix, AZ 85051
(602) 939-5344

✳✳✳✳

Mprint

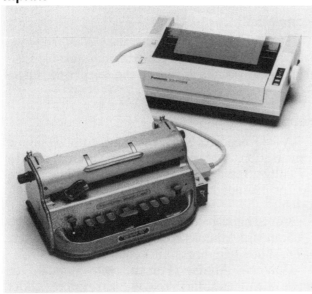

With Mprint a braillist can produce a well-formatted printed report, memo, letter, or any document for a sighted person and simultaneously produce and retain a separate braille copy. Three major benefits are gained from MPRINT:

The braillist can proof the inkprint copy by referring directly to the braille copy;

The braillist can retain a separate braille copy as a file document;

The braillist gains confidence and assurance that print materials produced are accurate.

Mprint is a microprocessor-based system that reads a stream of braille characters from a Perkins brailler, translates those characters into the corresponding ASCII characters, and transmits those characters to a standard serial or Centronics parallel printer.

The braillist can enter information in Grade I and/or Grade II contracted braille and Mprint au-

tomatically expands the Grade II braille into full ASCII text for simultaneous printing from the connected printer. Alternatively, the user can print the Grade II characters directly for learning, checking, and reviewing.

At school, Mprint can help a blind student taking a test for a sighted teacher; the student can take the test and proof it in braille, hand in the printed copy to the teacher, and retain the braille copy for future reference.

At work, a blind receptionist can take telephone messages for sighted co-workers. Blind secretaries can write memos, reports, and prepare documents for sighted co-workers and retain their own braille copies.

MPRINT can be a useful tool in all situations where blind and sighted people communicate in writing.

VTEK
1625 Olympic Blvd.
Santa Monica, CA 90404
(800) 345-2256 Continental U.S. & Hawaii
(800) 338-4898 Canada
(213) 452-5966 Alaska and Puerto Rico

✳✳✳✳

OTHER SOURCES OF WRITING AIDS:

ABBEY MEDICAL
ACCESS TO RECREATION, INC.
ALIMED INC.
AMERICAN FOUNDATION FOR THE BLIND
CLEO INC.
FLAGHOUSE, INC.
HOYLE PRODUCTS, INC.
INDEPENDENT LIVING AIDS, INC.
J.A. PRESTON CORPORATION
LS&S GROUP, INC.
LUMEX
MADDAK, INC.
OPTION CENTRAL
SCIENCE PRODUCTS
THERAFIN CORPORATION

For additional information, including addresses and phone numbers, see CATALOGS.

TELEPHONE COMMUNICATION

Command Telephone System

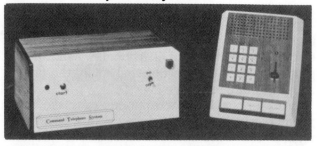

The Command Telephone System requires no physical action to receive telephone calls. The speakerphone component lets you listen and respond to incoming calls from several feet away. The command module activates the speakerphone when the telephone rings and disconnects the speakerphone when the conversation is ended. A ring adjustment lets you select the number of rings before the system goes to work for you. Modular connections are provided for quick installation.

C.T.S.
5600 N. Antioch Road
Kansas City, MO 64119
(800) 635-7323

✳✳✳✳

AT&T National Special Needs Center

The AT&T National Special Needs Center serves the communications needs of persons nationwide with hearing, speech, motion, or vision impairments. A number of special products are made available.

Handsets for Hearing and Speech Amplification

AT&T handsets amplify speech or sound, making it easier for a speech- or hearing-impaired person to enjoy everyday phone conversations.

Handsets plug easily into any modular telephone. Adjustable controls on the receiver let you set the volume of the incoming voice. Speech amplification models let you be heard without voice strain. Prices range from $34.95 to $84.95.

In-Line Amplifier

An alternative to amplification handsets, the In-Line Amplifier attaches directly to the handset cord, boosting the volume of incoming voices as much as 20db. Ideal for hearing impaired people, noisy environments, or poor line transmission. Price: under $40.00.

Portable Telephone Amplifier

The Portable Telephone Amplifier attaches easily and securely onto most telephone handsets, providing amplification up to 20db directly from the receiver. The volume is adjustable. Price: about $25.00.

SignalMan™ Control Unit

The SignalMan™ alerts the user to an incoming call by causing a lamp to flash an unmistakable ON-OFF signal with each ring of the telephone. Price: about $40.00.

Headsets

AT&T headsets allow for hands-free telephone conversations and are ideal for people who have difficulty gripping a receiver or holding one to the ear for extended periods. The volume is fully adjustable and a switch hook, for switching from headset to hand-held receiver, is provided.

Standard Model (For use with standard single or multi-line telephones) Price: about $60.00

Universal Model (For use with standard or electronic single line telephones) Price: about $80.00

Telecommunication Devices for the Deaf

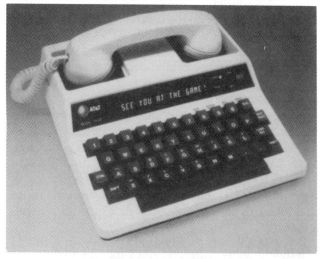

State-of-the-art TDDs from AT&T make it easy to stay in touch, by saving and sending printed messages over phone lines. All TDDs have a four-row typewriter style keyboard and large, bright fluorescent display with blinking cursor for easy readability. Models with printers use upper and lower case printing to set off incoming and outgoing messages. Several models are available, with prices ranging from $249.95 to $649.95.

Directel™

Directel provides full telephone service for people with severe motion impairments. A "puff" activator switch uses a breath of air to place, receive, and disconnect calls. Simply blow into the plastic mouthpiece and the Directel connects the user to a telephone operator who dials the call. Directel can be fitted with a variety of special switches, microphones, and headsets to accommodate an individual's needs. Price: about $500.00.

AT&T
National Special Needs Center
Suite 310
2001 Route 46
Parsippany, NJ 07054-1315
(800) 233-1222
(800) 833-3232 (TDD Users)

****

Speakerphone (Able-Phone 2000)

The Speakerphone provides fifty-three number auto-dialing, including single button auto-dialing for twenty user programmed numbers and single button emergency auto-dialing for police, fire, and ambulance. For easy manual dialing, the Speakerphone is equipped with a large keypad. If falsely triggered, the unit automatically hangs up. Like the Able-Phone it is controlled by whistle tone, and it can be configured with other switches. Wireless remote control is optional, with a no-pressure-re-quired touch switch.

Able-Phone

The Able-Phone by DQP offers cordless communication with true hands-free operation. The adjustable whistle tone conforms to individual capabilities, and an automatic "O" is provided for operator dialing. The Able-Phone can be configured with other switches such as leaf, blow, and touch. It can be attached to wheelchair, bed, or belt and can be operated by respirator dependents.

DQP
14167 Meadow Drive
Grass Valley, CA 95945
(916) 477-1234

****

OTHER SOURCES OF TELEPHONE COMMUNICATION AIDS:

ACCESS TO RECREATION, INC.
ALIMED INC.
AMERICAN FOUNDATION FOR THE BLIND
CLEO INC.
INDEPENDENT LIVING AIDS, INC.
LAUREL DESIGNS
LS&S GROUP, INC.
MADDAK, INC.
RADIO SHACK
SCIENCE PRODUCTS
THERAFIN CORPORATION

For additional information, including addresses and phone numbers, see CATALOGS.

MOBILITY

WALKING

Autosupport

The Autosupport Prince of Wales cane is made of specially formed aluminum sections that have been heat treated for strength and durability. It is self-opening by actions of a heavy duty elastic cord, and can be folded into a carrying case which fits conveniently into pocket or purse. The classic curved wood-tone handle fits 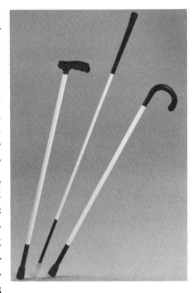 comfortably in the hand. The Autosupport is finished in durable white epoxy with a red anodized tip section. It is available in lengths of 33 to 36 inches, and weighs less than 11 ounces. Also available reflective. If you prefer, the Autosupport can be purchased with a sculptured hardwood pistol grip handle.

Cable Cane

The Cable Cane uses the patented, plastic sheathed stainless steel cable system and adds a uniquely designed tension handle with a non-slip, nylon coated pistol grip. The index finger points down the shaft, while the middle finger in its own slot grips the cane firmly. Epoxy painted sections are specially form- 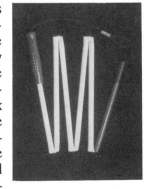 ed on both ends to ensure a rigid structure when assembled. When not in use, the Cable Cane folds to a compact 10 inches. Lengths range from 34 to 54 inches. The finish conforms to all white cane laws.

Autofold

The Autofold is a high quality, self-erecting cane. Heavy duty tension cord provides exceptional durability. Like the Cable and Autosupport Canes, it is made of specially formed aluminum sections, with lengths from 34 to 54 inches, adaptable to all heights. It has a retaining strap and comfortable rubber grip. The cane folds to a compact 10 inches and stores in a convenient polyvinyl case. The finish conforms to all white cane laws. Available reflective.

AUTOFOLD
208 Coleman Street Ext., P.O. Box 1063
Gardner, MA 01440
(508) 632-0667

✳✳✳✳

Mowat Sensor

The Mowat Sensor is a small, hand-held device which warns the user about approaching obstacles. Used like a flashlight, it sends a narrow beam of high frequency sound into the environment, which is reflected off anything in its path. The reflected signals received by the sensor are exhibited in the form of vibrations. The rate of vibration depends on the sensor's distance from the obstacle. It has two distance settings; one for indoor, cluttered environments and the other for outdoors. The Mowat Sensor should be used in conjunction with a long cane or a dog guide and provides valuable information regarding obstacles above knee height which can often be quite dangerous to a visually handicapped person. It also simplifies finding one's way through a parking lot or locating clear pathways or doorways. This is particularly useful for the person who occasionally travels in unfamiliar environments. The Mowat Sensor is priced at under $700.00.

Note: Several hours of instruction by an orientation and mobility instructor are necessary to enable a visually handicapped person to achieve proficiency in the use of the sensor.

HUMANWARE, INC.
6140 Horseshoe Bar Road, Suite P
Loomis, CA 95650
(800) 722-3393
(916) 652-7253

****

Deluxe Walk-A-Cycle™

"I am writing to you at this time relative to the Walk-A-Cycle™ which has been utilized by several of my patients with Parkinson's disease. This has given them a new freedom both in and out of doors, with the feature of voluntary braking reducing greatly the danger of falling backwards or forwards, the seat arrangement serving them well, particularly in times when they have been in 'off' condition and unable to move much on their own or when they have been fatigued from exertion. Usual walking devices do not have ready braking or for that matter a place to rest when needed. It is obvious that the device should prove very practical for patients with limb girdle weakness due to muscular dystrophy or atrophy, and I am enthusiastic about its potential. It also might prove to be of value for patients with weakness due to spina bifida and those with hemiplegia or tetraplegia."—Dr. Henry A. Peter, M.D., Dept. of Neurology, University Hospital, Madison, WI

The Walk-A-Cycle's™ 26" wheels roll over sidewalks, pebbles, lawns, or carpets. A sling seat provides a ready resting place. Wheel governors allow you to adjust wheel resistance, while the hand brakes provide added control. With the addition of other options, the Deluxe Walk-A-Cycle™ can be custom designed to fit your needs. Prices for the Deluxe Walk-A-Cycle™ start at around $700.00. Options available include:

Large Basket Car Carrier
Small Basket Storage Cover
Cane Holders AM-FM Radio
Crutch Attachments One Hand Brake Operation

Stroke Arm Rest Tray

AMERICAN WALKER, INC.
797 Market Street
Oregon, WI 53575
(608) 835-9255

****

Wheeled Walker

The Wheeled Walker has wheels on all four legs. However, it will not run away with you since gentle pressure on the handles will automatically lock the back wheels. It's available in a variety of child and adult sizes for users as small as 3' 2". A Basket and Dining and Writing Tray are both available as accessories. For added convenience the Wheeled Walker doubles as a seat. Price: about $250.00.

BALLERT INTERNATIONAL, INC.
3677 Woodhead Drive
Northbrook, IL 60062-1816
(800) 345-3456
(708) 480-0390

****

OTHER SOURCES OF WALKING AIDS:

ABBEY MEDICAL
ALIMED INC.
AMERICAN FOUNDATION FOR THE BLIND
ARJO HOSPITAL EQUIPMENT, INC.
CLEO INC.
CONSUMER CARE PRODUCTS
FLAGHOUSE, INC.
INDEPENDENT LIVING AIDS, INC.
J.A. PRESTON CORPORATION
KAY PRODUCTS INC.
LS&S GROUP, INC.
LUMEX
MADDAK, INC.
MARSHALL MEDICAL
OPTION CENTRAL
RIFTON
ST. LOUIS OSTOMY AND MEDICAL SUPPLY
WINCO INCORPORATED

For additional information, including addresses and phone numbers, see CATALOGS.

WHEELCHAIRS

The Yorkhill Chair

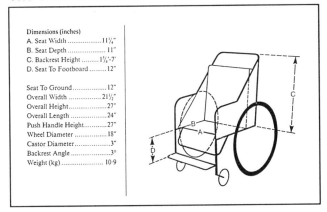

Dimensions (inches)
A. Seat Width .... 11¼"
B. Seat Depth .... 11"
C. Backrest Height .... 1¾"-7"
D. Seat To Footboard .... 12"

Seat To Ground .... 12"
Overall Width .... 21½"
Overall Height .... 27"
Overall Length .... 24"
Push Handle Height .... 27"
Wheel Diameter .... 18"
Castor Diameter .... 3"
Backrest Angle .... 3°
Weight (kg) .... 10·9

This light compact chair is designed for use by the spina bifida child of between two and six years of age. The cushion extension acts as a leg rest for use with calipers, and the molded semicircular tray is useful for mealtimes or as a play table. The chair is immobilized by the rear foot operated prop stand, and the rear 18" wheels (without handrims) are designed so that the child can propel him/herself around the classroom or home, independently.

The Newton Manual

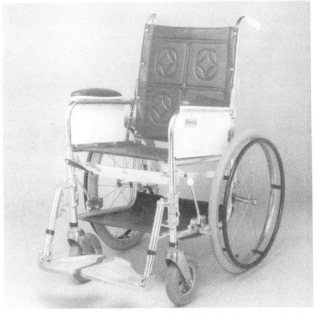

The Newton Manual wheelchair is one of the lightest all-purpose wheelchairs. The frame is maintenance-free polished anodized aluminum with welded joints. A special triple over-center linkage system makes the chair highly portable and easy to fold, and provides carefully designed support. The backward tilt ensures a comfortable and secure sitting position.

A push-button release quickly removes the padded armrests for sideways transfer, such as to bed, car, etc. The foot rests are die cast aluminum and especially shaped and lipped to prevent slipping. A parcel shelf under the seat provides valuable space for carrying small packages. Several models of this chair are available, along with a variety of accessories.

The Badger Powered Wheelchair

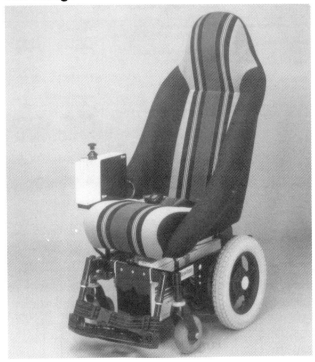

The Badger is a high performance wheelchair that doesn't conform with conventionally accepted wheelchair appearance. Design concepts permit a number of different seat options which make it suitable for both indoor and outdoor use, and it is transportable. As a child's chair, it can be considered a growing chair. Its performance and maneuverability set it apart in competitive electric wheelchair sporting events. In fact it was a silver medal winner in the 1986 World Cerebral Palsy championships.

MK II Elan

The Elan powered wheelchair is ideal for indoors or out. Its independent rear suspension gives a comfortable ride and smooth acceleration. The Elan's joystick control may be fitted on the right- or left-hand side, and gives fingertip control of speed and direction. In addition, the control is fitted with a variable speed range selector. The chair brakes automatically when the joystick is released. Also, the Elan is equipped with a drive disengagement device in the rear hub to allow the chair to be pushed by an attendant if necessary.

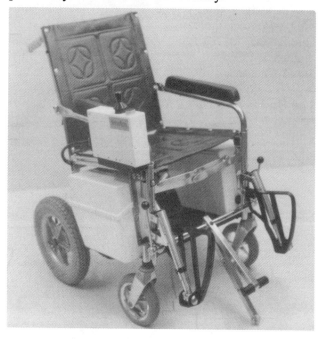

Avon Deluxe

The support system for the Avon Deluxe chairs was designed with the help of physiotherapists to give corrective positioning to children and adolescents suffering from a flaccid spine or scoliosis. The complete system (which is available in kit form for existing chairs) consists of adjustable thoracic and pelvic pads, and a fully adjustable head support. The Avon Deluxe offers a wide range of options and accessories, and supports can also be specially made to suit individual requirements.

NEWTON WHEELCHAIRS U.S.A.
21209 Lago Circle, 12E
Boca Raton, FL 33433
(407) 483-7184

Note: Newton also makes chairs, especially for wheelchair athletes, that are light, fast, maneuverable, and "built to take it."

✳✳✳✳

Iron Horse One

The Iron Horse One is designed as a durable, low-maintenance chair for the active user. In putting this chair together, the designers used nuts, bolts, screws, and other major components (i.e. bicycle wheels) that are available in well-supplied hardware stores and bicycle shops. Any basic household tool box is likely to have all the tools necessary to work on the "Horse," with the exception of two Allen wrenches. These are provided with the chair, along with a user's manual explaining the basic maintenance tasks and how and when these should be done.

The Iron Horse has a range of standard features designed to contribute to and enhance the lifestyles of active wheelriders.

The front and rear wheels of Iron Horse One have patented suspension systems. The rear wheels are suspended on Iron Horse's "Eagle Wings." These use a die-cast, coil spring mechanism to provide up to two inches of shock absorption for a 200 pound rider. The 7" front casters are mounted on a similar die-cast assembly, called the "Falcon Fork," providing 3/4' of travel absorption (for the same 200 pound person). The rear wheels have roller-bearing hubs, vinyl-coated handrims with extensions, and come with 26" bicycle tires for expanded tread choices. The Iron Horse One offers 8" pneumatic or 7" hard rubber front tires.

The Iron Horse frame is made of 1", 18 gauge, nickel-chromium coated, polished stainless steel. The folding frame is designed with a "Dos Equis" folding mechanism. This double-X not only provides a firmer chair, but locks into place when unfolded. The incline of the seat back is factory-set at five degrees open from vertical (95 degrees) for rider comfort. With the front of the chair raised another five degrees, the rounded shoulder syndrome common to wheelchair riders is eliminated. Also, the frame has non-detachable folding footrests, comes with swing back armrests, and has detachable anti-tip bars.

Because this chair is designed for the active user, components will become worn and need repair or replacement. The wheelrider's manual also presents an extensive list of troubleshooting hints to assist in spotting problems before they occur. With the design concerns for locally-available parts, potential breakdowns can be avoided and parts replaced in the wheelrider's own community.

In the event that the damage is too major for the user to handle, Iron Horse offers a toll-free number to discuss the problem with company staff, order original parts, or arrange for repair or replacement by Iron Horse. This company guarantees a 48 hour turn-around time on in-house repairs.

The founder of Iron Horse Productions is George "Sandy" Duffy, Jr. Sandy, as a result of a vehicle accident, became a paraplegic (T9) in 1969. Prior to his accident, Sandy had led a very active life, including many outdoor hobbies and pastimes. As he progressed through his rehabilitation program, Sandy was exposed to many of the standard wheelchair designs. Resuming an active life after the rehabilitation process meant accepting the limitations those chairs imposed.

Sandy couldn't understand how people could continue to design wheelchairs where the only shock absorber was the user's own flesh and spinal column. Sandy was looking for a chair that contributed to his lifestyle rather than constrained it. Sandy is part of the generation of wheelriders who believe their lifestyles can be as active, mobile, and recreational as they want them to be.

IRON HORSE PRODUCTIONS
2624 Conner Street
Port Huron, MI 48060
(313) 987-6700
(800) 426-0354

✳✳✳✳

Zippie & Zippie TS

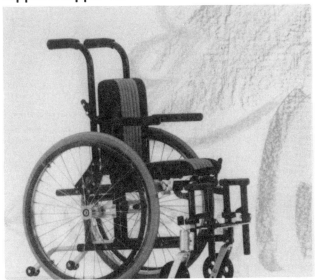

Zippie is just for kids. It offers adjustability, portability, and durability, and is designed with a growing system that makes size changes easy and inexpensive. The solid seat and back can be modified to accommodate additional support accessories. Swing away footrests guarantee 90/90/90 degree positioning.

The Zippie TS provides a Tilt-In-Space frame option that maintains a 90/90/90 degree posture while reclining within a 30 degree range. For optimum positioning, the cable trigger mechanism positively locks into place from 90 to 120 degrees to provide maximum flexibility.

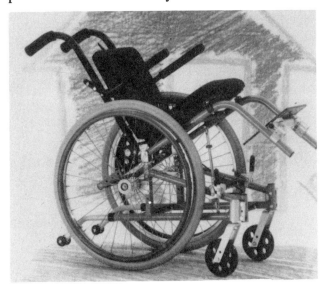

Quickie™

The Quickie™ wheelchair's lightweight construction, bright frame colors, and aesthetically pleasing design shift the emphasis from the cold institutional image of the past to a positive and independent image for today. Every chair can be customized to fit a user's body size and personal needs. Its modular frame with a lock-out folding seat provides a combination of rigid-chair performance and fold-up portability. The modular frame concept also gives each user the freedom to change quickly and inexpensively the dimensions of his chair by simply substituting interchangeable parts. The chair can grow or change, right along with a child, or can accommodate an adult's changing needs.

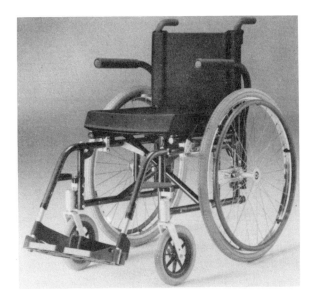

The Quickie™ 2 can grow or shrink in length and width by simply changing front frame components, cross-braces, and upholstery. Other features of Quickie™ wheelchairs include low mount out-of-the way brakes, adjustable center of gravity and caster angle, plus many accessory options that allow each user to customize his chair. For easy traveling, the Quickie™ 2 folds up and fits neatly behind a car seat, or by popping off the wheels, it can even fit in the overhead rack of an airplane.

MOTION DESIGNS, INC.
2842 Business Park Avenue
Fresno, CA 93727
(209) 292-2171

****

Primary 500 Series

The Primary 500 Series by Safety Rehab is a custom-designed stroller for the physically involved child, ages one to five.

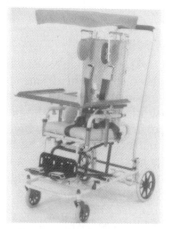

Positioning units on all of the Primary 500 Series Strollers are removable. When used in a car, they meet the head and knee excursion limits set by test requirements of Federal Motor Vehicle Safety Standards #213 with the safety-approved harness system. The Model 501 also offers a uniquely-designed highchair feature. The Model 502 is the primary series stroller providing the maximum in adjustability. The child's growth and changing positioning requirements are easily accommodated by multiple support pads.

All Primary 500 Series Strollers include: removeable positioning unit with stroller base, easy-to-clean vinyl upholstery, 30 degree tilt-angle in space, adjustable height arm pads, adjustable height and depth footplates with ankle straps, washable/removable birchwood tray, sunscreen mesh canopy top, support pad options, "Cheery Teddy Bear" applique.

900 Series Transporter

The 900 Series Transporter offers multi-support devices and support styles. The 900 Series is easily converted to an all-terrain transporter with a sturdy detachable "outdoor" base. The wider 912

base with its large wheels (8" front, 12" rear) allows safe outdoor mobility. The 910 "Ventilator" base is for the child who is ventilator dependent. The base is detachable—complete with platform and securing straps—and can accommodate both the ventilator and a battery. The 906 "Wheelchair" base, with either 20" or 24" wheels, allows maximum maneuverability.

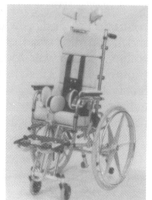

900 Series features include: thirteen (the 910 has nine positions standard) positions (between 0 and 45 degrees), easy reclining lever, two position arms, adjustable angle seat, three adapter bushings on arm tubes for placement of optional support pads, a variety of optional bases, and more.

SAFETY REHAB
SYSTEMS, INC.
147 Eady Court
Elyria, OH 44035
(800) 421-3349
(216) 366-5611 (Inside Ohio call collect)

****

Gendron

The Gendron line of standard wheelchairs consists of thirty-three basic models, each offering a variety of accessories and dimensions. In addition Gendron offers a wide selection of footrests, legrests, seat widths, reclining backs, and removable arms for many of the standard models. When a standard chair is not adequate to meet the user's size or physical condition, Gendron can design and build a special chair to meet the particular requirements of the individual.

X2 Series 6500

Gendron's X2 Series 6500 folding wheelchair is designed and built exclusively for the large person. The unit is available with a 20" wide seat (6500-W2), a 22" wide seat (6500-W3), or a 24" wide seat (6500-W4). The specially designed X-Brace is constructed of 11 gauge 1 1/4" square tubing providing the necessary support for the large individual. The opening and closing of the chair is guided by four telescoping side-frame members instead of the conventional two telescoping members. Seat tubes constructed of thirteen gauge tubing provide for positive attachment of upholstery, and additional support is achieved by means of two struts attached to the X-Brace and forward extremity of the seat tube. The upholstery is reinforced with a special Textilene liner. Offset 8" swivel casters contain four machined, radial flanged, full race, bearing assemblies to provide ease of maneuverability and long service life. Twenty-four inch rear wheels are mounted on 5/8" axles and four machined, full race, radial flanged bearings, each with a load rating of 560 pounds. Fluted handrims, toggle brakes, hook-on footrests, and stainless steel clothing guards are standard features. All eight combinations of Gendron's Footrests/Legrests are available for the X2, plus the "Mono-Post" adjustable height, removable desk or full arms. Many standard accessories are also available for this series.

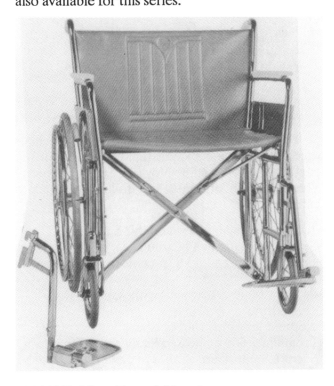

"2811" Folding Travel-About

The 2811 is a compact folding travel-about offering a low seat to floor height of 18". The unit has four 8" casters; two swivel and two fixed. User operated lever brakes lock the two rear wheels for exit and entry. The chair folds to a compact 10" and weighs just 30 pounds without the footrests.

GENDRON, INC.
Lugbill Road
Archbold, OH 43502
(800) 537-2521
(419) 445-6060 in Ohio

****

Kelly™

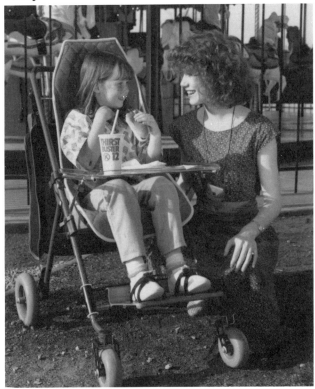

While it looks like a conventional stroller with its bright color and clean, smooth lines, Kelly™ is designed exclusively to meet the special needs of a mildly involved child.

Kelly™ has a firm back and seat. The recommended 90 degree angle is maintained at the seat, knee, and footplate, and good midline positioning is achieved by Kelly's™ natural side support. A shoulder harness, abductor, tray, and headrest are also available. An adjustable-height footplate is standard equipment, and can be fitted with footstraps to improve posture even further.

With just one frame, children from eighteen months to twelve years can continue to use their Kelly™. Interchangeable back/seat systems are available to provide a wide range of back height, seat width, and seat depth configurations.

The Kelly™ comes complete with: frame with height-adjustable footplate, firm back and seat with fire-retardant, machine-washable quilted cover, and lap belt. Optional accessories include a tray, shoulder harness, swingaway abductor, recline adjustment, angle-adjustable footplate, footstraps, head support, sunshade, raincape, and carrying bag. Price: about $500.00.

Travel Chair

The versatile Ortho-Kinetics Travel Chair can be used as an adaptive wheelchair, school chair, or as a high chair for eating or play.

For car travel, the chair fits right on the passenger seat with the child restrained by the three-point auto harness. To secure the chair, it is recommended that an additional Department of Transportation approved lap belt be used around the chair frame.

The Travel Chair has been independently tested to conditions similar to Federal Motor Vehicle Safety Standard 213. The Travel Chair tests were run in both the car seat and bus transport positions with D.O.T. approved restraint belts for the chair and the child. All tests were completed successfully.

The Travel Chair is a one-piece system which is easy to get in and out of a car since the base is not separated from the back and seat; no bending or kneeling is necessary. It can also be safely tied down and transported in a bus or van by utilizing the new Q'Straint™ system. The child and the chair are separately and securely fastened with no dependence of one on the other. This provides the same degree of safety available to automobile passengers.

Care Chair III

Designed for teenagers or smaller adults, the Care Chair III offers most of the same features and accessories as the travel chair. Accessories exclusive to the Care Chair III are swingaway elevating legrests and 20" wheelchair wheels. Like the Travel Chair, the Care Chair III can be used in an upright position at a table or with an optional tray for eating.

Optional equipment includes: wheelchair wheels, support pads, shoulder harness, headrests, abductors, seat wedge, carrying bag, swingaway and individually adjustable footrests, neckrest, and head support cushions.

ORTHO-KINETICS, INC.
P.O. Box 1647
Waukesha, WI 53187
(800) 558-7786
(800) 522-0992 in Wisconsin

✳✳✳✳

CONTEMPORARY HEALTH SYSTEMS

Contemporary Health Systems offers a large variety of wheelchairs—more than thirty models —including: Qualine Wheelchairs, Qualine Special-ty Wheelchairs, Qualine "Ovation" Lightweight Wheelchairs, Fineline Lightweight Wheelchairs, and Econoline Wheelchairs. They also provide an assortment of options and accessories.

Qualine Voyager Series—FullBack™

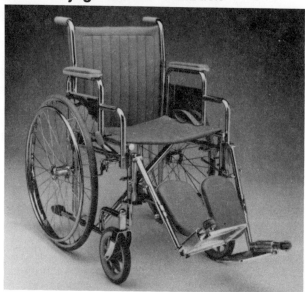

The Fullback™ is a stainless steel full recliner wheelchair with a choice of removable desk or full length arms. All Qualine Voyager Series Fullback™ Wheelchairs incorporate the following standard features:

- 1.2mm thick stainless steel tubing
- Sealed precision ball bearings
- Patented "Perma-lok" 8" precision molded front casters
- 24" adjustable rear wheels with stainless steel handrims
- Non-marking gray rubber tires
- Premium grade embossed leatherette with non-stretch interliner
- Accessory Pouch incorporated in back upholstery
- Padded upholstered armrests and calf pads on elevating legrest models
- Roller bumpers, heel loops included with swing away footrest
- Fully reclines from 90 to 180 degrees
- Detachable back
- 5/8" rear wheel axle and bearings on 20" seat width recliners
- Stainless steel side panels
- Attendant tip pedal
- Lever release arm locks on detachable arm models
- Choice of color: Navy Blue, Dove Gray

CONTEMPORARY HEALTH SYSTEMS,
INC.
1900 135th Street
Gardena, CA 90249
(800) 247-7773
(213) 719-1000 in California

✻✻✻✻

Enduro

Designed and developed for children, the Enduro is a growing pediatric wheelchair. Constructed of Titanium tubing, the frame is approximately four times stronger than aluminum yet weighs only 17 3/4 pounds including front rigging.

It offers a totally integrated seating system together with a chair that grows in width and depth, plus standards such as 90 degree footrests, solid insert seat and back, and adjustable seat height.

Enduro "Optima"

The Enduro "Optima," introduced in 1987, is a lightweight, children's orientation-in-space wheelchair. Combining the growth, mobility, and durability of the standard Enduro, the Enduro "Optima" incorporates an orientation feature which allows correct positioning of the seat and back while angling the entire fixed seat, back, and footrest position from 90 to 135 degrees.

Enduro "Encore"

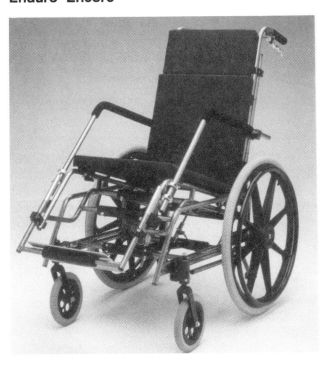

The Enduro "Encore" is an orientation-in-space wheelchair built for the adult population.

Enduro Adaptive Seating

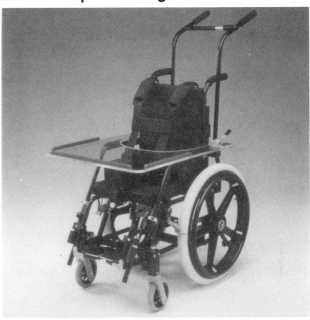

Enduro Adaptive Seating is based upon a linear/planar system that attaches directly to the seat and back. Most component parts are adjustable and easily removed so they can be used on new seating when there is a growth change. Because Wheel Ring makes all of its own brackets and fixtures, special custom seating can also be provided.

WHEEL RING, INC.
199 Forest Street
Manchester, CT 06040
(203) 647-8596

✻✻✻✻

Impulse

The Impulse manual wheelchair is custom designed to meet specific needs and specifications. The Impulse is tailor-made to fit the user exactly. Active users know what they want in a wheelchair, and Impulse allows them to design the chair from the ground up. "We believe the time to adjust to a chair is before it's built, not after you get it home." The Impulse is not a "production" wheelchair. Each unit is built by Everest and Jennings from the specifications submitted by the dealer.

Specifications:
• Seat Height Front—17" to 21"
• Seat Height Back—13 1/2" to 21"
• Back Height—7" to 18 1/2"

- Wheel Camber—0 to 7 degrees
- Back Angle—2 degrees forward/3 degrees backward
- Weight—beginning at under 20 pounds
- Seat Depth—14" to 18 1/2"
- Seat Width—12" to 18 1/2"
- Standard Equipment:
- Wheel Locks
- Anti-Tippers
- Quick Release Axles
- 5" solid casters
- 24" spoked wheels with sew-up tires
- Folddown Back

EVEREST & JENNINGS
3233 E. Mission Oaks Blvd.
Camarillo, CA 93010
(805) 987-6911

****

The Bounder™

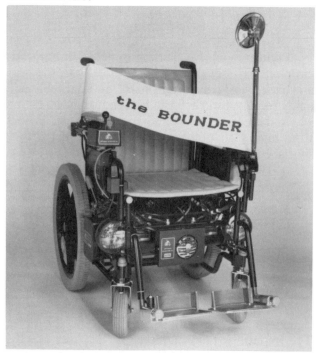

The Bounder™ is a power wheelchair by 21st Century Scientific, Inc. offering standard features that include: precision proportional control of chair speed by means of a two-axis joystick; a 1/4 HP permanent magnet motor with no gear box and no mechanical play in the drive train; spring actuated electro-mechanical brakes that will hold the chair on grades, even if the power is lost; an electric braking system that includes two driver accessible switches, jerk brake, brake alarm, and internally adjustable time delays to ensure precise stops on hills and lift gates; sliding dual group 27 battery box for increased range and ease of battery maintenance; a top speed of 8.5 MPH (models with increased hill climbing capability and slower top speeds are also available).

21st's Tuffy frame has extra tube members, numerous gussets, and durable semi-gloss black powder coat (silver powder coat and chrome are also available). The front caster assemblies include MSE Davis suspension forks, 8 x 2.00" pneumatic front tires and tubes, and anti-flutter stem bearings (8 x 1.75 pneumatic and semi-pneumatic front tires and tubes are available options). The rear wheels are 20" x 2.125" "mag type" with removable 12" pulleys, safety reflector, and precision 12" bearings. Thorn resistant rear wheel inner tubes are standard. The clutches for tensioning drive belts are easily adjusted, and the extra large V belts themselves are available at auto parts stores. Many major components of the Bounders™ are compatible and interchangeable with E&J Power Drives. Accessories for the Bounder™ include an Electric Leg Bag Emptier, a Detachable Rear View Mirror, an Electric Horn, and a Lighting Package.

Bounder™-16-DLA (16" wide) Price: under $6000.00
Bounder™-18-DLA (18" wide) Price: under $6000.00

21ST CENTURY SCIENTIFIC, INC.
7629 Fulton Avenue
North Hollywood, CA 91605
(818) 982-2526

Note: 21st Century Scientific, Inc. offers a variety of power wheelchair parts and accessories.

****

The A-Bec Performers

The Performer "40" series has versatile power chairs that are lightweight, eminently portable, and don't need vans for transporting. They are equipped with direct drive motors and 24 volt electrical systems. Its proportional controller smoothly accelerates with speeds up to 5 MPH. The inductive joystick, with no wearing parts, is light to the touch, requiring only 3 ounces of pressure. To ensure complete control, anti-tremor dampening slows the reaction time on the joy stick for users with hand coordination needs. As soon as you release the joystick, the Performer eases to a complete stop. A Four-Stage Progressive and

Regenerative Braking System is standard equipment. The sporty aluminum magwheels are specially-treaded for traction on outdoor terrain, yet are gentle on indoor floors. Extra large footplates are designed for proper placement and comfort. Swing-away foot rests and leg rests are optional. In a few seconds, the Performer can be folded to a slim 14" wide, and placed in the back seat or trunk of your car.

Other A-BEC wheelchairs include the Targa, offering high-powered performance and a full spectrum of features, and a line of All-Purpose power portables.

A-BEC MOBILITY INC.
A Sunrise Medical Company
20460 Gramercy Place
Torrance, CA 90501
(800) 421-2269
(800) 262-1331 in California

****

Beachmaster

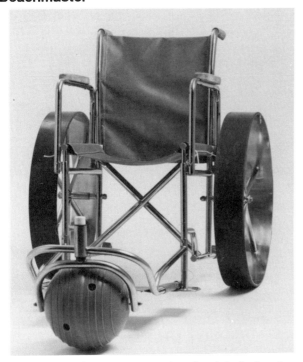

The Beachmaster aquatic wheelchair has been used for a variety of different applications, some rather imaginative: as a "launching pad" for ocean, lake, or pool swimming; for surf fishing; for "strolling" on the beach; in structured rehabilitation; or simply as a way of taking in the sun and enjoying the salt air.

Made of non-corrosive materials throughout, the Beachmaster employs a rugged stainless steel frame. It has 4" wide stainless steel wheels and uses non-absorbent fabric for seat and back. The patented wheel design permits the chair to be pulled atop soft sand or grass surfaces. With the rider seated in the chair, a companion rolls it into the water, up to about waist deep. The rider can then swim out, exercise and swim back into the chair. For pool use, the chair can be rolled down a ramp or lowered via a poolside lift. The wheels can be rubberized to protect pool surfaces, and stainless steel casters are used in front. The company's most recent innovation is the "beach ball" on the front of the chair. This allows the chair to be propelled forward either by the rider or a companion.

BEACH WHEELS, INCORPORATED
1555 Shadowlawn
Naples, FL 33942
(813) 775-1078

****

Electro-Lite

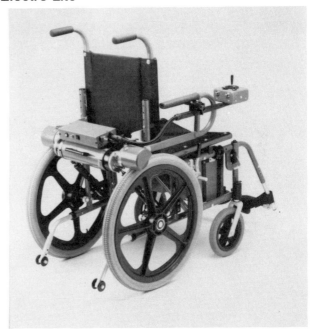

The Electro-Lite Power Chair by Damaco is "ultra-light." The entire chair, including batteries, weighs less than 100 pounds. And the whole system can be transported in the back seat or trunk of an automobile.

The Electro-Lite offers quick free wheeling capability and two maximum speed levels, HI (5 1/4 mph) and VARIABLE (less than 1 mph to 5 mph). Its swing-away arms are desk length and adjustable and the footrests, also swing-away, feature the distinctive "quad POP release."

DAMACO
20545 Plummer Street
Chatsworth, CA 91311
(800) 432-2434
(818) 709-4534

****

OTHER SOURCES OF WHEELCHAIRS:

ABBEY MEDICAL
ACCESS TO RECREATION, INC.
ADAPTIVE PRODUCTS
J.A. PRESTON CORPORATION
ST. LOUIS OSTOMY AND MEDICAL SUPPLY

For additional information, including addresses and phone numbers, see CATALOGS.

WHEELCHAIR PARTS AND ACCESSORIES

"Bye-Bye Decubiti®. . ." Wheelchair Cushions

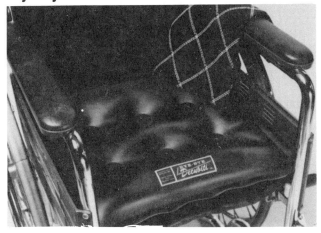

Available in a variety of designs and sizes to fit all wheelchairs, these 100% natural rubber cushions can aid in the prevention of decubitus ulcers by providing pressure equalization, and offering ventilation and shock absorbency. Inflated by mouth or low pressure pump, they may be adjusted for fullness to accommodate individual comfort and stability requirements.

These cushions are odorless and clean—if soiled they can easily be washed, dried, and returned to use. They are also completely autoclavable. They may be used in bed, bathtub, shower, boat, or stadium. Covers of either fleece or double-knit stretch fabric are available. The wheelchair cushions, in a variety of sizes, are priced under $60.00. The covers are $25.00 or less.

Lumbo-Posture Belt

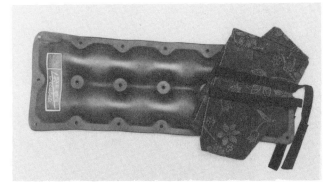

Like the BBD Wheelchair Cushions, the Lumbo-Posture Belt is made of 100% natural rubber. It's available in two sizes, each incorporating fleece/velour covering (used either side up) with elastic straps and Velcro attachments. Inflated by mouth or hand pump, it can be fastened around the seat back, secured around the waist, or placed wherever needed for posture control or pressure absorption. Both the cover and rubber pad are washable and easily changed. Price: under $60.00.

KEN MCRIGHT SUPPLIES, INC.
7456 South Oswego
Tulsa, OK 74136
(918) 492-9657

✳✳✳✳

Heel Loop Flipper (Patent No. 4463985)

Heel loops engaging the footrest hanger when the footrest is turned up create several problems: the wheelchair doesn't fold flat, the heel loop is crushed, the chair's occupant must lean forward to push the heel loop out of the way, the heel loops break down because of the necessity for repeatedly forcing the chair to fold flat.

The Heel Loop Flipper automatically flips the heel loop forward when the footrest is turned up, resulting in up to a 3" savings in folded wheelchair width. The footrest slips over the footrest hanger tube and locks with a twist of the wrist or a turn of a screwdriver. Price: about $20.00.

CHUCK CHEVILLON & ASSOCIATES, INC.
413 N. Mannheim Road, Suite #2
Bellwood, IL 60104
(312) 544-0080

✳✳✳✳

Safe Seat™

The Safe-Seat™ is a battery-operated, dynamic cushion for wheelchairs. The contoured resting surface is locally divided into equal stationary and movable areas. When the air bladder inside the seat inflates, the movable surface rises slowly and supports the occupant; when the air bladder deflates, the surface descends slowly, and the occupant's weight smoothly transfers back onto the stationary surface of the seat.

The Safe-Seat™ operates automatically, cycling about fifteen times each hour. The sitting pressure is completely relieved on all resting areas of the skin during each cycle as the occupant's weight transfers fully from the stationary surface to the movable surface and back again to the stationary surface. Cooling air circulates on the resting areas of the skin during each weight transfer, carrying heat and moisture away from the skin.

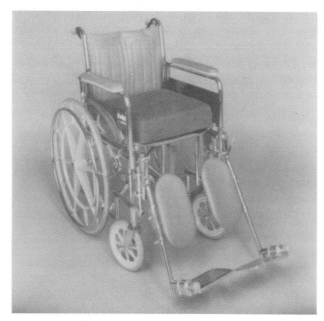

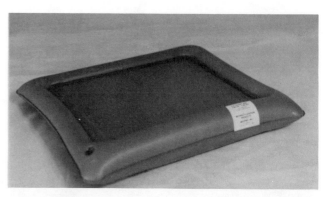

The seat starts to cycle as soon as it senses the occupant's weight. It stops when the occupant transfers off the seat. Molded of high density polyethylene, it is lightweight, sturdy, can be immersed in a tub, scrubbed, and hosed. All of the electrical components are contained in an inconspicuous black canvas bag which hangs from the wheelchair handles.

Safe-Seat™ operates on 12 volt battery power. A NICAD battery pack and battery charger are provided for manual wheelchair users. An electric cord with plug is provided to operate the cushion from an electric wheelchair battery.

Safe-Seat™ (wheelchair battery powered) Price: under $500.00

Safe-Seat™ (self-powered) Price: under $600.00

D.A. SCHULMAN, INC.
7701 Newton Avenue N.
Brooklyn Park, MN 55444
(612) 561-2908

✳✳✳✳

Chair Flotation Cushion

The patented design of the Spinal-Tech Chair Flotation Cushion effectively conforms to body contours, creating a comfortable seating environment for the user. The cushion consists of two separate parts: an inner chamber which can be filled with air, water, or gel and an outer air frame. Both are constructed from heavy duty heat-sealed vinyl.

The inner chamber, when filled with air, becomes an extremely lightweight flotation cushion weighing just two pounds. When filled with water or gel, the cushion weighs about twelve pounds. The inner chamber is constructed with a series of baffles to help maintain stability. The air frame which surrounds the inner chamber serves as a safety liner. Price: about $30.00.

SPINAL TECHNOLOGIES
859 Route 130
East Windsor, NJ 08520
(609) 443-8083
(800) 257-5145
(800) 222-0258

✳✳✳✳

Fold-A-Way Table

The Vireo Fold-A-Way table permanently attaches to the majority of basic-style wheelchairs and can be manually operated by the user. It can be mounted on either the right or left hand side, and can be tilted on an angle and adjusted up or down. The Table is constructed of moisture-resistant finished wood, with heavy duty coated aluminum cast brackets and stainless steel hinges. The same clamp that installs the table can be modified to fit most chairs.

Vireo Wheelchair Cylinder Holder

Vireo's chrome plated cylinder holder can be attached without tools to the left side of a wheelchair and won't interfere with the chair's normal operation. Accommodating both D and E size cylinders, it eliminates the need for a separate cart.

Vireo Wheelchair IV Pole

The Vireo Wheelchair IV Pole facilitates mobility without assistance. A unique clamping device allows the pole to be easily installed on either side of a wheelchair. Made of chrome plated steel tubing, this 4 pound pole extends from 32 to 62 inches.

VIREO INC.
P.O. Box 560
Annawan, IL 61234
(309) 935-6151

✳✳✳✳

Camera Holder for Wheelchairs

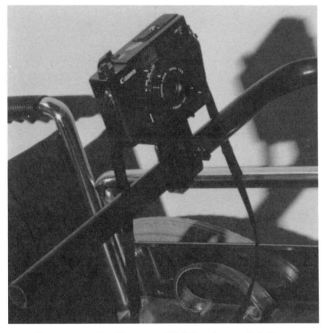

Ostergaard's Camera Holder is useful for amateur photographers, students, snapshooters, anyone who wants to take pictures. It attaches to your wheelchair and enables you to take the camera off your lap. It is fully adjustable.

OSTERGAARD ENTERPRISES
P.O. Box 15268
Fresno, CA 93702
(209) 275-4695

✳✳✳✳

Torso Support

Grandmar's Torso Support can be made to fit an automobile, wheelchair, or Geri chair. It gives the user total midline positioning while allowing unrestricted breathing. In the wheelchair version, a 2" webbing strap attaches to the back screws of the wheelchair; in the removable version, it slips over the hand grips. A second strap, 4" padded or 2" webbing, passes around the chest. This strap has side stays attached and is joined to the chair strap. Price: under $30.00.

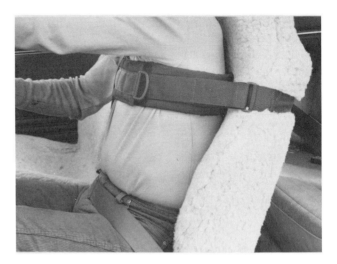

Stump Support

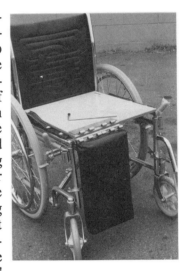

The Stump Support is a padded extension that fits onto the existing hardware of an elevating footrest, in place of a calf pad. It allows an amputee to have the use of a stumpboard that is easily swung out of the way, or removed when the wheelchair is being folded. The Support is made up of a ure-thaned marine grade ply insert, with a 2" cushion, T nuts, and a drop hook. Under $30.00.

Other Grandmar products include: Transfer Boards, Wedges, Cushions, Bags, Folding Lap Board, Contoured Head Rest, Torso Support, Foot Rest Covers, "Special Fittings," and a variety of wheelchairs.

GRANDMAR INC.
5675 "C" Landregan Street
Emeryville, CA 94608
(415) 428-0441

✳✳✳✳

Damaco D88VS

The lightweight Damaco D88VS is a portable power system that can snap on and off a manual wheelchair with no alterations to the chair. It features variable speed settings and you can select where the speed adjustment is installed, either at the manual controller or at the rear.

The D88VS can go anywhere you go with your foldable manual chair. Travel comfortably by plane, train, bus, car, even public transportation. The system is service supported by Damaco.

DAMACO, INC.
20545 Plummer Street
Chatsworth, CA 91311
(800) 432-2434
(818) 709-4534

****

Packa-Pouch

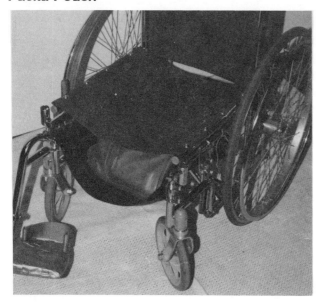

The Packa-Pouch is a waterproof, underseat carrier for wheelchairs. It easily attaches to manual, folding, and powered types, and is roomy enough for books, purse, papers, etc. Price: about $20.00.

IMAGES
P.O. Box 2152
Littleton, CO 80161-2152

****

Wheelchair Battery "Fuel" Gauge

The Curtis 900W24HW Wheelchair Battery "Fuel" Gauge provides a reliable, accurate indication of battery state-of-charge in an easy-to-read, empty-to-full type display. The gauge, in the words of one user, "provides peace of mind because I know I will not be stranded." By warning you before you reach "empty," the Curtis also prevents deep discharge damage to your battery and electrical

components. An adhesive mounting pad permits permanent mounting on the left- or right-hand arm. To prevent damage due to overcharging and minimize electric power costs, a charger control guide is provided.

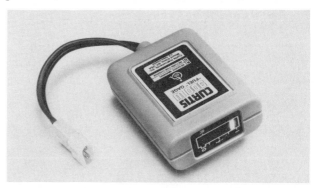

At the level of charge just prior to Empty, the Curtis provides a flashing-light alarm, the "reserve" alarm. At the Empty point, there is a second alarm—the two bottom-most bars on the LED display alternatively flash.

CURTIS INSTRUMENTS, INC.
200 Kisco Avenue
Mt. Kisco, NY 10549
(914) 666-2971

****

Pin Dot Seating Systems

Pin Dot offers six seating systems: Contour-U®, Plano®, EndoFlex®, Beadseat®, Quickfoam®, CP Seat, plus a complete line of interfacing components and accessories.

Contour-U®

Contour-U® offers total contact seating for persons with fixed, asymmetrical deformities. The cushions can be molded up to a depth of eight inches, providing control and support. They are custom made and are available in a virtually unlimited number of sizes (up to 24" x 28"). In addition, a broad range of accessories and interfacing hardware can be obtained.

Because of the custom contours, the user's weight is distributed over a large surface. This improves sitting balance and minimizes pressure on bony prominences. If a person is symmetrical, a modular cushion may be a cost-effective alternative to a Contour-U® cushion. For example, if an individual has a level pelvis but an asymmetrical spine, a Modular seat could be combined with a Contour-U® back. Such an approach can save time as well as money.

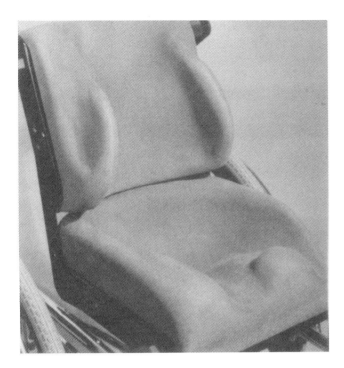

Endoflex®

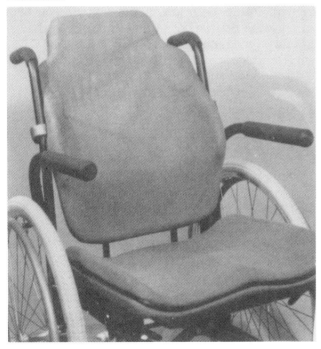

Endoflex® can prevent slouching, sitting fatigue, and low back pain. It allows the user to lean back, stretch, and shift weight. Its dynamic back extends, supporting the user when he moves. Yet the system neither raises the person nor pushes him forward because the framework is built right into the cushions. By simply unsnapping the cliplocks and pulling on the built-in handle, the user can eas-

ily fold the system in half. It weighs less than 14 pounds and can fit behind the seat of a car or in the overhead compartment on an airplane. In fact, it comes with a bag to protect the unholstery.

PIN DOT PRODUCTS
8100 N. Austin Avenue
Morton Grove, IL 60053
(800) 451-3553
(312) 470-7885 in Illinois

✳✳✳✳

Universal Wheelchair Electronics

If you've been having problems with wheelchair electronic breakdown or simply want to upgrade your older electronics, 21st Century Scientific's Universal Wheelchair Electronics can control nearly any 24V power wheelchair. It can be used on Marathon, Sprint, 3H, 3V, 3W, 3P, 3N, 32A, Arrow, Maxtra, Ranger, and Rolls IV chairs. The module is as quiet as a Marathon module, approximately the same size as a 3P module, is plug compatible with 3P, 3W, and 3V motors and hand controls, and has the same mounting holes as a 3P module.

21st's Universal Circuitry Module (UM1) supports both automatic and manual parking brake modes. It includes user accessible Brake Control and Brake Mode switches and comes with a circuit breaker-type battery cable that eliminates the fuse blowing problems sometimes encountered on chairs with fuse-type battery cables.

The Universal Hand Control (UCB 1) offers three mounting positions left to right, two separate low force toggle switches (one for on-off, one for hi-lo), a control stick assembly, rubber weather boots for both joystick and switches, and 0.95" diameter mini-ball knob.

Other features of Universal Wheelchair Electronics include: rugged 5/16" relay contacts, full-feature dynamic braking, complete parking brake control, jerk-brake, brake alarm, adjustable (joystick) sensitivity, adjustable reverse speed limiting, battery charger interlock, tri-mode low battery indicator, low battery speed reduction, low battery nudge, reverse polarity protection, high capacity output circuit, and easy servicing.

Electric-Leg-Bag-Emptier

21st's Electric-Leg-Bag-Emptier, for all 24V power chairs, allows the user to drain his or her own leg bag without assistance. It includes a 24V electric valve that mounts on the footplate and connects to the bottom of the leg bag drain tube, and a push-button switch that can be mounted anywhere on the wheelchair tubing. Both switch and valve include quick disconnect Anderson type connectors so that wheelchair footrests and arms can be easily removed after the system is installed. Note: Installation of the Electric-Leg-Bag-Emptier requires drilling of the footplate. Price: about $250.00.

Other products and services of 21st Century Scientific, Inc. include: Battery Chargers, Motor Kits, Battery Cables, Control Boxes, Tires and Tubes, Drive Pulleys, Fuses, Brake Kits, Battery Box Kits, Horns, Lights, Other Accessories and a "Wheelchair Electronics Rebuilding Program."

21ST CENTURY SCIENTIFIC, INC.
7629 Fulton Avenue
North Hollywood, CA 91605
(818) 982-2526

✶✶✶✶

The Uro-Matic

The Uro-Matic is an electronically operated urinary drainage device that works with a very small amount of electrical current supplied from a power wheelchair. The unit attaches to the foot plate and is linked by flexible tubing to a urinary drainage appliance worn under the user's clothing. The activating switch can be located anywhere on the power chair.

The Uro-Matic cleans easily with soap and water or appliance cleaners.

AHNAFIELD CORPORATION
3219 West Washington Street
Indianapolis, IN 46222
(317) 636-8061

✶✶✶✶

Patented Electronic Timer

The Lestronic II is a fully automatic charger. Plug it into the batteries and it turns itself on. The charger is designed not to respond to absolute voltages, but to the rate of change in on-charge voltage. As the batteries get closer to full charge the rate of voltage increase slows. When the rate of increase is at a level that indicates the batteries are fully charged, the electronic timer shuts the charger off.

LESTER ELECTRICAL OF NEBRASKA
625 West A Street
Lincoln, NE 68522
(402) 477-8988

✶✶✶✶

SBS

The roots of Storage Battery Systems, Inc. (SBS) reach back to 1915 and the introduction of the Baker Electric Car. As the electric car ultimately faded in popularity, SBS shifted its emphasis to the newly emerging forklift industry. Based in Milwaukee for more than sixty-five years, they have provided in-shop battery repair and warranty service for virtually every battery manufacturer in the United States.

SBS batteries feature 100% component inspection, heat seal covers, open venting at cell intersections, extra electrolyte capacity above the plates, an optical electrolyte level and state of charge indicator, unbreakable Daramic separators, bolt-on cables, and wide lug double wall tubular plates. The company offers both lead and gel wheelchair battery types in a variety of sizes, and also has Schauer and Lestronic II chargers.

An Electronic Level Sensor (ELS) that can protect your battery by alerting you of low fluid levels, is available as an accessory.

SBS
Storage Battery Systems, Inc.
P.O. Box 308
13664 West Silver Spring Drive
Butler, WI 53007
(414) 781-5800
(312) 543-4885 in Illinois

✶✶✶✶

Creative Rehabilitation Equipment

Creative Rehabilitation Equipment (CRE) is a custom shop that builds a wide variety of individual pieces which can be put together to form complete seating and positioning systems. By using CRE products, or CRE parts in combination with other manufacturers products, dealers can create customized systems for individual users.

CRE usually builds on a 1/2" AC plywood base. For extremely wide chairs or heavy weight, 3/4" AC can be ordered. A few things, like curved trunk pads and special headrests, are built out of plastic for the convenience of heat forming. All hardware fastening is done with machine screws and tee nuts.

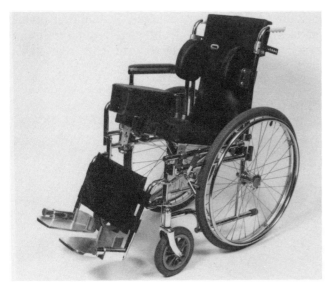

The foam is a dual density type, made especially for CRE. 1 1/2" foam is typically used on seatbacks and 1" on trunk pads, unless otherwise specified. Other foams can be ordered at additional cost.

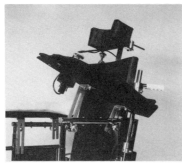

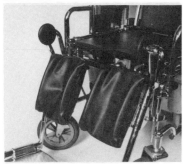

The board and foam units are enclosed in a premium grade Naugahyde. Approximately thirty-eight colors are kept in stock, ranging from standard wheelchair colors to the cheerful reds, greens, and yellows used on many of the children's units.

Recently, CRE developed a "Flip-Down Headrest." Unlike other headrests, it flips down and out of the way with just one hand. Since it stays attached to the chair, it can't be misplaced.

CREATIVE REHABILITATION
EQUIPMENT
513 N.E. Schuyler Street
Portland, OR 97212
(503) 281-6747
(800) 547-4611

****

OTHER SOURCES OF WHEELCHAIR PARTS AND ACCESSORIES:

ABBEY MEDICAL
ACCESS TO RECREATION, INC.
ADAPTIVE PRODUCTS
ALIMED INC.
ARCOA INDUSTRIES
CLEO INC.
COLUMBIA MEDICAL MANUFACTURING
CONSUMER CARE PRODUCTS
DANMAR PRODUCTS
DU-IT CONTROL SYSTEMS GROUP
J.A. PRESTON CORPORATION
KAYE PRODUCTS INC.
LAUREL DESIGNS
MADDAK, INC.
RAYMO PRODUCTS, INC.
ST. LOUIS OSTOMY AND MEDICAL SUPPLY
THERAFIN CORPORATION

For additional information, including addresses and phone numbers, see CATALOGS.

OTHER MOBILITY AIDS

"Foxy II"

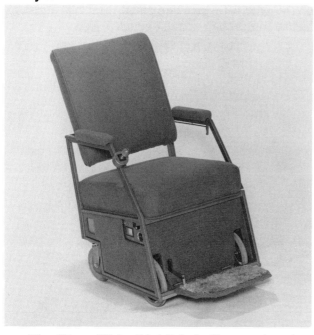

The "Foxy II" by Mobilchair Corporation, is a battery-powered easy chair with a 22 1/2" turning radius that allows access to most homes and offices without costly alterations. The overall width of only 20 3/4" is compact enough to fit through narrow doorways and between twin beds. "Foxy II" operates entirely under computer control for easy steering and smooth acceleration.

Standard features on the "Foxy II" include a power-driven footrest, a fold-down arm to facilitate lateral transfers, an on-board automatic battery charger, fully proportional speed control, and two large 1/4 h.p. motors for easy rolling through deep carpets, over door sills, and up ramps as steep as 10 degrees. "Foxy II" also has an automatic braking system that locks the wheels when the joystick is released or the power is turned off. Price: well under $4000.00.

MOBILCHAIR CORPORATION
7613 Convoy Court
San Diego, CA 92111
(619) 292-4865

****

Amigo RWD

Designed to enhance personal mobility, the Amigo RWD offers a variety of standard features including a 24V battery charger, 8" dual rear pneumatic wheels, gel filled front wheel, seat and brake locks, a varispeed drive head, arm rests, rear stabilizer wheel, and a five-year limited warranty. Price: about $2500.00.

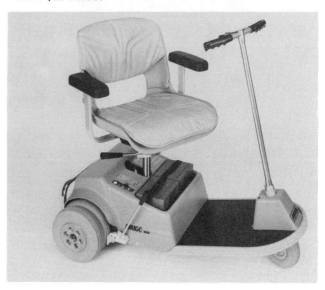

Amigo Supreme

The Supreme is a recent addition to Amigo's line of platform mobility aids. Easy to control and maneuver, the front wheel drive Supreme features an adjustable handle with user-friendly controls, power seat lift, flat free tires, battery charging gauge and on-board charger, automatic braking system, built-in horn, removable key switch, and a choice of four colors. Price: under $2250.00.

The following are some of the many accessories that are available for these and other units:

Baskets
Beverage Holder
Crutch Holders
Seat Cover (Sheepskin)
Cane Holder
Power Seat Lift

The Amigo Auto lift assembly, the Hitch-Hiker (for motorizing a manual wheelchair), and the Amigo Mini (in sizes for "little" people), can be obtained by special order.

AMIGO MOBILITY INTERNATIONAL
6693 Dixie Highway
Bridgeport, MI 48722-0402
(800) 248-9130
(517) 777-0910 in Michigan, Alaska & Hawaii

****

Gandy Pedal-Partner®

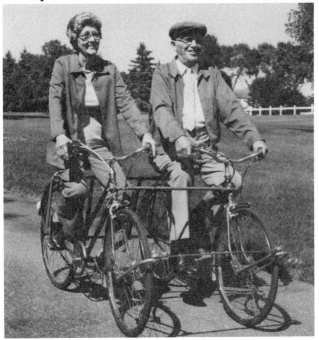

The Gandy Pedal-Partner® kit attaches two same-size bikes side-by-side for 4-wheel biking. The kit's base posts attach to the bike's front and rear axles and adjust in mounting to accommodate either wide fork "mountain" or "cruiser" style frames or the narrow front fork common to most 3, 5, and 10-speed bikes. Four tubular crossbars slide over the base posts and snap quickly and securely to them. A fifth bar joins the front tires and allows parallel turning, one person doing the steering.

Once installed, the Pedal-Partner® snaps together in moments for stable biking whether the rider is experienced or not, yet unsnaps for individual riding or for storage. Balancing is eliminated, making the unit ideal for senior citizens and many partially handicapped family members. A rear basket and attaching brackets are optional equipment. Price: about $100.00.

GANDY COMPANY
528 Gandrud Road
Owatonna, MN 55060
(800) 544-2639
(507) 451-5430

✳✳✳✳

Unitrol and Magnum

The Unitrol three wheeler is compact enough to permit excellent maneuverability in confined spaces and around stationary objects. The Magnum three wheeler provides top performance through soft soil and snow, on trails, and on steep inclines—places where many other units are unable to go.

Polished chrome steel tubing provides a frame around the 18" wide seat. Three inches of durable foam are covered with heavy gauge vinyl. The seat back can be adjusted forward and backward for maximum comfort. The 360 degree swivel seat locks in any position desired. Power and speed controls are designed for easy one-hand operation. All are mounted on the tiller at your fingertips, and can be operated equally well with right or left hand.

The steering mechanism is sealed ball bearing mounted. Easy one hand turns are possible and can be made in a 31" radius on the Unitrol (34" on the Magnum).

The optional power seat gives six inches of additional height. The seat belt increases safety and security.

VOYAGER INC.
P.O. Box 1577
527 West Colfax
South Bend, IN 46634
(800) 233-2682

✳✳✳✳

Pony II™

"Before we got Steve a Pony II™, he had virtually no freedom of movement and didn't play with the kids in the neighborhood. Now he's become much more developed socially. My advice to other parents . . . Try it, you'll love it."—Mrs. D.R.

The Pony II™ puts children at the eye level of their peers. And it doesn't look like a vehicle for the disabled. It only goes as fast as the throttle is squeezed, up to a maximum of 3.5 mph. There's also a speed limiter on the control box that can be set by either parent or therapist.

Braking on Pony II™ is automatic. When the thumb control is released, the vehicle comes to a complete stop. Its fully pneumatic non-marking tires provide an air cushioned ride over almost any type of surface. The rear wheels can be extended backward and outward for greater stability and better traction.

Pony II™ accommodates either one or two batteries. With two, it can travel up to sixteen miles on a single charge.

Pony II™ comes in two models: the 4312 for children age two to eight and the 4313 for children nine and older. As the child grows, the most costly components including the control, brakes, and complete power head, can be transferred from the small unit to the large, resulting in considerable cost savings. There are three different sized seats to choose from and four tiller sizes. In addition, the seat adjusts up and down and to and from the tiller.

Pony II™ disassembles quickly and easily without tools, and fits comfortably into the trunk of your car for trips, vacations, and outings. A number of options/accessories are available.

ORTHO-KINETICS, INC.
W220 N507 Springdale Road
P.O. Box 1647
Waukesha, WI 53187
(800) 558-7786
(800) 522-0992 in Wisconsin

✳✳✳✳

Sand-Rik™

"Our family had always gone to the beach together. When a stroke caused paralysis in the left side of my body, my life obviously changed. The beach vacations became fewer, and even these were difficult. Real participation was seriously limited. Resentment and negative feelings were involved. The Sand-Rik™ enabled me to access the beach with ease and with the regularity to participate in 'our' vacation. I was able to be on the beach with my new granddaughter and all my children."—C.D., West Point, VA

The Sand-Rik™ gives elderly and disabled persons easy access to beaches and other rough terrain previously inaccessible. You can go hunting, pond fishing, surf fishing, bird watching, or down a country trail. The Sand-Rik™ will go through mud, gravel, sand, and water.

The Sand-Rik™ is virtually maintenance free. It is weather, salt air, and rust resistant, and is equipped with rubber ATV tires and high-tech bearings for easy rolling. The adjustable chaise lounge has arm rests that unsnap and swing out of the way for easy transfer. Options include a collapsible canopy, flotation (for use in lakes, ponds, pools, or other calm water), a car carrier, a shoulder harness, and seat belt.

COMANCO
Rt. 8, Box 19EE
Mechanicsville, VA 23111
(804) 746-4088

✳✳✳✳

Creeper

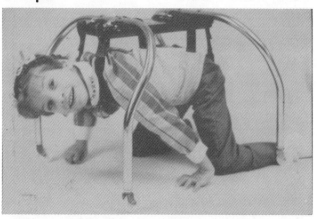

"This is our six year old little girl, Natalie. She was born with cerebral palsy. Though the doctors and therapists gave us little hope that she would ever creep or walk, we felt compelled to provide our daughter with the opportunity for normal development. We decided to try the Creeper six months ago.

"As a baby's walker enables the normal child to experience and learn the mechanics of walking, the Creeper enables our handicapped child to experience and learn the mechanics of creeping. Natalie did not possess the necessary coordination, balance, or arm, neck, and leg strength to creep; but through the Creeper's adjustable support and ease of movement, she has the opportunity to experience and enjoy the freedom of mobility. She first learned that by moving her arms and legs in the Creeper body movement occurs. Her skills for independent creeping continue to develop, which affords contented free time for us. It is a joy watching Natalie move in the Creeper, knowing she is comfortable, happy, and working towards a more independent and normal life. And best of all, she's beating the odds—Natalie's now trying to creep independently!"—G.P., Abilene, Texas

This device has been designed as a creeping aid for handicapped children in the age group of one to eight, weighing up to sixty-five pounds.

The child is suspended in a fully padded and flexible fabric sling, which is totally adjustable from the frame to give the optimum height for proper creeping.

The manufacturer recommends that the device be individually fit adjusted for the child by a physician, therapist, or similar health care professional, that it not be used for prolonged periods of time and/or without supervision, and that it should be used for children who weigh no more than sixty-five pounds. Price: under $250.00.

CUSTOM-AID™ CORPORATION
P.O. Box 3313
Abilene, TX 79604
(800) 654-5340
(915) 695-1640

A subsidiary of Proctor Brothers Manufacturing, Inc.

✳✳✳✳

Trike 324

"After designing a Trike for my own use, I started New England Handcycles with a single goal—deliver an excellent product to people who really enjoy it. And do they enjoy it! Our handcycles are in use all across the country, in Canada, and in Europe. Our customers range from nine year olds to teens, young adults to retirees and their stories range from the believable to the incredible."—Bill Warner

The Trike 324 was designed by Bill Warner, a Massachusetts Institute of Technology graduate. An avid cyclist before his spinal cord injury, Bill was determined to get back on the road. For the rider, the Trike opens up a new world. Bill has gone cycle touring in England and Bermuda. Other Trike riders participate in 10K footraces or tackle marathon courses.

The gearing consists of two derailleurs and gear clusters. The gears are switched via two levers as in a ten-speed bike. The result is a twenty-four speed system able to handle many types of terrain. On turns, the rider steadies the upper body with the hand-cranks, causing the Trike to center. Braking is accomplished via a hand-crank mechanism. Simply backpedal—a little to slow down, more to stop. An important safety feature is that the brake is entirely separate from the drive chain.

NEW ENGLAND HANDCYCLES, INC.
48 Bogle Street
Weston, MA 02193
(617) 237-7720

✳✳✳✳

Surry Tricycloped

The Surry is a convenient street-legal three-wheeled vehicle that averages 80 miles per gallon, can accelerate to 30 miles per hour, and is equipped with canted side rails for easy on and off. Both gas and brakes are controlled by hand, as is the lever that raises the wheelchair ramps behind you after entering. Readily serviced at any motor-cycle repair shop, the standard Surry comes with an electric starting system, a two gallon fuel tank, solid state ignition, easy operating hand brakes, and head and tail lights that come on automatically when the engine starts. Other amenities include bright chrome wheelchair stops, a short six foot turning radius, and automatic transmission. Price: well under $4000.00.

NATIONAL MEDICAL INDUSTRIES, INC.
1438 West Bannock Street
P.O. Box 3268
Boise, ID 83703
(208) 343-3639

✳✳✳✳

Tri-Wheeler™

Back in 1963 Ralph Braun, "driven by a personal desire for better mobility," invented the Tri-Wheeler™ in his cousin's farm shop. Numerous requests from other wheelchair users led to the founding of Save-A-Step Manufacturing Company the following year. By 1972, the company had grown to become the Braun Corporation. Today, Braun manufactures a full line of mobility products.

The Tri-Wheeler™ has an executive-style "extra-firm" foam-cushioned chair with "flip-up" armrests, that offers comfort and ease of transfer. Its wide-track pneumatic tires provide good traction on slippery surfaces. Having both indoor and outdoor capabilities, the Tri-Wheeler's™ cruising range is fifteen miles. Sealed gel/cell type batteries and twin electric motors are standard equipment as is a manual, palm-operated parking brake. The turning radius is 30". For greater access at home or in the office, a swivel seat base and vertical power seat are available. If unable to successfully operate the standard tiller control, Braun also manufactures the unit with a joystick.

THE BRAUN CORPORATION
1014 S. Monticello, P.O. Box 310
Winamac, IN 46996
(800) THE LIFT
(219) 946-6153 in Indiana

✳✳✳✳

The Bob Hall Racer

The Bob Hall Racer is a cage design frame with adjustable upholstery and leg straps. The racer offers over center steering that provides maximum steering range and prompt automatic spring return. It features 4130 aircraft tubing, cordura upholstery, electrostatic paint, and custom fitting with rigid construction. Front and rear wheel options include 12", 14", and 18" diameters, as well as 24", 26", and 700C rear wheels.

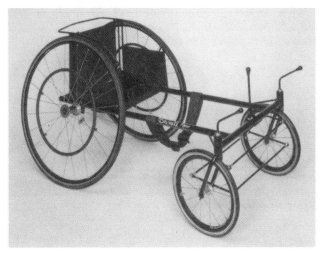

Hall's lightweight chair for everyday, tennis, or basketball use is called the Signature Chair. Its adjustable upholstery, rear wheel plate positioner, and minutely adjustable camber plate offer the potential for a good fit with the customized dimensions that you choose.

Models in the Team Hall Series include the Road Hugger, Trailing Arm, Aero Three-Wheel Racer, and Traditional Fork Racer. Prices range from $1475.00 to $2100.00.

HALL'S WHEELS
11 Smith Place
Cambridge, MA 02138
(617) 547-5000

✳✳✳✳

Sterling

The Sterling is a rear-wheel-drive vehicle that can take you places you previously thought you had to avoid, like gravel roads, bumpy walkways, mud puddles, and ramps. The fingertip control is bi-directional and allows one-hand operation for either forward or reverse movement. You can elect to go as fast as five miles per hour outdoors or limit your speed indoors with the speed control dial. A clutch lever disengages the drive train into neutral for free-wheeling. The Sterling's adjustable chassis permits the base to stretch by four inches to accommodate taller individuals. The body is made from high-strength, lightweight, U-V stabilized plastic. A "de-docking" mechanism unlocks the rear drive assembly making the unit easier to transport.

A built-in "fail-safe" unit ensures that the vehicle will not operate unless it is reassembled correctly and all plugs are properly locked. The control panel and adjustable steering tiller are positioned for easy handling. Control circuitry monitors the electronics. Should anything go wrong, the Sterling shuts off and a light on the control panel flashes. A battery charge indicator lets you know when it's time to recharge the batteries. Note: According to the manufacturer, the range between charges—with new batteries, on hard, level surfaces—is twenty-five miles. The height of the seat is adjustable, it can swivel 360 degrees, and the arm rests can be flipped up. The Sterling's turning radius is 51 inches, its load capacity 250 pounds. Price: well under $3500.00.

A-BEC Scoota Bug™

The lightweight and completely modular Scoota Bug™ disassembles without tools and fits into most auto trunks. The variable speed throttle, positioned for either right or left hand use, allows you to slow down or speed up to a maximum of four miles per hour. The reverse button lets you change directions and a freewheel device permits manual operation. The Scoota Bug™ is equipped with two-stage automatic brakes and twin battery packs (to provide 24 volts of power). The seat rotates a full 360 degrees and automatically locks at every quarter turn for easy transfer or desk access. The variable height seat adjusts to 15", 16", and 17". The turning radius is 33", the load capacity 200 pounds. Price: under $2000.00.

A-BEC MOBILITY INC.
20460 Gramercy Place
Torrance, CA 90501
(213) 533-0306
(800) 421-2269
(800) 262-1331 in California

✳✳✳✳

Handicycle

The Handicycle is a hand-driven tricycle for adults and children, designed for long distance riding. It's offered in three wheel sizes—16", 20", and 24", and is available in red, yellow, black, or blue (built and painted at the time you order).

Features of the Handicycle include an adjustable bucket seat, coaster brake, parking brakes on each rear wheel, leg rests with straps or foot rest with heel stop, and an easy-to-adjust chain. All parts are "bicycle" for easy maintenance.

Other cycles by the For Fun Cycles Corporation include the Duo-Cycle, manufactured and engineered especially as a recreational vehicle for two riders; the Single Cycle, an adult tricycle with an optional canopy for protection from the sun; and the Cargo Cycle, with a payload capacity of 500 pounds (plus the rider).

FOR FUN CYCLE CORPORATION
966 N. Elm Street
Orange, CA 92667-5471
(714) 997-1952

****

OTHER SOURCES OF MOBILITY AIDS:

ABBEY MEDICAL
ACCESS TO RECREATION, INC.

ADAPTIVE PRODUCTS
CLEO INC.
CONSUMER CARE PRODUCTS
FLAGHOUSE, INC.
GUARDIAN
J.A. PRESTON CORPORATION
KAYE PRODUCTS INC.
KAYE'S KIDS
MARSHALL MEDICAL
RADIO SHACK
RIFTON
SUNRISE MEDICAL
TASH, INC.
WINCO INCORPORATED

For additional information, including addresses and phone numbers, see CATALOGS.

CHAPTER SIX

TRANSPORTATION

VEHICLE RAMPS, LIFTS, AND CARRIERS

EZ-Access™: Portable Wheelchair Ramp

The lightweight EZ-Access™ Ramp bridges the gaps over steps and curbs. Two ramps extend to over five feet in length, locking securely into place with special snap button catches. Holding over 350 pounds of weight, the ramps are made of extruded anodized aluminum. The two ramps weighing only seven pounds each simply collapse and are stored in a pouch on the back of the wheelchair. Price: about $150.00.

EZ-Access™ Telescopic Vanramp

Like the EZ-Access™ Ramp, the EZ-Access™ Vanramp bridges gaps over steps and curbs, but also makes vans and mini-vans more accessible. The two ramps extend over seven feet in length, and are capable of holding 600 pounds. After use they can be collapsed for easy storage. The two together weigh only fourteen pounds. Price: about $300.00.

HOMECARE PRODUCTS
P.O. Box 58997
Seattle, WA 98138
(206) 251-9183

✳✳✳✳

Side-Door "Swing-Out" Ramp

The Side-Door "Swing-Out" Ramp by Vartanian is offered for full size and mini vans. Utilizing a coil spring counter balance for easy deployment, it can handle weights of up to 650 pounds. Side-Door "Swing-Out" Ramps are available for sliding or bay doors.

Flat Floor Wheelchair Ramp

Flat Floor Wheelchair Ramps are also offered for full size and mini vans, and can be used for side or rear door applications.

Portable Folding Ramps—The "Roll Away" Ramp

Vartanian's Portable Folding Ramps offer mobility with versatility. Equipped with a reinforced center hinge, zinc plated for rust resistance, and designed to accommodate up to 650 pounds, the "Roll Away" ramp allows transfers without carrying.

Portable Non-Folding Ramps

Useful for home, travel, or permanent applications, lightweight Portable Non-Folding Ramps are available in an assortment of sizes from three feet.

Telescopic & Straight Bar Wheelchair Tie-downs

Vartanian also produces Telescopic and Straight Bar Wheelchair Tie-downs, available for all standard wheelchairs.

VARTANIAN INDUSTRIES, INC.
P.O. Box 636
Switzgable Drive
Brodheadsville, PA 18322
(717) 992-5700

✳✳✳✳

Chair Topper

The Chair Topper is one of the many products developed by Ralph Braun and the Braun Corporation. Designed to fit a wide range of vehicles, the unit automatically folds and stores a conventional folding wheelchair inside an attractive, watertight fiberglass cover—with a touch of the convenient, hand-held control. A compact 57" long, 51" wide, and 22" high, the Chair Topper features a universal mounting system for easy installation.

THE BRAUN CORPORATION
1014 S. Monticello, P.O. Box 310
Winamac, IN 46996
(800) THE LIFT
(219) 946-6153 in Indiana

****

Automate Wheelchair Carrier

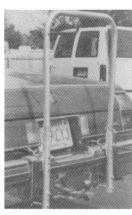

The Automate Wheelchair Carrier is designed to fit any and all types of cars. Made of heavy-gauge, lightweight aluminum, it can be attached to a "traditional" steel bumper with a simple wrap-around chain mounting. For late model cars with molded bumpers, it can be mounted to a standard light duty hitch. To use the carrier: tip the folded wheelchair back, hooking the front of it on the lower hanger. Then, rotate the back to position it on the upper hanger. Fasten the chair with tiedowns and cover both chair and carrier. When not in use, simply pull the release pin and lift the carrier out of the sockets, which remain on the bumper.

Options:
- Bumper Mount Price: under $100.00
- Hitchmount Price: about $125.00
- Washable Cover Price: about $40.00

AMERIMED, INC.
1605 DeSoto Road
Sarasota, FL 34234
(813) 351-8103
(800) 433-1099

****

Kar Kady

Kar Kady was developed by a family needing a simple, reliable way to transport a wheelchair outside of their car. Kar Kady does the lifting. Its spring-assisted action raises your wheelchair and locks it securely into place on the back of your car. It can be installed quickly and easily on any standard trailer hitch, with no major vehicle modifications. Both the trunk and gas tank remain accessible without having to remove the wheelchair. A protective cover is also available. The EZ Lift Kar Kady is priced under $300.00 and the Kar Kady Weatherproof Cover is priced at about $60.00.

EZ LIFT AND CARRIER CO.
10609 Boedeker
Dallas, TX 75230
(214) 363-4820

****

The Buddy System™

The Buddy System™ wheelchair carrier mounts on a standard trailer hitch by tightening one screw. Made of durable lightweight steel, it is equipped with adjustable front wheel wells and can accommodate all standard, non-electric wheelchairs. For convenience and safety while loading or unloading it tilts toward the curb. A specially designed T-handle latching system makes it easier for you to disengage the carrier when you load or unload your wheelchair. The spring on the T-handle latch is coated stainless steel packed with a special lubricant designed for both hot and cold climates. The Buddy System™ can be inverted to 90 degrees when your car is parked or not in use, or quickly removed and stored in the trunk. Price: under $400.00.

INNOVATIVE SPECIALTIES, INC.
Route 1, Box 75
Harriman, TN 37748
(615) 882-3080

****

Mac's Van Lift

This lift is especially appealing when there is more than one wheelchair occupant. When interior space is at a premium, an outside liftgate naturally leaves more room inside. It also allows the wheelchair to travel straight in and straight out of the van, without having to turn at all. The platform is a large 45" in length, 48" in overall width, with a ramp width of 30". The lift has a load capacity of 750 pounds, so an aide can ride up, or down, with the wheelchair. The no-skid surface is "see through," so you can easily identify any obstacles beneath the platform. A positive stopper on the ramp remains up at all times to keep the wheelchair from accidentally rolling off the platform. A spring assist is provided to help in folding up the platform. The remote control is mounted on the inside of the door. The lift doesn't block the rear windows or tail lights, and the bumper remains intact for a good appearance. Mac's Outside Rear of Van Lift is priced at about $1650.00 with installation and manual backup priced at about $150.00 and $200.00 respectively.

Tiger Lift

The Tiger Lift mounts on any class "2" or "3" trailer hitch, and can be mounted on any car, truck, or R.V. (Some cars may require air shocks). It is constructed out of durable, square steel tubing. It was designed to accommodate a wide variety of electric wheelchairs. The platform is 24 1/2" in width, 48" in length, and extends 31" from the bumper. It weighs 75 pounds empty and has a load capacity of 155 pounds. The surface is diamond cut steel mesh. Controls are located at a convenient level, including a key lock to prevent tampering. Price: about $1500.00 with installation under $100.00.

MAC'S LIFT GATE, INC.
2801 South Street
Long Beach, CA 90805
(213) 634-5962

****

Bruno Scooter-Lifts™

The Bruno Scooter Lift™ (VSL-700, 800, and 900) was designed for mini-van and full-size van installations. It can be used at the side door opening or at the rear. A special adaptation will also allow its use in the side door of a Chrysler Vista station wagon and the Nissan Stanza wagon with sliding doors. The Scooter Lift™ is for the user who needs to have his or her scooter picked up fully assembled, including seat and tiller.

The latest design model of the VSL-700 is rated to lift scooters and/or wheelchairs that weigh up to 200 pounds and includes a special release mechanism that allows the unit to be pushed in by hand if the lift develops a motor or electrical malfunction, or the vehicle's battery goes "dead."

The Scooter-Lift™ Jr. (ASL-300 FWD and ASL-400 RWD) is a trunk lift that works in auto trunks, hatchback autos, and the rear of station wagons when used in conjunction with a sub-base. It will pick up and stow a disassembled scooter, without the seat and vertical tiller or with a folding tiller in the lowered position. The Scooter-Lift™ Sr. (VSL-500) is equipped with pick-up "C" arm that enables it to pick up a fully assembled scooter.

Bruno Curb-Sider™

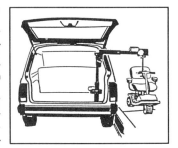

The Scooter-Lift™ Curb-Sider™ (VSL-600) was specially designed for vehicles such as the Chevy S-10 Blazer, Ford Bronco, Jeep Cherokee, and any vehicle with a tailgate or with a narrow rear door opening (hatchback types).

Bruno Wheelchair Lifter

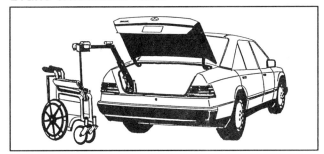

The Bruno Wheelchair Lifter (AWL-100), a manual folding wheelchair lift, is fitted with a special "docking" device and "T-bar." The chair starts out in the vertical position, and changes to the horizontal, making it easy to enter a vehicle's trunk or hatchback area. A van model (AWL-150) is available that stores the wheelchair in a vertical position.

Bruno's OutRider™ & Out-Sider™

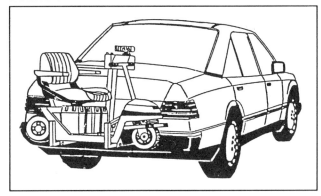

The Out-Rider™ Pick-Up-Lifter mounts behind the cab of a pickup truck at the driver's side. It is designed to pick up a manual wheelchair or a three-wheel scooter. This lift works well for a person who transfers from the wheelchair to the pickup truck. It is completely electric, and has both motorized "up/down" and "in/out" features, making it fully automatic.

The Out-Sider™ features an automatic holddown device. It also has a self-leveling platform that is self locking when folded into the vertical stored position. A built-in weight distribution feature transfers some of the weight forward, and at the same time tilts the lift upward to allow more vertical height clearance from the ground.

Other additions to the Bruno line of product options include a Seat-Lift and an automatic door operator for a Nissan Stanza Wagon.

BRUNO INDEPENDENT LIVING AIDS
430 Armour Center, P.O. Box 84
Oconomowoc, WI 53066
(414) 567-4990

****

Ricon S-1000

The unique, fully-automatic S-1000 offers a split platform that folds out of the doorway opening for easy access to your vehicle when the lift is in the stored position. When the lift is lowered the user can leave the platform by either the front or the side.

The S-1000 has a double hand rail, an exclusive inboard safety flap and an easy to use manual backup system. Its all-steel construction and electro-hydraulic power assure smooth, reliable operation in any climate.

Other Ricon lifts include the fully-automatic Mini-Rider™ that fits most popular minivans, the Classic™ offering rear or side door installation for full-sized vans, the Econo-Rider with a fold-in-half platform that gives unobstructed window visibility, and the all-electric, fully automatic Golden Boy Swing Lift™ that allows you to get in and out of tight parking spaces in a jiffy.

Ricon Accessories include the "RiControl™" automotive hand control, a "Six-Way Power Seat," and "Door Operators" for sliding and swinging doors.

THE RICON CORPORATION
11684 Tuxford Street
Sun Valley, CA 91352
(800) 322-2884
(818) 768-5890 in California

****

Pulsar Digital Remote Controls

Pulsar Remote Controls are compact, can be installed in minutes, and offer single button operation. As described by the manufacturer, Pulsars have "a built-in safety circuit which enhances the safety and function of your lift and has been tested without failure for two years before being put into production."

The Pulsar II makes Ricon's "R-30" and "Minirider™" lifts operate sequentially and automatically. It will also operate Jure and other single switch units.

Pulsar II is available with built-in single key or magnetic switching.

PULSAR DIGITAL SYSTEMS
P.O. Box 2706
Culver City, CA 90230
(818) 609-1584
(818) 996-0822

****

Braun Lift-A-Way™

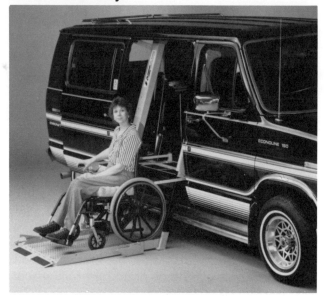

The Lift-A-Way™ Fully Automatic lift provides independent mobility through total command of raising, lowering, folding, and unfolding functions. The Semi-Automatic "Lift-A-Way™" raises and lowers at the touch of a button and its see-through platform is easily folded and unfolded by an attendant. Both Fully and Semi-Automatic models are available to fit the side or rear doors of most domestic and foreign full size and mini-vans. The gravity down system uses gravity to gently lower the platform, saving 40% of the battery drain. The box header construction provides strength and rigidity while maintaining normal headroom.

Braun "Swing-A-Way"™

The need for increased vehicle access for both wheelchair user and able-bodied passengers led to the development of the fully automatic "Swing-A-Way™" Wheelchair lift. Its rotary design moves the lift platform from the van interior to the ground in a smooth, steady motion.

The Swing-A-Way™ is available in two models. The Front Post model, for full size Ford and Chevy slide door vans, offers a compact design providing complete access to the vehicle's interior. The Rear Post model, for full size Ford and Chevy slide door or swing door vans and full size Dodge swing door vans, is available for those seeking more front passenger room. An optional Automatic Door Operator for slide door applications and an Outside Control Station provide instant access. A Manual Back-Up System is standard.

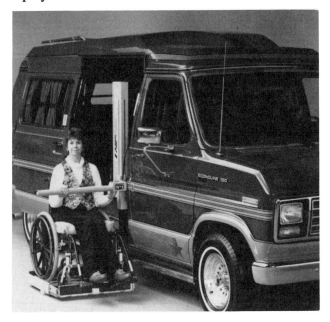

THE BRAUN CORPORATION
1014 S. Monticello
P.O. Box 310
Winamac, IN 46996
(800) THE LIFT
(219) 946-6153 in Indiana

* * * *

Lectra Aid™

The Lectra Aid™ is a lift that was designed with "RVing" in mind. It attaches next to the door, lifts you up (to the desired level), and swings you in—either in an aluminum chair or on an aluminum platform.

Lectra Aid™ operates with a reversing 12 volt D.C. motor and is powered by the RV battery. In can be installed on most RV's with a minimum of modification to the RV. Weight is restricted to 250 lbs. For persons over that another product, the "Lectra Aid™ Super Lift," is available.

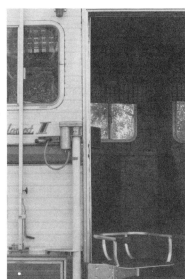

When traveling, the platform or chair assembly can be removed and stowed in the RV.

SFH PRODUCTS, INC.
1801 E. Medlock
Phoenix, AZ 85016
(602) 265-7370

* * * *

OTHER SOURCES OF RAMPS, LIFTS, AND CARRIERS:

ADAPTIVE PRODUCTS
WHEELCHAIR CARRIER, INC.

For additional information, including addresses and phone numbers, see CATALOGS.

DRIVING CONTROLS

RiControl

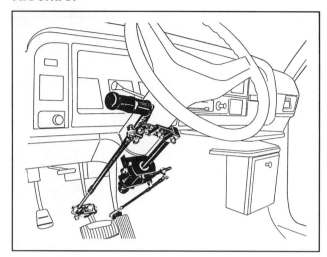

The RiControl Automotive Hand Control offers sturdy, all-steel construction with aircraft ball joints and attractive black anodized finish. When you want to accelerate, simply pull the hand control toward the seat and rim of the steering wheel. To brake, push the control directly toward the brake pedal. This is the most natural way for accelerating or braking. You can also apply both the brake and accelerator at the same time which is sometimes helpful when starting on a grade. The RiControl can be mounted on either the right or left side of the steering wheel and is fully adjustable.

THE RICON CORPORATION
11684 Tuxford Street
Sun Valley, CA 91352
(800) 322-2884
(800) 263-2356 in Canada
(818) 768-5890 in California

✳✳✳✳

Rotary Hand Operated Driving Control (CT-100)

By combining a twist-style throttle with a thrust-style braking mechanism the CT-100 gives the driver independent, simultaneous, one-hand control of both throttle and brake for ready adaptation to most driving situations. By replacing traditional mechanical foot pedal linkages with a cable hook-up directly to the carburetor throttle mechanism, the control provides more clearance for operation, as well as ease of entry and exit.

Right Angle Hand Operated Driving Control (CP-200 II)

The CP-200 II combines a pull-style throttle with a push-style braking mechanism to provide easier operation for persons with reduced upper body strength and mobility. Together, the CP-200 II and the CT-100 give the driver independent, simultaneous, one-hand control of both throttle and brake for ready adaptation to most driving situations. The CP-200 features minimal obstruction for driver entry and exit, universal mounting, and simplified installation. Acceleration and deceleration are achieved through direct cable hook-up to the carburetor.

Pneumatic Hand Control

The Wells-Engberg Pneumatic Hand Control consists of only a few basic components that are easily installed by a competent mechanic in most vehicles. The system was designed to provide ease of operation, reliability, and low maintenance under normal use conditions. It eliminates mechanical linkages, and there is no obstruction under the steering column to hinder entrance or exit. Acceleration and braking are described as "virtually effortless," with sufficient feedback for sensitive control. And it allows accelerator choke-trip before the engine is started—a necessity for cold climates.

Other driving aids from Wells-Engberg include a "Left-Foot Gas-Feed," a "Parking Brake Handle," and a variety of steering devices.

WELLS-ENGBERG CO., INC.
P.O. Box 6388
Rockford, IL 61125
(800) 642-3628
(815) 874-5882 in Illinois

✳✳✳✳

One Lever Hand Controls/Left Foot Gas Pedal/Dual Brake Controls

Kroepke Kontrols can be installed in most American and foreign cars. They are made of steel and forged steel parts. There are no bulky castings or sharp projections. Many of the Kroepke installations do not require holes to be drilled because they are custom designed to fit your car. According to the manufacturer, "They can be installed by any capable mechanic at your dealer or service station in only two hours time." Inasmuch as car interiors are not marred, their resale values are unaffected. Kroepke Kontrols do not interfere with the normal operation of the automobile.

KROEPKE KONTROLS, INC.
104 Hawkins Street
Bronx, NY 10464
(212) 885-1100, (212) 885-2100
(212) 885-1547

✳✳✳✳

Supergrade IV Hand Control

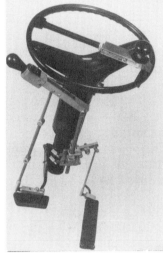

The "Supergrade IV Hand Control" fits any American made vehicle, (even with tilt steering) and most foreign made vehicles. One of the only adaptation parts which may be needed is a #118 Special Brake Bracket, where the normal brake bracket interferes with the steering column. The other bracket that may be needed is a #121 Column Mount Bracket (four types are available), which should be used in the event that the regular angle mount bracket is unable to clamp onto the steering column. Handicaps, Inc. reports that a qualified installer can put in the control in 2 1/2 to 3 hours, depending on the vehicle.

HANDICAPS, INC.
4335 South Santa Fe Drive
Englewood, CO 80110
(800) 621-8385 ext. 248
(303) 781-2062

✳✳✳✳

"Slim Line Control"

The Slim Line control is a strong, compact unit. The main body is built of heavy wall steel tubing, heli-arc welded, and chrome plated. The handle is contour shaped for maximum driver room. The adjusting bars are steel, threaded full length and cadmium plated. There are no cables or gears to clog or wear out. The control attaches to the underside of the dash, on the right side of the steering column, the main support bar extending through the fire wall. The control lever extends across and under the steering column, then upward to a point near the turn signal lever, as the operator desires.

The linkage to brake and throttle is direct. With proper transfer parts from Gresham, this control can be removed and reinstalled in another car.

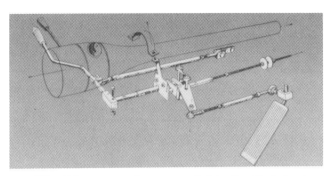

Slim Line controls are available for "left brake & throttle or throttle only," "right brake and throttle or throttle only," and "brake only."

Steering and Other Driving Aids

Gresham steering aids include a "Quad Grip With Pin" (developed with the cooperation of the Orthotics Departments of the University of Michigan Medical Center and the Institute of Rehabilitation Medicine, New York University Medical Center), "Flat Quad Spinner" (for a quadriplegic with flat extended hand), "Spinner Knob," "Tri-Post Spinner," and "Upright Quad Spinner."

Gresham also offers a "Hand Dimmer Switch," "Left Foot Accelerator," "Hand Operated Parking Brake," "Left Hand Shift Lever," "Right Hand Turn Signal Switch Lever," "Quad Grip," "Key Holders," and "Dual Brake Controls for Driver Education Vehicles."

GRESHAM DRIVING AIDS
P.O. Box 405
30800 Wixom Rd.
Wixom, MI 48096
(800) 521-8930

✳✳✳✳

"Monarch Mark 1-A"

The "Monarch Mark 1-A" may be used for either right or left hand installation. The brake is applied by pushing the control handle directly toward the brake. The accelerator is activated by moving the handle toward the seat, at a right angle to the brake movement and parallel, or nearly parallel, to the rim of the steering wheel. Generally, the weight of the driver's hand and arm is sufficient to maintain a desired speed. Both the brakes and accelerator may be applied at the same time if necessary (as when starting or maneuvering on severe grades).

The operating handle is fully adjustable after installation. The accelerator can be adjusted to provide any desired ratio of leverage. This design allows for movement of the accelerator pedal by the non-handicapped driver without movement of the control handle. A "Brake Only" option is available as is a "Toggle Type Dimmer Switch" and a "Horn Button."

A variety of other driving aids are also available from MPS.

MPS (MANUFACTURING AND PRODUCTION SERVICES CORPORATION)
7948 Ronson Road
San Diego, CA 92111
(619) 292-1423

＊＊＊＊

Mobility Products and Design (MPD) Hand and Quad Controls

MPD's 3500 Series Hand Controls are easily adjustable and don't interfere with normal foot pedal operation. They're available for right or left hand driving and provide maximum hand support. The 3700 Push-Pull Quad Control meets the needs of most C4/C5 quads, post polio, muscular dystrophy, and other related disabilities. It offers all-mechanical positive connections to the gas and brake. MPD driving controls are all-aluminum and are available to accommodate a variety of needs.

MOBILITY PRODUCTS AND DESIGN, INC.
A Division of Crow River Industries, Inc.
3200 Harbor Lane
Minneapolis, MN 55447
(800) 843-3893

＊＊＊＊

Joystick Driving System

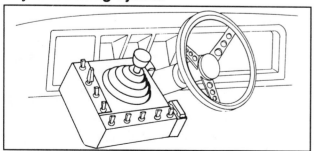

Ahnafield Corporation's Joystick Driving Control is a reliable system for severely disabled drivers. It can be used by one-handed individuals or persons with severely limited use of both hands and arms.

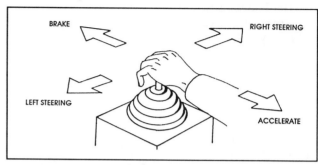

The driver controls the vehicle with a two-axis joystick. Moving the joystick left to right steers the vehicle; pushing it forward applies the brake; and pulling backward activates the throttle.

The control can be mounted on the left or right side at any position required by the driver and can be installed in a Dodge, Chevrolet, or Ford van. The standard steering wheel, brake pedal, and accelerator remain as a functional part of the vehicle for use by able-bodied drivers.

Driving Consoles

Ahnafield's consoles are designed to enhance the appearance of the vehicle interior. The control panel nomenclature is engraved and back-lighted for easy reading.

The consoles can contain any number of functions with many different types of switches available. They can be located anywhere convenient for the driver—on the left or right side, on the hand control, or in any combination.

Remote Start

Ahnafield's Remote Start is a radio transmitter that starts a vehicle within a hundred-foot range from indoors or outside. It measures engine conditions and automatically selects the proper starting procedure for a cold or warm engine as required by the vehicle's manufacturer. It will automatically restart if the engine stalls. If the engine refuses to start, the system will shut down to save battery drain. A fast idle release automatically taps the gas pedal when needed to reduce engine speed and choke setting. This saves fuel and reduces exhaust temperatures. The Remote Start activates all preset accessories such as heater, air-conditioner, radio, etc.

Reduced-Effort Steering Modifications

Ahnafield's reduced-effort steering modification enables drivers with hand and/or arm weakness to steer a vehicle. Approximately two to three pounds of effort are needed to control standard factory-installed power steering. With this modification less than 8 ounces are necessary. (These figures may vary depending on tire size and model of car or van.)

Reduced steering modifications are available for all American vans and most American and foreign-made cars with factory-installed power steering. According to Ahnafield, factory power steering units can be equipped with reduced-effort steering modifications and returned within twenty-four hours of receipt.

Reduced-Effort Braking Modifications

Ahnafield braking modifications enable drivers with little strength in their hands and/or arms to brake the vehicle by reducing the effort needed. The system can be used on all American vans and most American and foreign-made cars with factory installed power brakes. Heavy-duty tandem power brakes are needed for reduced effort braking modification on full-size General Motors cars, full-size Chrysler (Dodge and Plymouth) cars, half-ton Chevrolet (G10) vans, and Dodge/Plymouth (B100) vans.

Foot Steering

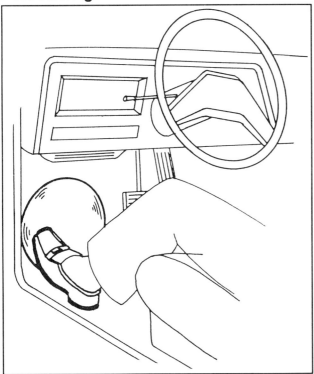

The Ahnafield Foot Steering System is designed for individuals with limited or no use of their hands and arms. A special floor mounted device

provides complete steering capabilities with the foot. It can be installed on cars, vans, and trucks.

Other accessory controls can be repositioned to complement the Foot Steering System. These controls include ignition, turn signals, gear shifter, head-lights, windshield wipers/washers, emergency flashers, heat/air conditioner, power seat, power locks, and power windows. Remote accessory controls are relocated for each individual's driving needs. A power door opener is also available.

Back-Up Systems

Ahnafield Back-up Systems for Reduced and Zero Effort Steering and Braking Systems function as a safety check, automatically supplying needed power to operate the systems in the event of an emergency (i.e., engine failure).

AHNAFIELD CORPORATION
3219 W. Washington Street
Indianapolis, IN 46222
(317) 636-8061

✳✳✳✳

Programmable Electronic Consoles

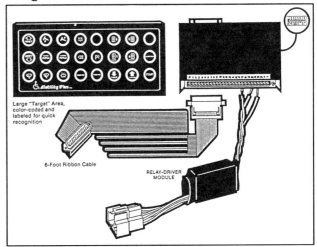

Programmable Electronic Consoles are offered in two configurations. The twelve-function panel is for lights, ignition, and other electronic operations, whereas the twenty-three-function panel covers just about every driving application except for the gas and brake. Both can be mounted within easy reach.

The target areas are color coded and labeled for fast recognition. The soft touch membrane switches respond instantly and are easy to see at night (luminescent).

Each switch carries a two-way option. The

latching option provides on/off operation for lights and similar activities. Momentary allows operation of the starter, setting the heat and cooling ranges, etc. These dip switches are set at the time of installation. Servo connections for heaters, gear shifts, and air conditioning are also available.

The consoles come complete with OEM plugs for easy connection to the original harnesses. Repairs (if necessary) are made with modular replacements.

MOBILITY PLUS, INC.
A Division of John D. Crafts, Inc.
10 Birch Street
Lisbon Falls, ME 04252
(207) 353-5503

✳✳✳✳

OTHER SOURCES OF DRIVING CONTROLS:

ADAPTIVE PRODUCTS

For additional information, including the address and phone number, see CATALOGS.

VAN CONVERSIONS

Strap-Lok (Model 1202)

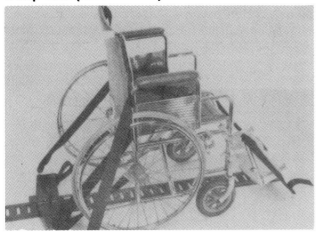

The "Strap-Lok" is a simple way of restraining a wheelchair and its occupant. A single track bolts to the vehicle floor and allows a wheelchair to be securely "buckled in place" at two points on the track with four straps to the frame of the chair.

Vacuum Gas & Brake Systems (8000 Series)

CCI's 8000 Series Vacuum Gas and Brake Systems (VGB) are situated for optimum ease of operation. Both push/pull and side-to-side controls are available in either right or left hand models. The VGB Systems don't disable the original controls. Proportional feedback allows the driver to feel the actual braking and delivers much greater control. The vacuum canister holds a working reserve which allows up to six braking maneuvers if the engine is not operating. The first electrical backup is built into the VGB handle and continues to deliver smooth braking in the event of control cable failure. The second is a simple push-button operation located on the Vacuum Monitoring and Warning System.

This System includes a two-function switch. In the Manual position, the parking brake is set by simply depressing the push-button contact. In the Automatic position, the same push-button acts as the second brake backup.

CREATIVE CONTROLS, INC. (CCI)
32450 Dequindre
Warren, MI 48092
(313) 979-3500

✳✳✳✳

Tie-Down Systems

Mac's Tie-Down Systems are made of strong nylon straps and self-locking clasps. These durable products are designed to fit all manual wheelchairs and are available in two styles, the "Hook and D-ring straps" and the "Tie-down Bars." Each system is equipped with an 8' leather belt. It is available with either a floor bolt-in assembly or easy to remove track fittings.

MAC'S LIFT GATE, INC.
2801 South Street
Long Beach, CA 90805
(213) 634-5962

✳✳✳✳

Cam Lock Rear Wheel Tie Down

The Braun Cam Lock Rear Wheel Tie Down locks the rear wheels of a wheelchair in place by simply backing the chair into the tie-down. An audible "clicking" sound and a visible "LOCKED" symbol are your assurance that the rear wheels are locked in place. The chair is released by stepping on the release levers. The Cam Lock Tie-Down is adjustable to accommodate most wheelchairs (adjustable to 26" maximum, 3" minimum width) and is available in Floor Mount (14686A) or Rail Mount (14792A) styles.

Manual Slide Bar Tie Downs

Braun's Manual Slide Bar Tie Downs are designed to lock the rear wheels of a wheelchair in place with the movement of a single lever. Constructed of heavy gauge steel, these tie-downs are available in Floor and Rail Mount styles. Both are offered in two widths to accommodate most wheelchairs. The dimensions listed are the maximum widths of wheelchairs which will fit in these tie-downs.

Rail Mount (15138A)—28" maximum, 17 3/4"
    minimum.
Rail Mount (12346A)—25 1/2" maximum, 14 3/4"
    minimum. Floor Mount (15137A)—28" maximum, 17 3/4" minimum.
Floor Mount (12345A)—25 1/2" maximum, 14 3/4"
    minimum.

THE BRAUN CORPORATION
1014 S. Monticello
P.O. Box 310
Winamac, IN 46996
(800) THE-LIFT
(219) 946-6153 in Indiana

****

Freedom Edition Motorhome

The Freedom Edition Motorhome is unique in the fact that it is designed as a wheelchair accessible recreational vehicle. It includes such features as a wider aisle, roll under sinks, an accessible bathroom, and a Crow River wheelchair lift with a fold-in-half platform. The vehicle can also be equipped with hand driving controls and six-way power seat for total driveability. The body can be transferred from chassis to chassis, so, according to Peter Galietta Sr., President of Healthcall Rehabilitation Equipment and Supply, "you can easily realize thirty-five years of usefulness from it."

HEALTHCALL REHABILITATION
EQUIPMENT AND SUPPLY
311 N. Western Avenue
Peoria, IL 61604
(309) 676-6054

****

Mini-Top

The Pop-Top Company has manufactured retractable tops for camper vans since 1965. Their Mini-Top is intended to provide the extra headroom needed by persons who are confined to a wheelchair while riding in a van. The Mini-Top can be a practical alternative to a dropped floor or full raised roof (the Mini-Top provides the headroom only where it's needed).

The tops are pre-fitted to match the roof contour of the van, and all materials needed for the installation are included. According to the manufacturer, total installation is less than three hours, including trimming out the existing ceiling to fit to the Mini-Top.

POP-TOP COMPANY
1895 Blase Nemeth Road #6
Painesville, OH 44077
(216) 354-5231

****

Drive-Master Corporation

Drive-Master Corporation has been developing and installing driving and mobility aids for over thirty-five years. It was founded in 1952 by the late Alan B. Ruprecht, a paraplegic who began by designing special equipment in his garage for his own use.

V16 Low Effort Braking Modifications

V25 No Effort Braking Modifications

Standard factory power brakes require 20 foot-pounds of pressure to operate. The low-effort braking modification reduces the pressure required to 11 foot-pounds. The no-effort braking modification reduces the pressure required to 7 foot-pounds or less. (These statistics will vary slightly depending upon model of van or car.)

Modifications are available for all American vans and many American and foreign cars with factory power brakes. Full-sized General Motors and Chrysler (Dodge/Plymouth) cars and 1/2 ton Chevrolet (G10) and Dodge/Plymouth (B100) vans must have heavy duty (tandem) power brakes for no-effort braking modifications.

V26 Backup System For Braking

The V26 backup system provides emergency, power assisted braking in the event the factory power brake system fails due to engine failure or low vacuum. It is available for all American vans and most American full and mid-sized cars with factory power brakes. A test circuit is included so the system may be checked prior to driving. Audio and visual alarms alert the driver to factory power braking failure. The backup system for braking is activated when the engine vacuum drops below a safe level, which can be the result of engine stalling, a broken vacuum line, or other vacuum leak.

V15 Low Effort Steering Modifications

V23 No Effort Steering Modifications

Standard factory power steering requires approximately 40 ounces of effort to operate. The low-effort steering modification reduces the effort needed to 20-24 ounces. The no-effort steering modification reduces the effort needed to 8 ounces or less. (These statistics will vary slightly depending upon model of van or car and tire size.)

Modifications are available for all American vans and many American and foreign cars with factory power steering.

Horizontal Steering

The Drive-Master horizontal steering system is customized to meet the needs of the high-level spinally injured and all others who experience limited arm strength and range of motion. It is most often used in conjunction with vacuum servo hand controls. The system is fully adjustable in all planes and telescopes for maximum driver comfort. It eliminates the arm-lifting motion needed to steer conventionally, and can be installed on any tilt or non-tilt steering column. An optional interchangeable system allows conventional steering as well.

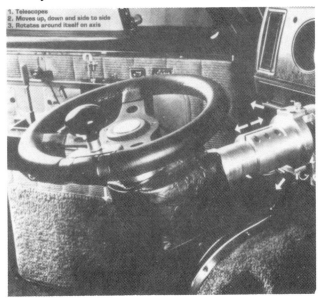

V24 Backup System For Steering

The V24 provides emergency power steering, allowing the driver to steer the vehicle out of traffic without a loss of control. It starts operation instantaneously in the event of factory power steering failure. The backup system for steering is available for all American vans and most American full- and mid-sized cars with factory power steering. A test circuit is included so the system may be checked prior to driving.

Note: Some states require backup systems for all wheelchair drivers.

DRIVE-MASTER CORP.
16 Andrews Drive
West Paterson, NJ 07424
(201) 785-2204

****

Power Seat Base

The Ricon 6-Way Power Seat Base facilitates a driver's self-transfer from a wheelchair to the driving seat and, once there, allows for optimum driving positioning. The Ricon 6-way power base makes this procedure completely automatic. It provides twelve inches of front-to-rear travel; nine inches of height adjustment; and a full 90 degrees of swivel from the straight-ahead driving position to the transfer position.

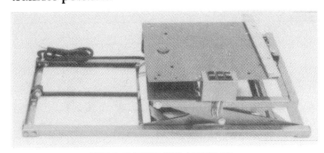

THE RICON CORPORATION
11684 Tuxford Street
Sun Valley, CA 91352
(800) 322-2884
(800) 263-2356 in Canada
(818) 768-5890 in California

****

Viking

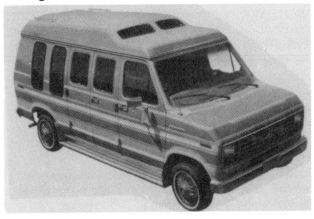

Viking offers a full line of van tops and interior headliners in a wide range of sizes and styles for most full size and mini vans. There is also a unique line of van accessories to complement the Viking tops, including: luggage racks, "Sport Rails," TV antenna kits, "Sport Step," trim kits, camper top windows, and running boards.

VIKING FORMED PRODUCTS
P.O. Box 319
Middlebury, IN 46540
(219) 825-8401

534 Hwy. 78
Loganville, GA 30249
(404) 466-2251

3715 N. Frontage Road
Lakeland, FL 33809
(813) 686-1116

****

The Roadrunner™

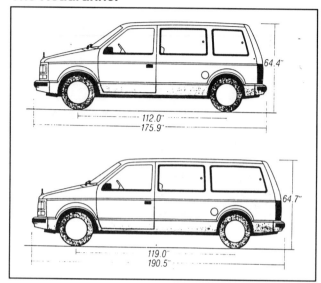

Because of its patented electrically powered automatic door/ramp system and 10" lowered floor, the Roadrunner™ from Independent Mobility Systems (IMS) requires no lift. Push one switch and the door opens, the vehicle "kneels," and a ramp deploys. Since there is no lift, all occupants can enter and exit through the 53 1/2" side door opening without lift obstacles or lift cycle delays. With its "easy move" driver and passenger seats, you can ride up front or drive, or even accommodate two wheelchairs. Because IMS uses Chrysler's narrow-profile minivans, you can go virtually anywhere a car can. The Roadrunner™ operates with virtually all chairs and most adaptive driving systems.

The Traveler™

Designed for commercial service, the Traveler™ offers a 10" lowered floor, with a manual swing-away ramp and door, multiple wheelchair tie-down positions, passenger assist handles, and non-slip flooring.

INDEPENDENT MOBILITY SYSTEMS
3900 Bloomfield Highway
Farmington, NM 87401
(800) 622-0623
(505) 326-4538 in New Mexico

****

Celebrity Coach

Celebrity Coach specializes in providing both consumer and commercial handicap transportation.

From furnishing a semi-automatic attendant operated wheelchair lift to a fully appointed conversion van with raised roof, raised doors, power pan (elevated floor), horizontal power seat, fully automatic wheelchair lifts with automatic door operators, manual and electric wheelchair tie-downs, hand controls, and special driving accessories, Celebrity can add any special adaptive equipment that you may require. All of their van conversions are available on Ford, GMC, Chevrolet, and Dodge chassis.

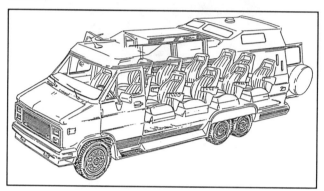

Celebrity Coach Limousines are offered in two models; the "Transporter" Series with seating to eleven passengers and the "V.I.P." with a divider wall and custom wet bar. The coaches are stretched 48 inches and are available on either a Ford or Chevrolet chassis. The "stretch" includes a full length, custom molded reinforced raised roof and stretched running boards.

CELEBRITY COACH, INC.
700 E. Main Street
Larksville, PA 18651
(717) 779-9505

****

Handi-Van, Inc.

Handi-Van, Inc. offers three products nationally: a Chrysler Mini-Van with a 10" drop floor (from the firewall to behind the rear door), a space-saving Automatic Platform Lift (that fits Ford Aerostar, Dodge Mini-Ram, Chevrolet Astro, Plymouth Voyager, GMC Safari, and Dodge Caravan without door or body modifications), and a Ramp that swings out to allow better van access to walking passengers.

HANDI-VAN, INC.
8250 Eastwood Road
Mounds View, MN 55112
(612) 786-5235

****

HDS (Handicapped Driving Systems, Inc.)

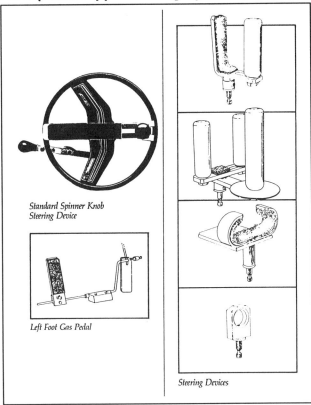

Standard Spinner Knob Steering Device

Left Foot Gas Pedal

Steering Devices

HDS offers complete conversion packages. Hand controls, steering devices and various extensions, ramps, semi-automatic and fully-automatic lifts, tiedowns, and a variety of special products are available. Vans can be modified to allow for increased headroom and taller door openings. Raised fiberglass tops in different heights can be modified with raised side or rear doors for maximum clearance for equipment or wheelchair users. Lowered floors can provide increased headroom and door openings without increasing the overall height of the van.

HDS–HANDICAPPED DRIVING
SYSTEMS, INC.
12273 Nicollet Avenue
Burnsville, MN 55337
(800) VAN-6176
(612) 894-1914 in Minnesota

****

New Era

New Era is an authorized Ricon, Drive Master, and Crow River dealer that specializes in adapting vans. Available modifications include raised roofs and doors, hand controls, steering devices, power transfer seat, lifts, left foot gas pedal, and lowered floor.

NEW ERA TRANSPORTATION, INC.
810 Moe Drive
Akron, OH 44310
(800) 325-9649
(800) 325-9647 in Ohio

****

Freewheel Vans, Inc.

Freewheel Vans, Inc. offers a wide selection of van conversion styles, including original designs, or will customize a van to your requirements and specifications. A variety of lifts, ramps, extended tops, hand controls, wheelchair tie down systems, wheelchair carriers, trunk loaders, adaptive driving devices, and other equipment is available. Located just west of Denver in the foothills of the Rocky Mountains, Freewheel can arrange to have customers picked up at nearby Stapleton International Airport and brought to their facility.

FREEWHEEL VANS, INC.
4901 Ward Road
Wheat Ridge, CO 80033
(303) 467-9981

****

Access Custom Conversions

Access Industries, Inc. provides van conversion services and handles a full line of mobility equipment including electric three-wheel scooters, trunk lifts, ramps, and porch and stairway lifts. They operate their own fabrication shop for all body modifications, as well as shops for adaptive equipment installation, customizing, and painting. They offer such options as lowered floors, raised roofs and doors, rotary lifts, platform lifts, power door operators, hand controls, and driving systems.

ACCESS INDUSTRIES, INC.
2509 Summer
Memphis, TN 38112
(901) 323-5438

****

OTHER VAN CONVERSION RESOURCES:

ABBEY MEDICAL

CLEO INC.
GUARDIAN
LUMEX
MADDAK, INC.
ST. LOUIS OSTOMY AND MEDICAL SUPPLY
SUNRISE MEDICAL

For additional information, including addresses and phone numbers, see CATALOGS.

CHAPTER SEVEN

HEALTH AND FITNESS

EXERCISE AND MASSAGE

Row-Cycle

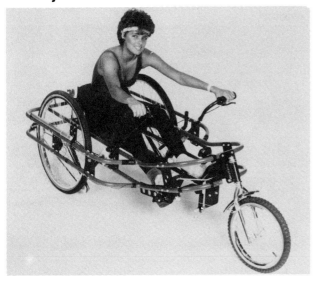

"The advantage to our use of the Row-Cycle is that if the paralyzed muscles fatigue, individuals can still use the non-paralyzed muscles in the upper part of the body to move the Row-Cycle around. In addition, both the paralyzed and non-paralyzed muscles can work together, providing a very good workout. We think that this can not only be used in rehab, but in addition will provide a potential new sport. . ."—Dr. Jerrold S. Petrofsky, Chief Executive Officer, Casa Corazon, Lake Forest, California

The Row-Cycle is a rowing machine that eliminates the "boredom factor." It is a three-wheeled vehicle propelled by rowing action and steered by tilting the seat. Although the seat is also able to slide on a channel, it can be secured for the wheelchair user. The feet are held on a platform by Velcro straps and, in conjunction with the rowing arms, aid the user in feeling stable. In addition, the cushioned backrest is adjustable. Although a seat belt is standard equipment, the manufacturer reports that some users include a second belt to give added support to the upper trunk. Both the

three-speed shift stick and hand brakes are located on the rowing handles. One of the two available models of the Rowcycle is specifically for quadriplegics or those with balance and/or dexterity problems. The Row-Cycle is constructed of high quality, ultra light aircraft aluminum enabling it to be carried on a standard bicycle rack. Its three-speed transmission allows speeds up to 20 mph and provides the ability to climb steep grades. There are several adjustments which can increase performance and permit one size to be used by a six year old or a sixty year old. As reported in the December 1987 issue of _Sports 'n Spokes_, "the Rowcycle will not move backward—a slight inconvenience until the rider gets used to this limitation." Parts are warrantied for a year, the frame for a lifetime.

ROW-CYCLE
3188 N. Marks, #120
Fresno, CA 93722
(209) 268-1946
(800) 227-6607

✳✳✳✳

Upper-Max Exerciser

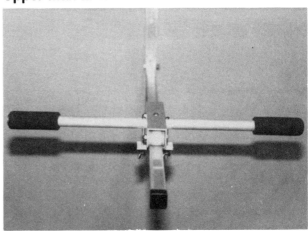

The back and forth pushing and pulling motion of the "Upper-Max" strengthens arms, shoulders, chest, and upper back while increasing heart rate and blood circulation. The mounting bracket is attached to a stud and remains on the wall, but the lightweight exerciser can easily and quickly be removed for out of the way storage when not in use. Five height adjustments make finding a comfortable exercise position easy. Resistance is also adjustable from zero to the desired amount. Exercising with the "Upper-Max" is convenient for quadriplegics, paraplegics, stroke patients, and other wheelchair users.

For those with little or no hand grip, "Holding Mitts" are available. The Upper-Max Exerciser is priced at under $75.00 with the Holding Mitts available for under $20.00.

THE CREATIVE SHOP
P.O. Box 7
Leoma, TN 38468

＊＊＊＊

Swell Relief™

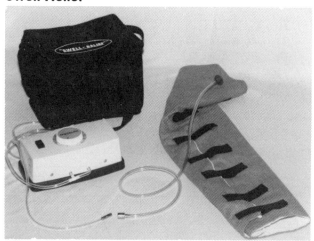

Swell Relief™ is a programmable intermittent compression pump and inflatable sleeve which reduces swelling of the limbs. Swell Relief™ repeatedly squeezes the limb and then relaxes it. Excess fluid is gently circulated back into the body as the sleeve applies controlled pressure. When the sleeve is relaxed, the blood returns to the limb to nourish the cells. The design of the sleeve permits arm bending and hand use, as well as size adjustment. Quick-disconnect allows the user to leave the room without removing the sleeve. A zippered black nylon bag with carrying straps stores the pump and sleeve for everyday use or travel.

Federal regulations require that use of these systems be authorized by a physician.

Pump Price: about $450.00
Sleeve Price: about $100.00

Bag Price: about $35.00

D.A. SCHULMAN, INC.
7701 Newton Avenue N.
Brooklyn Park, MN 55444
(612) 561-2908

＊＊＊＊

The Saratoga Cycle—Accessible Aerobic Fitness

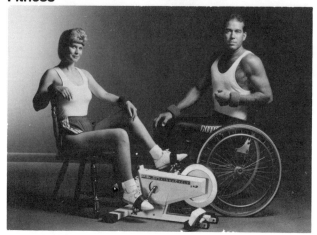

The Saratoga Cycle has been designed by a quadriplegic to be used easily without the need for body transfers or set-up help from someone else.

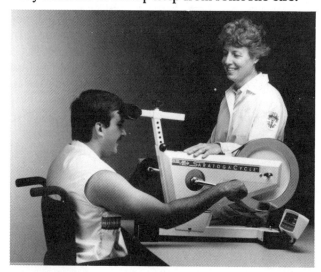

The Cycle can be used for arm exercise when fitted with handgrips and placed on any table top, and for leg exercise when the handgrips are exchanged for foot pedals and the unit is placed on the floor.

Unique features include three handgrip styles for people with full, limited, or even nonexistent hand grasp; an adjustable padded forehead rest; zero to full, easily adjustable resistance; a solid, balanced flywheel; and an electronic exercise computer.

Saratoga Cycle:

- with foot pedals and toe loops Price: about $950.00
- with standard handgrips Price: under $1000.00
- with limited grasp handgrips Price: under $1100.00
- with all three options Price: about $1100.00

SARATOGA ACCESS & FITNESS, INC.
6 Birch Street
Saratoga Springs, NY 12866-3834
(518) 587-6974

✱✱✱✱

F 7000 Foot Training Appliance

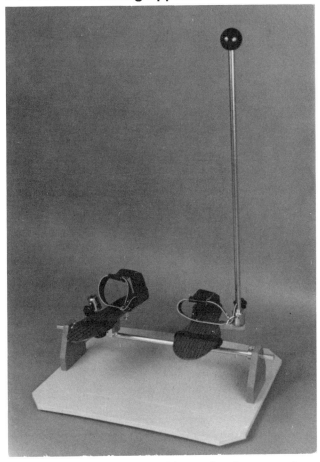

The F 7000 is designed for active foot exercises. It can be used for therapeutic or training purposes, as well as under water. The therapeutic movements include all natural turning and swinging movements of the ankle.

Ballert Wobble-Board

The Ballert Wobble-Board is made to give "safe and effective exercising in the clinic as well as in the home, provided the instructions are followed."

It is a strongly constructed circular wooden platform supported on a precisely designed hemisphere. As described by Ballert, the radius has been chosen to give the optimum exercise effect. The top surface is "anti-slip" and warm to the touch. The material contains an anti-fungal compound and can be easy cleaned.

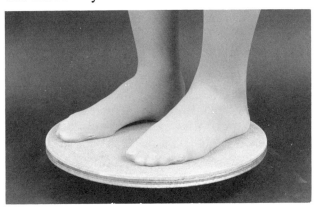

A 5000 Finger Healing Appliance

The A 5000 is an appliance for passive finger training to regenerate mobility, strengthen finger muscles, and relax hand muscles.

The fingers are placed in the "lifting movement device" and raised 30mm in succession. Pulling movements, of up to 40mm longitudinally for each finger, can be continuously added. Also, the A 5000 can typically be adapted to impediments of a single finger. Finger rails are included, so that distended fingers can be placed in the lifting device.

To use the "splaying device," the middle finger is placed in a resting position and the forefinger and third finger are splayed in a position of about 16 degrees. With each movement they are brought to an angle of 12 degrees in spread-out position. The thumb and small finger are placed in a splayed position of 30 degrees in front of the center line and are moved outwards in a spread-out position of 20 degrees with each movement. The finger movements can be infinitely adjusted from resting position up to a sequence of about 360 movements per minute.

Other finger movement and training appliances that are available from Ballert International, Inc. include the H 6000 Finger Movements Appliance and the H 6500 Finger Training Appliance.

BALLERT INTERNATIONAL, INC.
3677 Woodhead Drive
Northbrook, IL 60062-2450
(800) 345-3456

****

Wheelercise™

The video "Wheelercise™" created and developed by Maura Casey, Licensed Physical Therapist, consists of a beginner (ten minute) and advanced (twenty minute) workout. It offers a total upper body aerobic workout right from the wheelchair. The video works on shoulder depressors, triceps, biceps, medial-lateral and anterior-posterior sitting balance, rib isolation all the way down to the fingers and wrists (with wrist rolls). "Wheelercise™" is currently being used by many rehabilitation hospitals and recreation centers nationwide.

"Exercising on a regular basis helps increase your cardiovascular fitness level, increase your joint flexibility to make your upper body work better for you. Remember to get a medical clearance from your doctor before starting any exercise program."—Maura Casey, Casey-Diperi Enterprises

CASEY-DIPERI ENTERPRISES
P.O. Box 723
Butler, NJ 07405
(201) 492-1352

****

"Wheelchair Workout with Janet Reed"

"Wheelchair Workout with Janet Reed," written by Janet Reed, was the first program of its kind. It offers an opportunity to improve both the physical and emotional qualities of life by providing a way of feeling better, looking better, and enjoying oneself.

Janet Reed became a paraplegic in 1977 after being thrown from a horse. The idea for this project began in March 1983, after a friend asked her to dance from a wheelchair.

She designed the exercises after extensive research and testing under the supervision of Claire Hermann, an experienced registered physical therapist. The program has been endorsed by physicians and other professionals working with the disabled.

The benefits of the program are manifold: improved cardiovascular circulation, reduced stress, and better muscle tone. "People in wheelchairs can lead fuller lives by being physically fit. Regular exercise is especially important for the wheelchair-bound, because of the many health-related problems occurring due to their limited body movement."

"Wheelchair Workout with Janet Reed" can be done from an Amigo motorized wheelchair, other wheelchair, or sturdy chair. It consists of an audio cassette tape with a thirty-minute exercise program narrated by Janet Reed to the original contemporary music, "Move It" by Nolan Church, Jr. The tape's opposite side features the upbeat unnarrated music. The "Wheelchair Workout" also includes a 43-page Information Manual with easy-to-follow instructions and illustrations for the forty-seven different movements and other pertinent information.

WHEELCHAIR WORKOUT WITH JANET REED
12275 Greenleaf Avenue
Potomac, MD 20854
(301) 279-2994

****

OTHER SOURCES OF EXERCISE AND MASSAGE AIDS:

ABBEY MEDICAL
ACCESS TO RECREATION, INC.
ALIMED INC.
CLEO INC.
COLUMBIA MEDICAL MANUFACTURING
DANMAR PRODUCTS
FLAGHOUSE, INC.
HAUSMANN INDUSTRIES
J.A. PRESTON CORPORATION
KAYE PRODUCTS INC.
KAYE'S KIDS
LS&S GROUP, INC.
MADDAK, INC.
RIFTON
SNITZ MANUFACTURING
ST. LOUIS OSTOMY AND MEDICAL SUPPLY
THERAFIN CORPORATION

For additional information, including addresses and phone numbers, see CATALOGS.

POSITIONING

Padded Knee Control

"When I'm wearing it, not only do my knees stay together in a more comfortable position, but nothing slides off my lap! What a joy to have a lap again."—P.P. Oak Brook, IL

This comfortably padded leg belt can aid in improving posture and relieving hip pressure. Either buckle or Velcro closures are offered.

"The belt is great, lets me do more without having to worry about my feet falling off the foot rests when my legs jerk."—B.K. Council Bluff, IA

Price: under $20.00.

DVA HELPS
1425 East 22nd Avenue
N. Kansas City, MO 64116

✳✳✳✳

Stand Aid

"My wife has multiple sclerosis and has lost the use of her legs. She spends approximately seventeen hours each day in bed, and seven hours in a wheelchair. We purchased a Stand Aid primarily for the physical and psychological benefits from being able to stand.

"Approximately two months ago I discovered I had a hernia which would necessitate an operation ... This meant no more lifting and helping my wife from bed to chair, chair to bed, etc. We had to have help and hiring someone full time or asking a friend or relative to fill in was out of the question. In essence, we needed a mechanical device that would do everything I did. I'm happy to say the Stand Aid came to our rescue. We no longer consider this equipment just an aid to standing. In our case, it is an integral part of our pattern of living. We could not do without it.

"An added, unexpected advantage deals with the use of the Stand Aid in our motor home. The RV is the only means we have for travel. Built by Shasta Industries, our RV is equipped with a platform wheelchair lift and an aisle wide enough to accommodate a wheelchair ... This piece of equipment (Stand Aid) fits nicely in the aisle, allowing my wife to be picked up out of the wheelchair and placed in bed. Also, she can be taken directly to the bathroom, which is located at the end of the aisle in the rear of the RV.

"We recommend it highly for anyone in our circumstances."—F.P.A.

Stand Aid's Power Lift raises you from your chair or bed with the flick of a switch. Powered by a rechargeable battery, it puts standing within reach. The unit's support belts are adjustable, as is the table (adjustable both vertically and horizontally).

The Power Drive Control features: forward, backward, right, and left turning—plus speed control—all in one single lever control module. Two 12-volt rechargeable batteries are required.

The manufacturer advises that a free videotape is available.

STAND AID OF IOWA, INC.
Box 386
Sheldon, IA 51201
(800) 831-8580
(712) 324-2153 in Iowa

✳✳✳✳

OTHER SOURCES OF POSITIONING AIDS:

ABBEY MEDICAL
ALIMED INC.
CLEO INC.
COLUMBIA MEDICAL MANUFACTURING
CONSUMER CARE PRODUCTS
DANMAR PRODUCTS
FLAGHOUSE, INC.
J.A. PRESTON CORPORATION
J.T. POSEY CO., INC.
KAYE PRODUCTS INC.
MADDAK, INC.
RIFTON
ST. LOUIS OSTOMY AND MEDICAL SUPPLY
THERAFIN CORPORATION

For additional information, including addresses and phone numbers, see CATALOGS.

POOLS AND BATHS

Ferno Ille

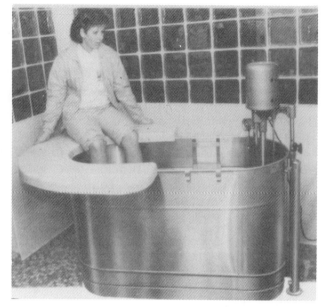

Ferno Ille manufactures hydrotherapy/patient handling equipment such as mobile, movable, and stationary whirlpools, Hubbard tanks, and stretcher and chair lifts.

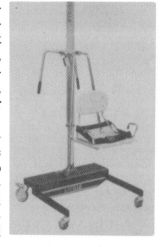

Ferno Ille hydrotherapy accessories are made by craftsmen who specialize in the fabrication of stainless steel specifically for hydrotherapy applications and users.

They include adjustable chairs, hose and valve assemblies, inside seats, tank top, headrests, hand grips, and other related products.

Most Ferno Ille products have passed extensive testing by both UL (Underwriters' Laboratories, Inc.) and CSA (Canadian Standards Association).

FERNO ILLE
A Division of Ferno-Washington, Inc.
70 Weil Way
Wilmington, OH 45177-9371
(513) 382-1451

∗∗∗∗

Easy Ladder & Transfer Tier

The "Easy Ladder" and "Transfer Tier" by Triad Technology, Inc. are two products in a continuing line of pool equipment designed specifically to meet the requirements of individuals with special needs. Triad's products are engineered to enable users to assist themselves to whatever degree possible, ranging from independent use through varying amounts of assistance. Both the "Easy Ladder" and "Transfer Tier" are durable, therapeutically planned products, yet by design are not clinical or mechanical appearing.

The "Easy Ladder" and "Transfer Tier" are completely removable, requiring no deck anchoring or modifications. They're lifted in and out, and to make it easier, there are dollies for each product. All pool depths and coping styles can be accommodated because each unit is custom trimmed at the factory. Construction is of fiberglass and stainless steel, and there are no moving parts to wear out or corrode.

Transfer Tier Price: under $2000.00
Easy Ladder Price: under $1500.00

TRIAD TECHNOLOGIES INC.
4000 Galster Road
East Syracuse, NY 13057
(315) 437-4089

∗∗∗∗

Removable Swimming Pool Parallel Bars

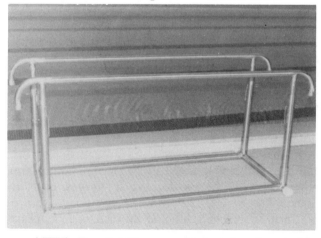

AFW's Parallel Bars are designed to be used in or out of the pool. They are free standing and adjustable, with a non-slip walkway. Made of #304 stainless steel, AFW assures that they will stand up in chemically treated water "for the life of the pool." Price: well under $3000.00.

Removable Access Ramp

AFW studies have shown that 90% of all swimmers enter and exit the pool by ramp regardless of their physical or swimming ability.

The AFW Ramp is made of the same stainless steel as the Parallel Bars, and is also intended to last for the life of your pool. The Ramp weighs 178 pounds and can be removed from the pool on its own wheels so as not to interfere with competitive swimming. Price: about $5000.00.

AFW COMPANY OF NORTH AMERICA
Exchange National Bank Building
North Union Street
Olean, NY 14760
(716) 372-2935

Jacuzzi

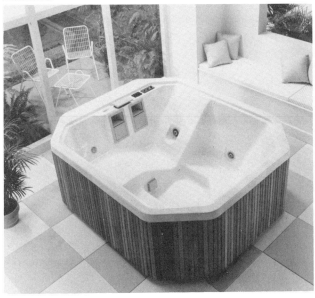

The key to the power of Jacuzzi whirlpool jets is not the pressure of the water, but the volume. Ordinary high pressure jets can actually hurt if you sit too close, and won't affect you at all if you just sit a couple of feet away. Jacuzzi Whirlpool Bath's patented high volume system creates a consistent air/water mixture that results in a soothing massage over the entire body. Each jet can be individually adjusted.

For easy filter cleaning without draining, Jacuzzis offer a top access filter. Silent air controls eliminate the "hissing noise" and provide precision adjustment for greater versatility of hydromassage. The fiberglass underpan resists water damage and deterioration, and the plastic wrapped foam insulation stays intact for the life of the spa. Jacuzzi's air channels are self-cleaning, draining completely every time thus preventing mold and bacteria.

JACUZZI WHIRLPOOL BATH
100 N. Wiget Lane
Walnut Creek, CA 94598
(415) 938-7070

****

OTHER SOURCES OF POOL AND BATH AIDS:

ABBEY MEDICAL
ALIMED INC.
AMERICAN FOUNDATION FOR THE BLIND
ARJO HOSPITAL EQUIPMENT, INC.
CLEO INC.
COLUMBIA MEDICAL MANUFACTURING
GUARDIAN
J.A. PRESTON CORPORATION
MADDAK, INC.
ST. LOUIS OSTOMY AND MEDICAL SUPPLY
SUNRISE MEDICAL

For additional information, including addresses and phone numbers, see CATALOGS.

OTHER HEALTH AND FITNESS AIDS

Porta-Lung™

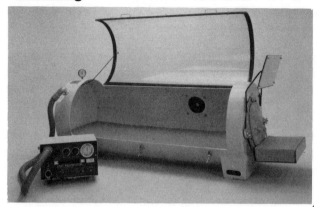

The Porta-Lung™ provides non-invasive ventilatory support designed specifically for the long-term respiratory patient who desires mobility not possible with the iron lung. The Thompson Maxivent or Monahan 170-C negative pressure ventilators provide "more than adequate pressure levels over the entire body." Both ventilators can be purchased from Porta-Lung™, Inc. and are included in the Porta-Lung™ Ventilating System. Service is available nationwide.

PORTA-LUNG™ INC.
401 E. 80th Avenue
Denver, CO 80229
(303) 288-7575

****

Hoyer Digital Scale

The digital electronic scale attachment from Ted Hoyer Company, Inc. offers many convenience and safety features and is designed for use with all Hoyer lifters.

The scale can be attached to a Hoyer lifter in minutes and will complete a self test when turned on. After the person is lifted, the digital display scale stabilizes and locks in his or her weight for an accurate reading. The display shuts off automatically after two minutes of continuous use, but the readout can easily be recalled if necessary. The unit provides precise digital readouts in both pounds and kilograms and is calibrated in tenths of a pound or kilogram increments. It will weigh up to 400 pounds or 182 kilograms.

Other features include a low battery indicator light and a flashing display that indicates when the weight capacity has been exceeded.

TED HOYER & COMPANY, INC.
P.O. Box 2744
Oshkosh, WI 54903

OTHER SOURCES OF HEALTH AND FITNESS AIDS:

ABBEY MEDICAL
ALIMED INC.
CLEO INC.
INDEPENDENT LIVING AIDS, INC.
MADDAK, INC.
ST. LOUIS OSTOMY AND MEDICAL SUPPLY

For additional information, including addresses and phone numbers, see CATALOGS.

CHAPTER EIGHT

RECREATION

SPORTS

Recreation Belt

"Before my wife 'Tody' had her stroke, which has left her with a brace on her left leg and no use of her left arm or hand, she was really an outdoor enthusiast. She loved to fish, hunt, work in her flower gardens, and every year in the late summer we would go berry picking and she would make jams and jellies, etc.

"As many of you know, it's a big transition from an active life like that to one where it's a daily struggle to get around and have the added dilemma of having to learn to do the simplest things with one hand.

"In order to try to resume a semblance of a normal life again, we would go fishing. She could cast the rod, but could not hold it to reel in. When she would get a bite, I would have to run over and reel in her fish. She was always luckier than me, and always had more bites. It came to a point, she felt she was being a burden out there and we felt she was making me work, when I was supposed to be enjoying myself.

"We were unable in all our efforts to find anything that would help us in any way.

"At about this point in time I suffered a bad accident that shattered my upper leg and broke some vertebra in my back, which meant several surgeries, and several years of being able to do almost nothing. So I have a little insight into what it's like to be handicapped. I learned one thing, however. The hardest job there is to be able to do nothing. This is when I put my mind to making something to try to help my wife be able to enjoy life more fully.

"Now with this device, she can go fishing, either bank or trolling. We go hunting but neither of us can walk too well, so it's mostly from the vehicle. She works in her flower garden, just hangs a small pail in the latching device to carry her tools, etc. We go berry picking, again hanging a pail in the latching device. She can put on and remove the belt by herself, and is virtually independent. And for all of us, that is the name of the game."

Persons who have lost the use of an arm can now enjoy sport fishing with the aid of the FreeHanderson Recreation Belt™. The harness and attached hardware allow the user to bait an hook, cast, troll, and reel entirely with one hand.

Developed by a Montana sportsman and his wife, following her stroke, the belt also has accessories for a camera mount and a rifle rest. It's also handy for carrying things like gardening tools, household items, craft supplies, or berry picking supplies.

Weight less than three pounds, either right- or left-handed. Price: about $150.00.

THE FREEHANDERSON COMPANY
P.O. Box 4543
Helena, MT 59604
(406) 449-2764

****

Royal Bee's Electric Retrieve Fishing Reels

"Being a one-handed fisherman, I thought I would always have to fish with live bait from a dock, pier, or boat. Royal Barton's electric retrieve reels opened up new opportunities that never existed before. The compact power pack and electric retrieve reel have given me the freedom to fish with live bait or lures or wade fish with the same capabilities as able-bodied fishermen. These electric retrieve reels were so impressive that the City purchased four reels for loan to disabled persons at no charge. With the purchase of these reels, their fishing experience can be enhanced." —Michael Gunning, Staff Liaison to the Mayor's Committee for Disabled Persons, Corpus Christi, Texas

One-handed fishing can be accomplished with the Royal Bee electric retrieve fishing system. The Royal Bee method of fishing is done by making your normal cast, then raising the rod tip to advance the bait. Then by lowering the rod tip, you retrieve the slack line electronically by pushing a button. Only three ounces of weight is added to the reel with the Royal Bee.

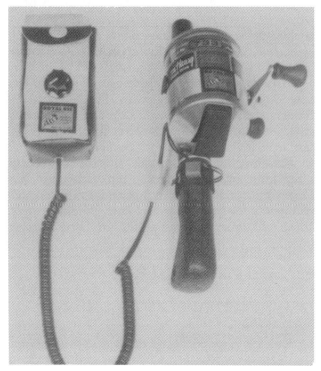

The system comes with 12 volt rechargeable battery and a variable speed control to adjust the speed of the retrieve according to the bait used. Available on both bait casting and spinning reels, it is also excellent for trolling with down riggers.

ROYAL BEE CORPORATION
703 Kihekah
Pawhuska, OK 74056
(918) 287-1044
(800) 331-7629

****

Van's EZ Cast

Van's EZ Cast was designed by Van who was injured in a football accident leaving him paralyzed from the neck down except for limited use of one arm but no wrist or finger movement. He had always enjoyed sports and he still wanted to participate in some form of outdoor recreation. He knew fishing would afford him that opportunity, as well as involvement with friends, so he developed a unique fishing system.

Van's EZ Cast works on the right or left arm of a wheelchair or lawn chair. All that is necessary is limited use of one arm. Two nylon clamps hold the

device in place. The two piece medium action graphite composite rod accepts any closed face spincast reel. By pushing the rod forward, the line holder automatically releases the line at the exact moment for a good cast. The unit includes rod, aluminum casting device, chair arm holder, two clamps, and a detailed drawing of a special splint for those with no wrist or finger movement. Price: about $80.00.

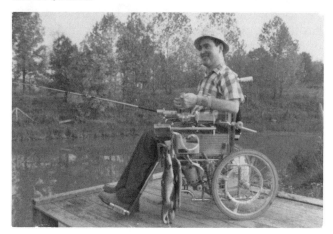

THE CREATIVE SHOP
P.O. Box 7
Leoma, TN 38468
(615) 852-2323

****

Bowling Ball Holder-Ring

The Bowling Ball Holder-Ring is a third hand for wheelchair bowlers. It can safely hold your bowling ball while you push to the foul line to bowl. The ring is made of 3/8" diameter steel and the attachment of heavy duty aluminum. A Tray Attachment converts the holder-ring into a handy tray for snacks or picnics, or a desk for classes 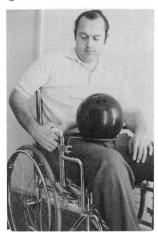 or letter writing. Price: about $25.00.

GEORGE H. SNYDER
5809 N.E. 21 Avenue
Ft. Lauderdale, FL 33308

****

AWC Active Life™ Glove

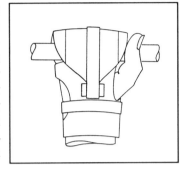

The AWC Active Life™ Glove assists the physically challenged individual in pursuing a better quality of life. For those with limited or no finger dexterity, it firmly adapts to major exercise machines providing a tight grip. In addition, it adapts to other sports and recreational equipment including fishing rods, ping pong paddles, and pool cues to mention a few.

Two types of AWC Active Life™ Gloves are available. The "single tunnel loop" gloves feature only one pile fabric strap attached to the leather mitten. The strap, when run through the single palmar loop to form a closed fist, enables the user to exercise on such machines as HydraFitness, Universal Gym, free weights, dumbbells, barbells, etc.

The "double tunnel loop gloves" feature two loop/straps. The smaller hook/pile strap enables the user to grip objects. The larger pile fabric strap reinforces the grip on the item being held by the smaller strap.

"Being a quadriplegic with no finger dexterity, I found what I had been searching for with the Active Life™ Glove. I can now do some of my favorite hobbies again. The Active Life™ Glove helped put the Act back into my life."—S.S., Wheelchair Athlete

PATTON MEDICAL GLOVE, INC.
P.O. Box 7100
Jacksonville, FL 32210
(904) 388-1182

✳✳✳✳

"Design For Integrated Recreation" (Videotape)

An 11.5 minute informational documentary explores the wide range of recreational activities made possible by creative design and the application of appropriate technology toward the attainment of recreational opportunities. This video was produced with funding from the Paralyzed Veterans of America's Spinal Cord Research Foundation in Washington, DC. It was produced and directed by Dan Woodard at the Stanford Instructional Media Department, Stanford, California.

Rehabilitation programs tend to place an emphasis on the development of independent living and vocational skills. Recreation is often provided in the form of entertainment. By developing modifications to existing equipment it is often possible for people with physical disabilities to participate in recreational activities in an integrated manner with family and friends. The development of new devices and systems is allowing people with varying abilities to play within existing sporting activities with others who may or may not have disabilities.

This tape presents a wide range of recreational opportunities, from gardening to sit-skiing, hand cycling, and flying, and is available for the cost of the tape cartridge and duplication. VHS tape priced under $25.00. 3/4" Sub Master about $30.00. Beneficial Designs gratefully acknowledges the Paralyzed Veterans of America for production of this tape.

"Arroya"

A seven-minute informational documentary on the Arroya VI downhill sit-skiing system is available in VHS, 3/4", and Betamax formats. The video was produced by the Rehabilitation R&D Center at the Veteran's Administration Medical Center in Palo Alto, California where the Arroya IV and V were developed.

Programs and ski areas initiating downhill sit-skiing will find the tape of interest and of use in educating lift, ski patrol, and ski area management personnel. It illustrates chairlift loading and unloading sequences as well as a variety of turning techniques including the kayak, spike, and swing methods. Sit-skiers are shown competing in slalom, giant slalom, and downhill skiing events at the 12th Annual National Handicapped Ski Championships which took place at Squaw Valley, California in 1983. VHS tape priced at under $20.00. 3/4" Sub Master priced about $30.00. Beneficial Designs gratefully acknowledges the Veterans Administration Rehabilitation Research and Development Center in Palo Alto for production of this tape.

"Winter Sports Workshop For Wheelchair Athletes"

This thirty-minute informational documentary is based on the 1987 Winter Sports Workshop for Wheelchair Athletes which was held in Engelberg, Switzerland in January 1987, where participants from all over the world gathered to share their skiing equipment for both nordic and alpine skiing for people with mobility limitations.

A Kiwanis Cup international competition for cross-country sledge events, for Men's 5K and 10K and Women's 2.5K and 5K events, was held prior to the workshop. During the workshop, nordic equipment was demonstrated along with a variety of poling and lane changing techniques.

Alpine mono-skiing was demonstrated by participants from all over the world, focusing on the development of the mono-ski. Particular attention was paid to the utilization of individualized and adjustable seating systems along with spring and dampening systems. As part of the workshop a demonstration/competition event took place in which participants had the opportunity to race in both the slalom and giant slalom. All of the equipment is illustrated in this video. In addition, instructors and staff from Torgon, Switzerland demonstrated their instructional teaching sequence progression, from initial entry and experience in the mono-ski, familiarization and balance drills for the beginner; to beginning and intermediate instruction techniques and skills, demonstrated on the hill. VHS tape priced at about $30.00.

BENEFICIAL DESIGNS INC.
5858 Empire Grade
Santa Cruz, CA 95060
(408) 429-8447

✳✳✳✳

OTHER SOURCES OF RECREATION PRODUCTS:

ACCESS TO RECREATION, INC.
AMERICAN FOUNDATION FOR THE BLIND
CLEO INC.
DANMAR PRODUCTS
FLAGHOUSE, INC.
J.A. PRESTON CORPORATION
LS&S GROUP, INC.
MADDAK, INC.
SCIENCE PRODUCTS
SNITZ MANUFACTURING
T.R.S.

For additional information, including addresses and phone numbers, see CATALOGS.

CRAFTS

Knitterella

Knitterella is an ideal knitting device for those who have difficulty knitting with needles. It is particularly suitable if you have trouble adjusting tension or have difficulty concentrating.

Knitterella is made up of two rows of pegs. It clips onto a table or board, and the rows of pegs can be swivelled towards or away from the user, for easy access. Wool is first wound round the peg by hand, and then the stitches are lifted over using a hand-held knitting hook. This process is repeated, and on the same principle as "French knitting," the knitting emerges.

The knitting aid was developed and designed at Loughborough University and is assembled at a disabled workshop in East London, England. The base of the device is made from Brazilian mahogany, and the ends are specially coated zinc castings. There are special rubber sleeves on the clips to protect table tops.

Learning to knit on Knitterella is much easier than with needles and good results start to emerge sooner. With Knitterella it is possible to pick up or leave a piece of work at any stage. Although there are forty-one pairs of pegs, only a few need be used and small items can be made using only the central pegs.

Flettevaeven

The Flettevaeven weaving loom can be used by persons with a wide variety of disabling conditions, and can apply any form of material, whether yarn or fabric remnants. It can be easily attached or detached from an ordinary table, and unlike many looms, takes up practically no space at all when not in use.

Knitterella Ltd. is a subsidiary of the Tana Trust, a registered charity.

KNITTERELLA LTD.
52 Warnford Court
Throgmorton Street
London EC2N 2AY, England

✳✳✳✳

"Speed Box"

"I found I was using the arm control without consciously thinking of what I was doing ... I find the device to be very sensitive to the slightest pressure, and I can 'walk it' around curves or to my stopping place on a seam almost one stitch at a time, if necessary."—E.J.H., Charlotte, North Carolina

The "Speed Box" arm-activated sewing machine control will adapt to virtually any machine. It is simply a matter of unplugging the existing control and plugging in the "Speed Box." The unit clamps on the right front of the sewing machine cabinet. The manufacturer advises that when ordering, the make and model of the machine on which the "Speed Box" is to be used should be specified. Price: about $125.00.

The "Speed Box" is now being used in North Carolina school systems.

TYSINGER SEWING & VACUUM CENTER
Route 9, Box 567
Highway 64 West
Asheboro, NC 27203
(919) 629-2825

✳✳✳✳

Tandy Leather

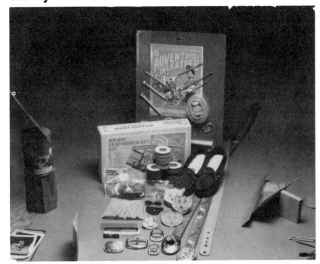

Tandy Leather offers an extensive line of leathercraft kits and supplies. You can shop in person (at one of over 300 stores nationwide), by mail, or by phone. The Tandy catalog includes a wide variety of products and is full of tips and hints for leathercrafters; there are how-to's, project ideas, books, even videotapes that can show you new ways to increase your enjoyment of the craft. Tandy reports that most mail and phone orders are shipped within twenty-four hours of receipt. They accept Visa, MasterCard, and Discover cards as well as C.O.D. orders.

TANDY LEATHER COMPANY
P.O. Box 791
Fort Worth, TX 76101
(817) 551-9770

****

OTHER SOURCES OF CRAFT AIDS AND SUPPLIES:

ACCESS TO RECREATION, INC.
AMERICAN FOUNDATION FOR THE BLIND
CLEO INC.
FLAGHOUSE, INC.
INDEPENDENT LIVING AIDS, INC.
J.A. PRESTON CORPORATION
OPTION CENTRAL
SCIENCE PRODUCTS

For additional information, including addresses and phone numbers, see CATALOGS.

GAMES AND TOYS

Blowdarts

Andrew Batavia, a researcher at the National Rehabilitation Hospital in Washington, DC, developed the activity, "Blowdarts," the idea being to play darts with a blowgun. As this does not require the use of one's arms or hands, "Blowdarts" can be a particularly useful recreational activity for persons with severe physical limitations. Set of 1 blowgun, 1 target, and 12 Velcro darts is priced under $40.00.

BLOWDARTS
AIB Unlimited, Inc.
P.O. Box 3635
Boynton Beach, FL 33424

✳✳✳✳

OTHER SOURCES OF GAMES:

ABBEY MEDICAL
ACCESS TO RECREATION, INC.
ALIMED INC.
AMERICAN FOUNDATION FOR THE BLIND
CLEO INC.
FLAGHOUSE, INC.

INDEPENDENT LIVING AIDS, INC.
J.A. PRESTON CORPORATION
LS&S GROUP, INC.
MADDAK
RADIO SHACK
SCIENCE PRODUCTS
SNITZ MANUFACTURING
THERAFIN CORPORATION

For additional information, including addresses and phone numbers, see CATALOGS.

✳✳✳✳

Toys that can accommodate the special educational, therapeutic, and recreational needs of exceptional children can be obtained from a variety of sources. The following companies offer a selection in their catalogs:

CONSUMER CARE PRODUCTS
DANMAR PRODUCTS
FLAGHOUSE, INC.
J.A. PRESTON CORPORATION
KAYE'S KIDS
MADDAK, INC.
PCA INDUSTRIES, INC.
SCIENCE PRODUCTS

For additional information, including addresses and phone numbers, see CATALOGS.

HOBBIES

The Magic Arm

The Bogen "Magic Arm" is a fully articulated arm with 90 degree pivotable and 360 degree rotatable ends, and an elbow that rotates 360 degrees. The unit is analogous to a human arm with a shoulder, an elbow, and a wrist except that you have considerably greater movement. In the relaxed position, you can move any of the joints to any desired position. A firm turning movement of the control handle located at the elbow joint locks all three joints firmly into position.

The "Magic Arm" may be just what you need to support a 35mm or 6x6 camera in tight quarters; for placement of small lights and flash heads; for gobos, reflectors, and flags.

Both ends have studs that fit into any standard 5/8" socket and the studs have flats for positive tightening. In addition, both ends are tapped: one is 1/4-20 and the other is for European threads so that they can be screwed onto tripods and light stands.

A flash shoe and a camera mount bracket are supplied. The plate can also be used to support the accessory fork and doubles as a holder for flags or extension poles. Price: under $75.00.

BENEFICIAL DESIGNS INC.
5858 Empire Grade
Santa Cruz, CA 95060
(408) 429-8447

****

CELESTRON

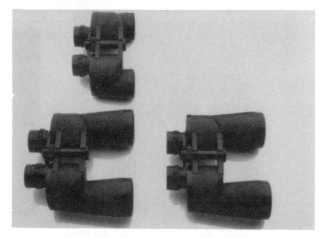

Whether your interest is bird watching, indoor or outdoor sporting events, hunting, concert/thea-ter, boating, travel, photography, nature study, surveillance, camping, astronomy, long distance microscopy or just general purpose, Celestron has a binocular or spotting scope that's right for you. Their binoculars have one of the largest power and aperture ranges available from the Mini 7x23 to the Giant 20x100. Their spotting scopes range from a compact 60mm (2.4") unit up to the impressive 350mm (14") diameter unit.

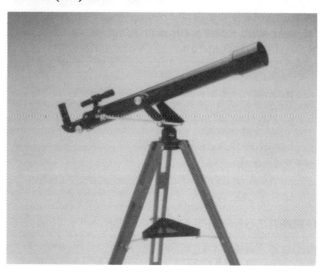

If your interest is serious astronomical study, or astro or terrestrial photography, Celestron offers a large variety of telescopes (all of which are camera adaptable).

CELESTRON INTERNATIONAL
2835 Columbia Street
Torrance, CA 90503
(800) 421-1526
(213) 328-9560

****

Walt Nicke's Garden Talk

"Walt Nicke's Garden Talk" is a readable catalog of gardening products containing over 300 useful items available from the Walt Nicke Co. Published twice yearly, it includes digging tools, edging irons, bulb planters, seed sowers, rakes and hoes, hand tools and trowels, weeders and gardeners' grips, pruners, pruning saws, scissors and shears, row covers, cold frames, propagators, pots, potted plant tools, pot labels, humidifiers, rain gauges, watering cans, hose nozzles, bronze faucets, water timers, shredders, chippers, compost bins, pest deterrents, scoops, spoons, knee pads, kneelers, boots and boot scrapers, books, bookplates, and subscriptions.

Easy Kneeler and Seat

"The two handles provide support for lowering your body onto the padded kneeling platform and make it easy to get up again. People who could not otherwise continue gardening can get down and work with the soil in comfort and safety. Also, you can turn the kneeler over and it becomes a handy seat. The frame is heavy gauge steel tube, painted green. The hardwood kneeling board/seat is clear-varnished and the foam pad can easily be switched from kneeling to sitting surface. The Kneeler/Seat is 22 1/2" long x 21" high x 11 1/2" wide. Weight 10 pounds. Price: under $50.00.

"As gardeners, we regularly use many of the products that we sell, and we talk and correspond with lots of our customers, so we are always happy to give you more information about a product or to help you make decisions."—Katrina Nicke

WALT NICKE CO.
36 McLeod Lane
P.O. Box 433
Topsfield, MA 01983
(508) 887-3388

✳✳✳✳

The "Baronet" Special Time and Labor Saving Garden Tools

The "Firm Grip Weed Puller" is designed and manufactured by Sheffield craftsmen to grip and pull out the most obstinate weeds in cultivated land. Intended for one-hand operation, the 34" long puller virtually eliminates the need to walk over flower beds.

The "Cut and Hold Flower Gatherer" is also designed for one-hand operation. With it, you can reach to the back of the flower beds or to the high rambler rose. The trigger is pointed down for flowers and up for fruit. With blades of finest Sheffield stainless steel the 31 1/2" gatherer has been shown and demonstrated on the B.B.C. TV "Gardening Club."

A. WRIGHT & SON LTD.
Midland Works, Sidney Street
Sheffield, S1 4RH, England

✳✳✳✳

OTHER SOURCES OF HOBBY EQUIPMENT AND SUPPLIES:

ACCESS TO RECREATION, INC.
T.R.S.

For additional information, including addresses and phone numbers, see CATALOGS.

MUSIC

Paiste Gongs, "Therapy-Oriented Instruments"

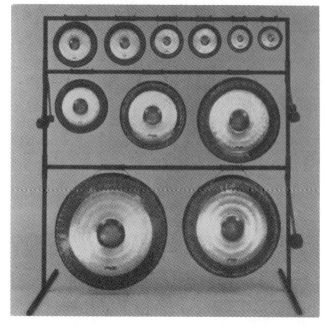

"Just as the gongs of the Far East are made for the far eastern ear, Paiste gongs are made for the western ear. (Generally speaking, far eastern gongs are more restrained, more diffuse and since they are intended for unaccompanied gong music in which note follows note, they are only very briefly sustained.) For people like us, who are accustomed to perceiving sound mentally, structured as music, the "European" gong liberates elemental forces, offering possibilities in therapy that are just beginning to be explored.

"The one characteristic of the gong which is of decisive importance in therapy (as found by institutions and individuals systematically working with Paiste gongs for some time) is its energy potential. This energy manifests itself acoustically as a both mentally and physically perceptible vibration, with an intensity capable of liberating emotions and of opening up new therapeutic approaches.

"Most of the therapeutic experience obtained until now, clearly indicates that the gong is an excellent working tool with catalytic effects on therapeutic activities if not (and the future may verify this) major influence on therapeutic success.

"The effective use of gongs in therapy requires the therapist to have a degree of knowledge and understanding of gongs that should not be underestimated. Seemingly small things of a technical nature, when mastered, can be extraordinarily useful in therapeutic work. The knowledge of how to grasp the mallet, where to strike the gong, and how to achieve a variety of desired effects makes it much easier for the player to develop the gongs full sonority and intrinsic character."

The MMB Horizon Series

The MMB Horizon Series is a new and ongoing monograph series bringing extensive coverage in many crucial areas of music therapy and allied professions. Individually authored, the monographs offer practical guidance and the most up-to-date research available. Titles include: "Accent on Rhythm—Music Activities for the Aged," "Fairy Tales—Musical Dramas for Children," "Music Therapy in Special Education—Developing and Maintaining Social Skills Necessary for Mainstreaming," "Music Therapy and the Dementias—Improving the Quality of Life," and "Guided Imagery and Music in the Institutional Setting."

MMB MUSIC, INC.
10370 Page Industrial Blvd.
Saint Louis, MO 63132
(800) 543-3771

＊＊＊＊

OTHER SOURCES OF MUSICAL INSTRUMENTS AND AIDS:

ABBEY MEDICAL
FLAGHOUSE, INC.
KAY'S KIDS
SNITZ MANUFACTURING

For additional information, including addresses and phone numbers, see CATALOGS.

TRAVEL/VACATION

WILDERNESS INQUIRY

Wheelchairs, dogsleds, and canoes may seem to have little in common, but they are seen together with increasing frequency throughout the wild places in North America. A relatively new field, integrated wilderness programming/travel holds great promise as a means to effect personal growth and positive change in lifestyles for anyone, especially people with disabilities.

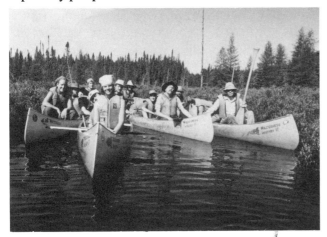

Since 1978 a non-profit organization called Wilderness Inquiry has conducted extended wilderness canoe and dogsled trips with physically disabled persons who are seeking to experience the rigors and solitude of wilderness camping.

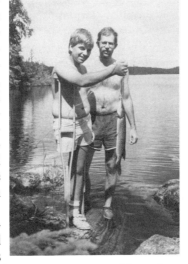

Children and adults from ages seven to eighty-two, including those with disabilities such as quadriplegia, paraplegia, spina-bifida, cerebral palsy, diabetes, multiple sclerosis, muscular dystrophy, blindness, deafness, and other conditions have all participated on these adventures.

Two features distinguish integrated wilderness programs from other types of adventure programs. First, they use wilderness as a medium to effect change in personal characteristics such as self-esteem, independent living skills, attitudes towards risk, and

perceived level of capability. These overall goals are not unlike those of many conventional therapeutic programs.

"Wilderness is technically defined according to the standard adapted by the U.S. Forest Service — at least five miles from the nearest road. Its qualities include remoteness, no man-made alterations, and a pristine and usually beautiful landscape. These and other characteristics create a natural setting that is conducive to effecting positive changes in awareness among many individuals."

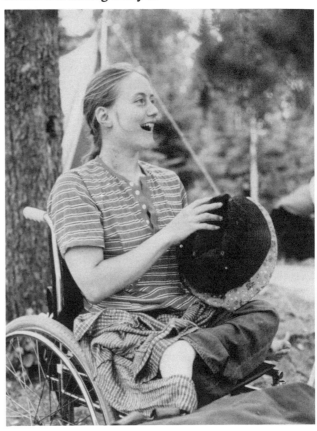

Second, these programs include a heterogeneous mix of people according to their disability and often their age. For example, a typical Wilderness Inquiry group includes two people who use wheelchairs, one who uses crutches, and two people with sensory impairments or other disability type that does not affect their mobility. Also included are non-disabled people. Instead of segregating people according to type of disability or age, these groups include a broad mix of people coming together to share an integrated experience.

Water based activities such as canoeing provide the means to travel great distances in the wilderness with relative ease. These methods of travel — canoeing, rafting, kayaking, etc. — are ideally suited for persons with mobility impairments as those who push their own wheelchairs generally have enough upper body strength to paddle one of these craft.

The greatest physical difficulty facing most disabled persons in these activities is with back support and balance. Usually, problems can be remedied with simple adaptations, such as a backboard or other gear specifically adapted by Wilderness Inquiry.

In addition to the many social benefits of integrated adventures, securing a mix in the abilities of participants also solves certain logistical problems. For example, people with balance problems often team up with wheelchair users in crossing trails and portages. The wheelchair provides a stable base of support for the person with balance problems, while they in turn provide an extra boost of power to get over rough terrain. These "symbiotic" helping relationships are encouraged on mixed ability wilderness adventures. The key ingredients to success are cooperation, trust, and allowing enough time for the task to be completed.

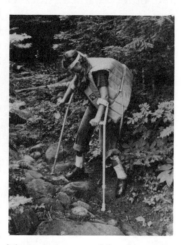

These activities allow integrated wilderness programs to achieve their goals of social and physical integration. "Group members are not segregated by their ability level, they are joined by their desire to experience the wilderness. Hard work and determination are often associated with wilderness travel, but they are balanced by the beauty, solitude, and the confidence gained in learning that one can enjoy a wilderness environment."

WILDERNESS INQUIRY
1313 Fifth Street SE, Suite 327
Minneapolis, MN 55414
(612) 379-3858

****

Access, North Carolina

"Access, North Carolina" is a cooperative program of the Division of Vocational Rehabilitation Services of the North Carolina Department of Human Resources that produces a vacation and travel guide for disabled persons. The pub-

lication, of about 300 pages, is available free of charge and includes: sites of general interest, snow skiing areas, waterfalls, national and state historic sites, outdoor dramas, national recreation areas, state forests and parks. Through the use of symbols and ratings, "Access, North Carolina" simplifies accessibility information.

Surveyors trained in accessibility visited and surveyed each tourist attraction in the state, using as a guide an eight-page checklist developed by a technical review panel. Each attraction was rated for accessibility in these areas: parking, entrance, interior, exterior, and restrooms. "Partially accessible" ratings were given if a feature of the attraction meets some of the accessiblility requirements but not all.

Pertinent information is also included about special accommodations such as wheelchairs available at the site, accessible telephones, water fountains, concession stands, and picnic tables. In addition, comments about site features that are not accessible are often provided.

NORTH CAROLINA DIVISION OF
TRAVEL AND TOURISM
Department of Commerce
Raleigh, NC 27611
(800) VISIT NC
(919) 733-4171

****

HANDICABS

Handicabs has been providing transportation for mobility impeded persons since 1973. Their radio-dispatched, air conditioned vehicles are specially equipped with ramps and lock downs. The traveler is rolled into the vehicle, the wheelchair is locked into place, and safety belts are secured before driving begins.

Handicabs provides the following categories of services (depending on the traveler's needs): Curbside Service; Door Through Door (special assistance service); Hospital, Nursing Home Entries, Discharges and Inter-Institutional Transfers; Two-Man "Non Emergency" Stretcher Service. In addition, they offer tours for the able-bodied visitor as well as the wheelchair traveler. There is no charge for the use of a Company wheelchair.

HANDICABS OF THE PACIFIC, INC.
Post Office Box 22428
Honolulu, HI 96822
(808) 524-3866

****

Skychair

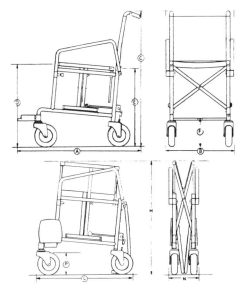

"The Newton Skychair has been designed and built by people in the business of making wheelchairs, (for people in wheelchairs ... in flight). It has many advantages including its light weight. It is inexpensive and simple to use. Furthermore, it is easily stored on board the aircraft to satisfy all the safety requirements and it fits within the parameters of existing aircraft without the need for modification."—Dr. Jim Dunlop, Senior Overseas Medical Officer, British Airways

This lightweight, folding chair has many new features which enable physically challenged passengers to be moved easily to and from seats—and then easy access from the seat to the chair. The swing-away armrests and fold-down back also allow easy access to toilet facilities on most aircraft.

Streamliner

The "Streamliner" can be used with the large wheels fitted as a normal wheelchair for in-terminal use and as a boarding chair. Where the aircraft doesn't carry the in-flight "Skychair," the large rear wheels of the "Streamliner" can be removed quite easily without the passenger leaving the chair.

NEWTON PRODUCTS
Meadway Works
Garretts Green Lane
Birmingham B33 0SQ, England
(021) 783-6081

****

Wheelchair Wagon Tours

Florida-based Wheelchair Wagon Service provides vans equipped with hydraulic lifts and raised roofs, for the elderly and the physically challenged. They offer transportation to and from the airport and all Florida attractions, as well as to doctors' offices, hospitals, homes, and nursing homes.

You can be assisted from your airline seat, escorted through the airport, taken—with your luggage—to the hotel of your choice; and visit attractions like Walt Disney World, Epcot, Sea World, The Kennedy Space Center, and Cypress Gardens.

WHEELCHAIR WAGON TOURS
P.O. Box 1270
Kissimmee, FL 32742
(407) 846-7175

****

Evergreen Travel Service

Evergreen Travel Service tours have gone around the world twice including visits to Nepal, India, South America, South Africa, and China. "In fact, every place except Prussia, and we go there this year."

Tours are available for the blind (they've been doing them for twenty-eight years), as well as the physically challenged ("Wings on Wheels"). They also operate tours for "Slow Walkers"—Seniors who have no disability but cannot keep up with the pace with a regular tour.

EVERGREEN TRAVEL SERVICE, INC.
19505(L)-44th Avenue W.
Lynnwood, WA 98036-5699
(800) 562-9298
(206) 776-1184

****

Whole Person Tours

Bob and Betty Zywicki are recognized worldwide as leading experts in travel for persons with physical disabilities. They have been operating Whole Person Tours since 1981 and publish *The Itinerary*, a magazine for travelers with disabilities. The Zywickis have conducted seminars and workshops throughout the U.S. and have been sought for their advice by editors of major newspapers and magazines, authors of travel books, and the U.S. and foreign travel industry. Bob, disabled for twenty-six years, travels the world in a wheelchair.

Their philosophy: "Abled-bodied or disabled, we're all Whole Persons, worthy of equality, dignity and respect." Whole Person Tours are planned to offer as much equality in sightseeing and enjoyment as trips for able-bodied persons. "If we don't find vehicles with lifts and accessible lodgings and sightseeing, we just don't go there!"

Accessible vacations with Whole Person Tours include: breakfast and most dinners daily, including banquets; licensed guides plus a Whole Person Tours escort; cruises; entertainment; wine tastings; a "Frequent Traveler Discount Program." All types of disabilities are accepted but, unless you are fully capable of taking care of all your personal needs—including propelling your own chair—you must be accompanied by an able-bodied companion.

WHOLE PERSON TOURS, INC.
P.O. Box 1084
Bayonne, NJ 07002-1084
(201) 858-3400

* * * *

OTHER SOURCES OF AIDS FOR TRAVEL AND VACATIONS:

AMERICAN FOUNDATION FOR THE BLIND
MADDAK, INC.

For additional information, including addresses and phone numbers, see CATALOGS.

EDUCATION AND VOCATION

WORK STATIONS

JOB ACCOMMODATION NETWORK (JAN)

The Job Accommodation Network (JAN) was established by the President's Committee on Employment of the Handicapped to provide information on practical accommodations that have proven successful in business and industry. It enables business to talk to business about ways to manage and lower disability costs. JAN also collects job accommodation information and makes it available to businesses seeking ways to enable persons having functional limitations caused by disabilities to be productive in the work environment.

Job accommodation ranges from installing a ramp for a person using a wheelchair to installing a telephone amplifier for an individual who is hearing impaired. Further, there are many accommodations that you may not have recognized, such as rearranging a work schedule for an individual with a heart condition.

The Network operates a toll-free number for information about ways to accommodate an individual with a disability. The call will be answered by a consultant trained to make it easy to find a suitable cost effective solution.

JOB ACCOMMODATION NETWORK
P.O. Box 468
Morgantown, WV 26505
(800) JAN-PCEH TTY/TDD

****

ABRAMS, STONE & ASSOCIATES

Human resource consultants; designers of programs and systems for training and evaluation.

ABRAMS, STONE & ASSOCIATES
P.O. Box 183
Stone Ridge, NY 12484

****

OTHER SOURCES OF AIDS FOR INCREASING JOB ACCESSIBILITY:

ALIMED INC.
AMERICAN FOUNDATION FOR THE BLIND
CLEO INC.
HAUSMANN INDUSTRIES
INDEPENDENT LIVING AIDS, INC.
J.A. PRESTON CORPORATION
LS&S GROUP, INC.
LUMEX
MADDAK, INC.
RIFTON
SCIENCE PRODUCTS

For additional information, including addresses and phone numbers, see CATALOGS.

TOOLS

SOURCES OF TOOLS DESIGNED TO ACCOMMODATE WORKERS WITH SPECIAL NEEDS:

ALIMED INC.
AMERICAN FOUNDATION FOR THE BLIND
ARCOA INDUSTRIES
DANMAR PRODUCTS
FLEETWOOD
INDEPENDENT LIVING AIDS, INC.
J.A. PRESTON CORPORATION
LS&S GROUP, INC.
MADDAK, INC.
RADIO SHACK
SCIENCE PRODUCTS
THERAFIN CORPORATION

For additional information, including addresses and phone numbers, see CATALOGS.

OFFICE EQUIPMENT

Staplex Model SJM-1

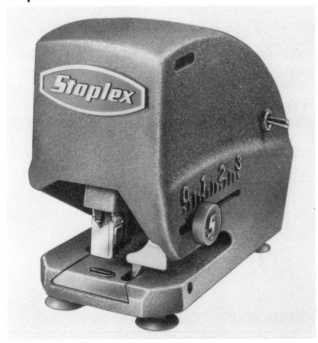

The Staplex Model SJM-1 Automatic Electric Stapler is designed for stapling up to 20 sheets of 20-pound paper or the equivalent. (The SJM-1 is widely used by people with disabilities for many office, graphic arts, and packaging applications.) Model SJM-1 features quick front loading with standard type 1/4-inch High Speed Staples and has an automatic depth selector knob for staple positioning. The SJM-1 staples automatically when work is inserted, and is also available with foot switch activators.

Made in the U.S., the heavy-duty Model SJM-1 is ruggedly constructed of cast duraluminum throughout. It is capable of doing a wide range of stapling operations in offices, printing departments, mailrooms, schools, banks, ticketing counters, etc.

The Model SJM-1 is one of seventy-five different electric staplers offered by the Staplex Company.

THE STAPLEX COMPANY
777 Fifth Avenue
Brooklyn, NY 11232-1695
(718) 768-3333

****

OTHER SOURCES OF OFFICE AIDS:

ACCESS TO RECREATION, INC.
AMERICAN FOUNDATION FOR THE BLIND
DU-IT CONTROL SYSTEMS GROUP
FLEETWOOD
INDEPENDENT LIVING AIDS, INC.
KAYE'S KIDS
MADDAK, INC.
OPTION CENTRAL
SCIENCE PRODUCTS

For additional information, including addresses and phone numbers, see CATALOGS.

CLASSROOM EQUIPMENT AND FACILITIES

Viewpoint Optical Indicator (VOI-6)

For many disabled people, a light-pointing device is an effective way to select locations on a manual communication board or objects in the environment. The VOI-6 is designed for mounting on the front, top, or side of the head. An angle adjustment is also possible once the unit has been mounted. The VOI-6 offers the user a direct selection approach of indicating choices as well as a means of training for those persons capable of progressing to higher level LED devices. At a distance of two feet, the VOI generates a light spot of approximately 5/8". The closer the selected item, the smaller the spot.

The Viewpoint System allows for the creation of low-cost communication aids. Manual boards may be effective for the user with limited head control. Price: approximately $400.00.

Training Aid 2 (TA-2)

The Training Aid 2 is designed for teachers and therapists to evaluate cause and effect awareness, potential control switch operation, and to train proper or requested physical movements. The Training Aid 2 is operated using one or two control switches. Two channels each have both power and switch outputs for turning devices on and off, such as radio, TV, appliances, or toys.

The TA-2 has an internal clock which allows training sessions to be a set length of up to twenty minutes. During each training session, internal counters record the activations of each control switch and the number of times that each reinforcement was turned on.

An accompanying Application Manual, developed by Phillipa Campbell, OTR, M. Ed., a researcher active in this field, has been developed to enhance the overall usefulness of the system and offer specific strategies for using the TA-2.

For individual users, the TA-2 may be used as a single environmental control, in which the user controls the off/on of one appliance. Price: under $600.00.

Versascan (VS-1)

Versascan (VS-1) permits the non-speaking individual to make selections on an overlay by advancing a lighted lamp to the desired location. Overlays can be handmade for activities involving colors, letters, mathematics, symbols, sight words, phrases, or telling time. The VS-1 can be expanded to as many as sixteen lamps (and overlay locations) as communication needs expand. Optional remote lamps enable the individual user to respond independently to various standardized tests, i.e., Peabody Picture Vocabulary Test and the Columbia Mental Maturity Scale. Price: about $800.00.

Prentke Romich and their network of consultants feel that it is very important for potential users, professionals, and consumers to have an opportunity to work directly with PRC products for evaluation purposes. Contact your local PRC consultant regarding the "rental" provision.

PRENTKE ROMICH COMPANY (PRC)
1022 Heyl Road
Wooster, OH 44691
(800) 642-8255
(216) 262-1984

✳✳✳✳

KIMBO EDUCATIONAL

Kimbo Educational specializes in movement oriented recordings, early childhood material, and fun listening. They currently offer more than 1500 titles in subjects areas that include balance and coordination, fine and gross motor skills, numbers, colors, feelings, language, and imagination. Most Kimbo recordings are accompanied by a Teacher's Guide that includes complete instructions and suggested activities. Among titles of special interest:

Fun Activities Perceptual Motor Skills (KIM 9071 or 9071C)
I Like Myself (KIM 0800 or 0800C)
Daily Living Skills—Housekeeping Tasks (KIM 8057 or 8057C)
Self Help Skills—Adaptive Behavior (KIM 8055 or 8055C)
Community Helpers—Vocational Awareness (KIM 8058 or 8058C)
Socialization Skills—Adaptive Behavior (KIM 8056 or 8056C)
Rhythmic Parachute Play (KEA 6020 or 6020C)
Seatworks (KIM 9100 or 9100C)
Fine Motor Skills For Secondary (KIM 7058 or 7058C)
For The Young At Heart! Fitness For Seniors (KIM 2047 or 2047C)

A catalog of Kimbo's records, cassettes, filmstrips, read-alongs, and videos is available.

KIMBO EDUCATIONAL
Division of United Sound Arts, Inc.
10 North Third Avenue
P.O. Box 477
Long Branch, NJ 07740
(800) 631-2187
(201) 229-4949 in New Jersey or outside the
continental U.S.

****

NATIONAL TECHNICAL INSTITUTE FOR THE DEAF (NTID)

NTID, one of the nine colleges of the Rochester Institute of Technology (RIT), is the world's largest technological college for deaf students. Created by Congress and funded primarily by the U.S. Department of Education, NTID represents the world's first effort to educate large numbers of deaf students within a college campus planned principally for hearing students. Together with 12,000 full- and part-time hearing students, nearly 1,200 college-age deaf students from all fifty states, the District of Columbia, and several U.S. territories study and reside on the RIT campus.

In addition to the academic programs based within NTID, RIT's deaf students also benefit from nearly 200 other technical and professional courses of study offered by RIT's other eight colleges.

NTID offers deaf students the opportunity to go to college in a hearing environment and thus make their transition to a hearing society easier and more effective.

NTID's mission is threefold: to provide technological and professional education for hearing-impaired students; to prepare professionals to work with the nation's hearing-impaired population; and to conduct research into the social, educational, and economic needs of hearing-impaired people.

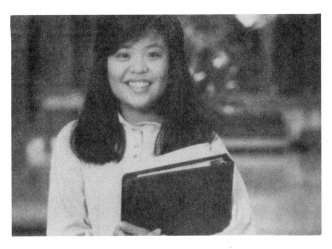

NATIONAL TECHNICAL INSTITUTE FOR THE DEAF
Rochester Institute of Technology
One Lomb Memorial Drive
P.O. Box 9887
Rochester, NY 14623-0887
(716) 475-6826 (Voice/TDD)

****

OTHER SOURCES OF CLASSROOM AIDS AND EQUIPMENT:

AMERICAN FOUNDATION FOR THE BLIND
CLEO INC.
FLAGHOUSE, INC.
INDEPENDENT LIVING AIDS, INC.
LS&S GROUP, INC.
PCA INDUSTRIES, INC.
SNITZ MANUFACTURING
TASH, INC.

For additional information, including addresses and phone numbers, see CATALOGS.

COMPUTERS

Vantage™

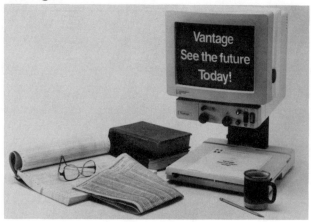

"Vantage™" has been described by Telesensory Systems, Inc. (TSI) as "an entirely new generation of CCTV. It displays a positive image, black letters on a white background, or, flip a switch and you read white letters on a black background. You can choose between black and white, green or amber screens. Reading materials or other objects can be magnified from 3 to 45 times. Brightness and contrast are easily adjusted, as are the focus and aperture. The movable reading table slides easily in any direction. Dual fluorescent lights brightly illuminate the text. Both margin stops and table drag can be set to your liking. Reading material of any type is easily viewed, from hand-written letters and prescription bottles, to calculator displays.

"Vantage™'s" 14-inch non-glare screen tilts up or down so you can adjust it to the perfect viewing angle. Underlines and overlines help you focus on the text you want. The "windowing" feature lets you block out all but one line.

"Vantage™" can be used as the monitor for "Vista," TSI's image enlarging system for IBM PC's and compatibles. The "Vantage™"/"Vista" combination means you have simultaneous access to enlarged computer information as well as written material. You can read both from the same monitor using a split screen.

Braille Interface Terminal (B.I.T.)

The Braille Interface Terminal is a powerful PC accessory combining computer software and hardware designed to provide complete braille access to off-the-shelf computer programs for IBM PC's, XT's, and AT's as well as most compatibles.

The Braille Interface Terminal hardware package contains a 20-cell braille display which serves as a window to the computer screen. A braille keyboard allows the user to enter data and commands for the computer from either the braille or PC keyboard. A joystick makes maneuvering the review window simple and efficient. A custom circuit board provides the interface to make the B.I.T. extremely fast.

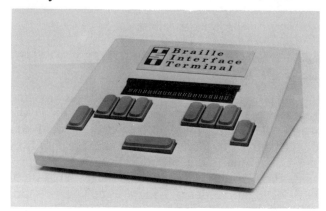

Overlay software provides a set of commands for access to off-the-shelf software. Review command moves the window to the beginning or end of a line, to the top or bottom of the screen, or to a specified line. If the user wants to find a particular section of text, a special "Find" feature makes the process fast and easy.

Lapvert

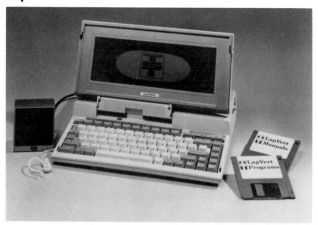

Unlike mosts PCs, the six-pound LapVert can be used immediately. Its customized programs provide automatic voice prompting and verification from the moment of startup. First-time users get practical success before toiling with "operating systems," "application programs," and "screen reading" commands. This benefits people who aren't crazy about computers and those who can't schedule or afford computer teachers. It also lets those classroom teachers and family members with limited computer skills assist blind students.

The LapVert combines the Toshiba T1000 computer with a proprietary speech synthesizer board using the well-known SC-02 speech synthesis microprocessor chip. Braille labels mark Special Function Keys F1-F10. Raised dots provide tactual orientation for seven other keys. For greater speed and flexibility, an optional 3/4-million characters of electronic memory can be added without increasing the unit's dimensions, which are those of a three-ring notebook two-inches thick. A 5 1/4" external drive is also available.

Other TSI Products

TSI's braille embosser, "Versapoint-40," brings desktop publishing to braille users, computer professionals, teachers and business people. Capable of putting a dot anywhere on the page, it opens a world of production possibilities.

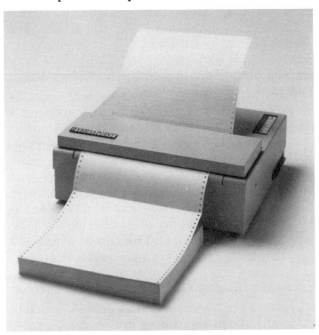

"VersaPoint" has the largest buffer of any embosser in its price range. It offers a speed of 40 characters per second, 6-dot or 8-dot braille, underline spacing, adjustable paper widths, tractor-, micro line-, and backward form-feed, preset configuration software, 11 solenoids, 6 computer braille translators, tactile graphics, vertical printing, and multiple copies.

The portable braille computer "Versabraille II+" (VB II+) features a built-in microdisk drive. It also offers battery-conservation circuitry to guarantee maximum battery life, a silent rubberbrane keyboard, user-friendly operating system, flexible com-

munication ports, and special applications software.

TSI's "VersaPoint Graphics" can create tactile graphics on IBM PC's and compatibles. Lorin Software's programs can create tactile graphics on the Apple IIe or IIc.

TELESENSORY SYSTEMS, INC.
455 North Bernardo Avenue
P.O. Box 7455
Mountain View, CA 94039-7455
(800) 227-8418
(800) 874-9009 in California
(415) 960-0920

✳✳✳✳

Freedom Writer

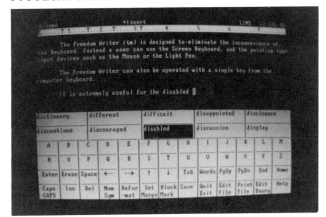

The "Freedom Writer" makes it unnecessary to type on a keyboard. Instead, alternative input devices are used such as a mouse, light pen, joystick, single key, single switch, or speech input. With the "Freedom Writer," it is unnecessary to enter every letter of the text you intend to write. Instead, the word and phrase dictionary is used; it can be set up to contain specific words that you most frequently need. No special hardware adaptations are necessary. The "Freedom Writer" can be used to write letters, reports, tutorials, essays, newsletters, small or large books, and computer programs or research papers.

Help U Type

The "Help U Type" program is designed for people who have difficulty in using the computer keyboard. "Help U Type" users include people who type with one or two fingers, a headstick, mouthstick, or keyguard. It works in the background with many thousands of standard programs on IBM PC, PS/2, and compatible computers.

The "Help U Type" features: word prediction,

one finger operation, repeat key defeat, user defined dictionaries, user defined macros, and automatic spacing.

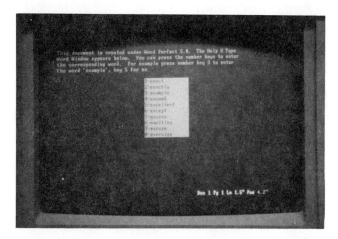

Free Demo disks are available for both "Freedom Writer" and "Help U Type."

WORLD COMMUNICATIONS
501 Glenmoor Circle
Milpitas, CA 95035
(408) 262-2870

✳✳✳✳

Large-Type Word Processing Programs For Poorly Sighted

The National Institute for Rehabilitation Engineering provides technical support for IBM-PC/XT /AT and compatible computers.

2X-4X Magnifying Personal Word Processor

This is a simple word processor, suitable even for young children. It is also suitable for people of all ages who may be learning disabled. The program saves, loads, and edits text, and is very simple to use. With ordinary computer display equipment (CGA, EGA, or VGA), the program allows the user to have either 2X or 4X magnification on the regular screen.

Disadvantages are limited editing functions and slow operation when text is longer than two pages. While often adequate for personal use, we do not recommend this program for business or professional use. No provision is made for automatic spelling checks. This program is often used for screening, testing, and training purposes, even for people who upgrade later to more advanced systems.

1X-2X Full-Featured Word Processor (Plus Optional Spell Checker)

With standard size monitors, this full-featured program allows the user to switch his display between standard size and double size. Printouts can be either, depending on the printer. Many poorly sighted people can use this program as is, or with various types of reading, telescopic, or microscopic glasses. Some people needing larger display characters use a larger-screen monitor. This is an excellent program for those who can use it. Good for non-disabled users, as well.

Multi-Font Graphics Word Processor

This is a commercial desktop publishing program for use with a graphics display system and most dot matrix printers. What You See is What You Get! If you select a 24 pt or a 36 pt font (included in the program) large type appears on the display and is printed on paper. One cannot display "large" and print "small"! A mouse is helpful but not required. This program is not compatible with spelling checker or thesaurus.

Display Magnification Utilities For Standard Software

A variety of different DOS utility software is available, ranging in price from $550 to $850, which allows a PC/XT/AT or PS/2 user to see the data from almost any standard software program, greatly enlarged on the screen. The programs can give from 4X to 20X screen magnification. Most of these utilities function in a "screen review mode" not giving magnification while entering data but only while reviewing data. This can be a problem, especially for users who are not good touch typists.

Hardware Display Magnification Systems

Using a plug-in board (hardware) plus matching software and a mouse control device, these systems work with almost all standard software and can give screen character enlargement of up to 80X, both in a screen review mode and in data entry modes. There is automatic tracking of the entry cursor, and automatic scrolling for reading lengthy text. This method is the most flexible and the most satisfactory for those using more than one program such as a special word processor.

Speech Output for Reading the Screen Aloud

These systems can be used alone by a totally blind person, and they are sometimes used, alone or in combination with display magnification, by partially sighted people. The lower cost systems are full-featured; they are suitable for most users.

Note: All software will work properly with IBM-PS/2 computers as well as with all PC/XT/AT computers and compatibles.

You can telephone The National Institute for Rehabilitation Engineering to discuss your needs and applications.

THE NATIONAL INSTITUTE FOR REHABILITATION ENGINEERING
P.O. Box T
Hewitt, NJ 07421
(201) 853-6585

✳✳✳✳

Hyper-Abledata

Hyper-Abledata is a desktop version of the Abledata database. Abledata is a government database of over 15,000 rehabilitation assistive device products. Hyper-Abledata was designed at the Trace Center with special interfaces that allow users with no database experience to operate the program and find desired product information. Hyper-Abledata occupies approximately 15 megabytes and runs under HyperCard on the Apple Macintosh computer (IBM versions are also being developed).

Hyper-Abledata is available on twenty-two floppy disks.

Hyper-TraceBase

Hyper-TraceBase is a multi-topic information database on communication, control, and computer access. TraceBase contains not only information on products, but also summary information, quicksheets on specific topics, funding notes, and bibliographic references. Hyper-TraceBase is a version of TraceBase that runs under Hypercard on the Apple Macintosh computer. Hyper-TraceBase is approximately two megabytes in size, and contains over 1300 product listings (IBM versions are also being developed).

TRACE RESEARCH AND DEVELOPMENT CENTER ON COMMUNICATION, CONTROL AND COMPUTER ACCESS FOR HANDICAPPED INDIVIDUALS
Room S-151 Waisman Center
University of Wisconsin
1500 Highland Avenue
Madison, WI 53705-2280
(608) 262-6966

✳✳✳✳

The Romeo Braille Printer (RB-20 & RB-40)

The Romeo is an extremely portable printer. It weighs in at only 31 pounds in its watertight aluminum case.

The Romeo prints at a speed of 20 characters per second (40 cps for model RB-40). During printing, it is actually quieter than many dot matrix and daisywheel printers. Using anything from 100 pound form-feed braille paper to ordinary paper, the Romeo is ideal for producing rough draft braille documents or more permanent materials. It can even emboss plastic or light metal foil. A specially designed die bar enables the Romeo to produce high-resolution graphics.

Sixteen configuration menus that tell the printer how to communicate with the computer and how to format the data being printed are stored in nonvolatile RAM. Thus, all changes that are made in these menus remain in memory even when the printer is turned off. Parameters are easily stored in these menus by using a numeric keypad. This eliminates the frustrating and time consuming procedures of using dip switches every time changes in parameters must be made.

The Marathon Brailler

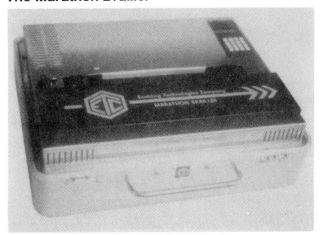

The Marathon Brailler is a high-speed portable braille printer, delivering high quality braille at a speed of 200 characters per second. Since it is equipped with both serial and parallel ports, it will interface with virtually any computer system or host device. There are sixteen configuration menus available, each storing a specific set of communication and formatting parameters in nonvolatile memory. Consequently, all selections will be retained when the unit is turned off. At the factory, eight menus are preset for popular microcomputer configurations. Menu and parameter choices are made by using a numeric keypad, eliminating the frustrating and time consuming use of dip switches. Users who do not read braille may verify menu selections on a built-in visual display. Also, individual parameters or entire menus may be printed out in braille. The Marathon is housed in an aluminum carrying case. Controls and connectors are located inside the case protecting them from inclement weather.

ENABLING TECHNOLOGIES COMPANY
3102 S.E. Jay Street
Stuart, FL 34997
(407) 283-4817

****

Screen-Talk Pro™

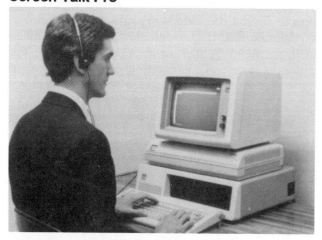

Screen-Talk Pro™ for the IBM PC and compatibles makes "non-talking" programs talk! All the tools needed to add voice inter-activeness to sophisticated programs such as Word Perfect and Lotus 1-2-3 are included with Screen-Talk Pro. Combined with virtually any of the popular voice synthesizers, Screen-Talk Pro™ can turn an ordinary PC into a full-featured "talking computer." Its features include:
- Completely interactive voice with DOS and other programs
- Review lines, words, and individual characters
- "Interruptability" for inertia-free operation
- 10 "voice windows" are always available
- Locates and identifies text strings, video attributes, and ASCII graphics
- ProKey enables custom macro design
- Extras included for Word Perfect, Lotus 1-2-3, and First Choice

Word-Talk™

Word-Talk™ is a staightforward, full-featured word processor for your Apple computer. It is well suited for use by students and professionals alike. A number of special features provide complete printed format control for visually impaired users. Its features include:
- Fully-integrated voice commands
- Supports most popular voice synthesizers
- "What You See is What You Get" design
- Global find and replace
- Block operations
- Printer commands
- Holds forty pages of double spaced text
- Compatible with other word processors
- Built-in "help"

File-Talk

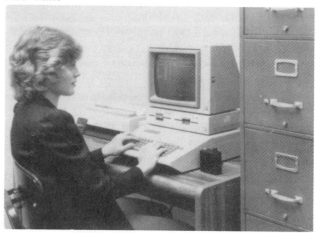

File-Talk is a talking database for the Apple. The program is completely memory resident for fast operation. File-Talk takes advantage of selected memory expansion cards for use with large files. Searches, sorts, and other operations are remarkably fast. File-Talk is ideal for home or business use. Its features include:
- Up to 250 fields
- 999 characters per field
- Instantaneous multi-criteria searches
- On-screen arithmetic
- Find and replace/global replace
- Rename/insert/delete fields
- Automatic sorting and re-sorting
- Compatible with Word-Talk files, or any other ProDOS files
- Mailing labels, form letters, and custom reports
- Supports most popular voice synthesizers
- Built-in "help"

Braille-Talk™

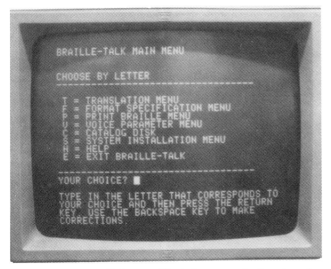

Braille-Talk™ is certified for translation by the National Library Service for the Blind and Physically Handicapped. With this program, anyone can produce accurate Grade 2 Braille. Any standard ASCII text file can be translated by Braille-Talk™. The resulting braille file is saved on disk. The braille file can be printed on any standard embosser. Among its features are:

- True Grade 1 or full Grade 2 translation options
- Format options
- Running headers and page numbers
- User expandable translation table
- Special control commands for printers
- Supports most popular voice synthesizers
- Built-in "help"

Large Print Dos (LP-DOS)

LP-DOS is a complete large print system on one disc. It is a software utility which enables you to run your IBM PC applications with enlarged text. Installation merely involves loading the program.

"I created Large Print DOS because I wanted a solution that I could use anywhere. Northeastern University has over 300 PCs available for general use and I can use LP-DOS on every one of them. This means that I am not tied down to a single machine. After work, I use LP-DOS on my PC at home. I use it to write letters to friends. I also use LP-DOS to create new versions of LP-DOS. I am constantly thinking of new features and receive many excellent ideas from my users."

The author of the program, M. Daniel Simkovitz, is a visually impaired electrical engineer. He is manager of Data Communications for the Computer Resource Center and Instructor in Computer Design for the College of Engineering at Northeastern University.

The Computer Aids "Solutions" catalog includes over forty items for the blind and visually impaired including systems, software, synthesizers and accessories.

"When I founded Computer Aids Corporation I did so with a clear vision—to ensure myself and other blind individuals every benefit made possible by the incredible technology of our times."—William L. Grimm, President.

Calc-Talk™

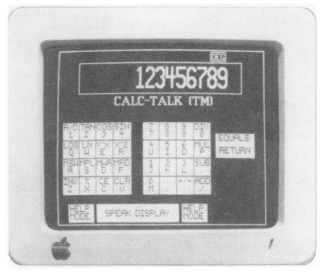

Calc-Talk™ turns the standard Apple keyboard into a 24-function scientific calculator with ten memories. Calc-Talk combines voice output with a nearly one-inch-high character display for low vision users. Its features include:

- Four functions of addition, subtraction, multiplication, and division
- Scientific functions including trigonometry, logarithms, exponents, and roots
- Speaks entries, functions, and answers
- Supports most popular voice synthesizers

COMPUTER AIDS CORPORATION
124 W. Washington, Suite 220
Fort Wayne, IN 46802
(219) 422-2424

✻✻✻✻

Computer Entry Terminal (CET-1 or CET-2)

The Prentke Romich Company's (PRC) CET is an alternate computer entry system for people who do not have the physical capability to access a standard computer. Head, brow, finger, or other body part movement may be used to make selections on the 128-location panel.

Speed of selection in computer operation is a key element in providing an effective alternate method of computer control. CET offers direct selection for those persons with good head control, as well as scanning for persons with switch control capabilities. This makes the CET appropriate for educational, vocational, or home settings where a person desires access to computer programs.

Each selection on the CET retrieves a single character, computer control function, or user-stored string of characters. This allows the CET user to perform every computer function using a control interface, the CET, and a keyboard emulating interface with a standard computer as if the standard computer was being used alone. (The control interface and keyboard emulating interface must be purchased separately.) PRC currently offers keyboard emulating interfaces for the IBM PC and XT, Apple II, II+, IIe, IIc, IIgs, and Franklin 1000.

The basic difference between the CET-1 and the newer CET-2 is in the amount of memory. The CET-2 offers a significantly larger capacity enabling it to meet the additional memory requirements of some newer programs.

Other computer related products offered by PRC include keyguards that can support the hand and allow the user to slide it across the keyboard without pressing any keys. PRC's keyboard emulators accept ASCII characters from an external device and enter them into the computer as if they were keystrokes on the keyboard. The ASCII characters could come from a PRC expressive communication aid such as "Express 3," "Minspeak 1," "Touch Talker," or "Light Talker".

PRENTKE ROMICH COMPANY
1022 Heyl Road
Wooster, OH 44691
(800) 642-8255
(216) 262-1984

****

Lyon VGA

Compatible with IBM PC and PS/2, Lyon Large Print provides a highly readable large print display of solid characters free of distortion. Now available in the Video Graphics Array (VGA) version, it can be used with IBM personal computers (PC, XT, and AT) and Personal Systems/2 Models 25, 30, 50, 60, and 80 and compatibles.

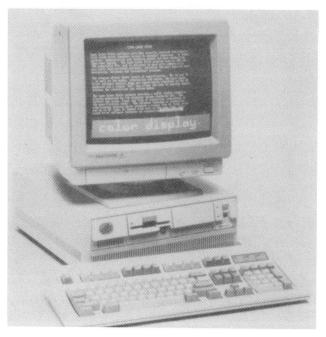

With Lyon's full color capability, users can set the foreground and background colors of the large print display independent of the application software. The program offers levels of magnification ranging from 3X to 9X, as well as two modes, interactive and review. All large print controls are clustered on the keyboard and keystrokes are logical and easy to learn.

Using only 23K of system memory (RAM), the program can be removed from RAM without having to warm or cold boot the PC. The VGA versions require no customized video adapter card. A Color Graphics Adapter (CGA) version is also available.

Speech Systems

Speech systems allow low vision and blind individuals to make full use of personal computers. They are ideal for rehabilitation centers, students, and business people who want to listen to what is displayed on the computer screen.

The Artic family of products distributed by VTEK provides clear synthesized speech capabilities available in five primary packages—Crystal, SynPhonix-215, SynPhonix-225, SynPhonix-245, and D'Light.

In addition, Artic Vision offers word processing, database, and communications applications and Business Vision offers the additional spreadsheet capability.

Artic speech products provide instantaneous responsiveness, user-tailored synthesized voices, externally adjustable pitch and volume control, high accuracy pronunciation, and excellent noise rejection. All use the same comprehensive command set, which provides easy movement between any two products, and they are compatible with VTEK products.

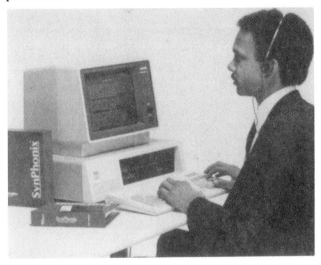

Artic D'Light

For the traveling professional or student in the classroom, D'Light is a talking laptop computer that weighs only 6 1/2 pounds. It combines the finest in phonetic speech synthesis with the power of a Toshiba T-1000 portable computer.

The D'Light package provides 512K of memory (optional 768K RAM available for about $400), and offers the TURBO-Pedal as an option. The TURBO-Pedal features two unique enhancement functions—fast forward and reverse speech scanning. In addition, two commonly used functions—suppress speech and enter review mode—may also be foot-controlled. The TURBO-Pedal increases efficiency significantly for many users. The speech access commands are identical to the comprehensive set used in the SynPhonix-215 for the IBM PC family and in the SynPhonix-225 for other Toshiba laptops.

The Braille Display Processor (BDP) ACT-I, ACT-II, AND ACT-III

The BDP ACT is a software transparent, paperless braille output device, that accesses most commercial ASCII text software without modification. With it, blind persons can use most software available to sighted people. No modification is needed. Insert the BDP ACT's own interface board

into any available expansion slot in compatible Apple, IBM, AT&T, or hardware-compatible, look-alike computers. The BDP ACT automatically converts ASCII code to braille.

The BDP instantly provides access to mainframe information when the PC is emulating a terminal.

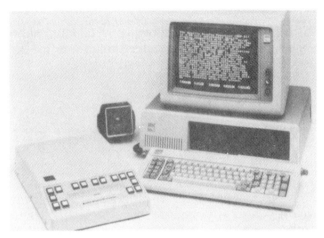

The BDP ACT outputs the computer display on a 20-cell refreshable braille display window in 6-dot braille. The user reads the information as it is displayed by the computer, retaining exact video screen format.

Computers were designed by the sighted for the sighted. If blind computer operators could see the screen as sighted computer operators do, their computer performance would be simple and efficient. The BDP ACT lets them see the screen. Blind operators move the braille display window to read any portion of the video display. Audio signals indicate the braille window's position in relation to the end of a line; end of a page; a blank page; and the top, bottom, left, or right margins of the video display. The Audio Cursor Tracking feature (ACT) enables the operator to use audible cues that guide cursor movement to the braille window. The blind computer operator literally sees the screen in braille.

VTEK
1625 Olympic Blvd.
Santa Monica, CA 90404
(800) 345-2256 Continental U.S. and Hawaii
(800) 338-4898 in Canada
(213) 452-5966 Alaska and Puerto Rico

RESOURCES

Trace Center
University of Wisconsin
314 Waisman Center
1500 Highland Avenue
Madison, WI 53706
(608) 262-6966

Information on Expressive Communication Aids, techniques and computer applications for the handicapped; also Trace Software Registry.

****

LIFT, Inc.
350 Pfingsten, Suite 103
Northbrook, IL 60062
(312) 564-9004

Not-for-profit contract programming company which identifies, trains, and hires physically handicapped for major corporations.

****

The Catalyst
Western Center for Microcomputers in Special Education
1259 El Camino Real, Suite 275
Menlo Park, CA 94025
(415) 326-6997

Contact Sue Sweeney, Editor. Subscriptions: Organizations—$20.00; individuals—$12.00.

****

Communication Outlook
Artificial Language Laboratory
Computer Science Department
Michigan State University
East Lansing, MI 48824
(517) 353-0870

State-of-the-art information regarding technology, to include computer applications. Subscriptions: $12.00.
"Assistive Device Bulletin Board"
Communication information network with electronic bulletin board of current information on new, commercially-available technology.

****

BIPED Corporation
Business Information Processing Education for the Disabled
26 Palmer's Hill Road
Stamford, CT 06902
(203) 324-3935

Non-profit educational program for computer programming and related informational processing skills for the disabled.

****

Closing the Gap
Route 2, Box 39
Henderson, MN 56004

Bud Hagen, Editor
Newspaper on computers and the disabled.

****

Apple's Office of Special Education Programs
20525 Mariani Avenue
Cupertino, CA 95014
(408) 973-6484 or (408) 973-2042

Through this office, Apple Computer, Inc. is involved with educational/human service organizations to help identify computer-related needs of the disabled.

****

IBM National Support Center for Persons with Disabilities
P.O. Box 2150
Atlanta, GA 30055
(404) 331-3206 or Voice (404) 238-3206

"The IBM Special Education Resources": This guide and other IBM-related information for disabled persons are available from this address.

****

OTHER SOURCES OF COMPUTER AIDS:

ABBEY MEDICAL
ACCESS TO RECREATION, INC.
DU-IT CONTROL SYSTEMS GROUP
LS&S GROUP, INC.
TASH, INC.

For additional information, including addresses and phone numbers, see CATALOGS.

CHAPTER TEN

CATALOGS

ABBEY MEDICAL

Orientation: Health Care Professionals

Contents: Physical Therapy; Physical Fitness and Rehabilitation; Ambulation and Gait Training; Wheelchairs and Accessories; Incontinence and Urinary Care; Furniture and Accessories; Bathroom Safety and Commodes; Occupational Therapy; Clinical Equipment; Orthopedic Equipment and Supplies; Respiratory Care.

Comments: Catalog of physical therapy and rehabilitation equipment for the healthcare professional. Contains over 500 products illustrated with black-and-white photos. Minimum order required.

ABBEY MEDICAL CATALOG SALES
13782 Crenshaw Blvd.
Gardena, CA 90249
(800) 421-5126
(800) 262-1294 in California
(213) 538-5551

✳✳✳✳

ABLEWARE

Independent Living from Maddak, Inc.
Orientation: General

Contents: Ambulation; Wheelchair Accessories; Tactile; Exercise; Recreation; Hot/Cold Therapy; Adapting Toys; Communication; Furniture; Bathroom and Toilet; Incontinence; Reading; Writing; Dressing; Grooming; Eating/Drinking; Hand Holds; Splinting; Kitchen and Household; Bed and Bedroom; Cushionings; Reaching; Therapists Testing and Treatment; Patient Care; Orthotics; Institutional.

Comments: Full-color catalog with black-and-white supplement containing over 600 products. $50.00 minimum order.

ABLEWARE
Independent Living From Maddak, Inc.
Pequannock, NJ 07440-1993
(800) 443-4926
(201) 694-0500

✳✳✳✳

ACCESS TO RECREATION, INC.

Orientation: Physically Challenged

Contents: Fishing Equipment; All-Terrain Vehicles; Four Wheel Drive Wheelchair; Recreational Wheelchair Attachments and Accessories; Swim Aids; Beach Vehicles; Exercisers; Sports Equipment (Archery, Pool, Table Tennis, Bowling, etc.); Craft Aids; Computer and Video Game Accessories; Environmental Controls; Books.

Comments: Catalog of adaptive recreation equipment for the physically challenged. Over 100 products ranging from a $10 Quad-Bee, a frisbee for quadriplegics, to a $6,000 all-terrain amphibious vehicle with hand controls.

"I understand the frustration of therapists and others like myself when it comes to finding the proper equipment to gain access to recreation. Individuals often don't have the resources to find equipment they need, and therapists are burdened with the endless searching through mountains of advertisements and catalogs. The Access To Recreation Catalog offers a single source for this specially designed equipment."–Donald A. Krebs, President, Access to Recreation, Inc.

ACCESS TO RECREATION, INC.
2509 E. Thousand Oaks Blvd., Suite 430
Thousand Oaks, CA 91362
(800) 634-4351
(805) 498-7535 in California

✳✳✳✳

ADAPTIVE PRODUCTS INCORPORATED

Orientation: Physically Challenged

Contents: Home Lifts and Household Modifications; Auto and Van Lifts; Driving Controls; Other Vehicle Modifications.

Comments: Catalog sheets from a number of manufacturers. Adaptive Products serves the disabled and elderly residing in the "Greater Chicagoland Metropolitan Area."

ADAPTIVE PRODUCTS
INCORPORATED
645 South Addison Road
Addison, IL 60101
(312) 832-0203

****

ALIMED INC.

Orientation: Health Care Professionals
Contents: Splints; Hand Exercisers; Edema
Control; Scar Management; Sensory Evaluation;
Hot/Cold Therapy; Arm Supports; Aids to Daily
Living; Splinting Materials; Back Supports;
Weights; Decubitus Ulcer Rx; Foot Orthotics;
Ankle/Knee Support; Clinical Tools; Infection
Control; Transfer Devices; W/C Cushions; Tumble
Forms; Clinical Furniture.
Comments: Catalog for health care profession-
als, with over 650 products. Illustrated with black
and white photos and line art. No minimum or-
der—$10.00 will be added to all orders under $50.00
to cover shipping, handling and insurance charges.

ALIMED INC.
297 High Street
Dedham, MA 02026
(800) 225-2610
(617) 329-2900 in Massachusetts

****

AMERICAN FOUNDATION FOR THE BLIND

Products For People With Vision Problems
Orientation: Blind and Visually Impaired
Contents: Calculators; Clocks/Timers; Communications; Education; Games; Health Care; Kitchen; Household; Measuring; Mobility; Personal;
Recreation; Tools; Watches; Writing.
Comments: Catalog contains over 250 products.
Ordering by organizations is basically the same as
for individuals. Prices are the same and no discount
is offered for quantity purchases. Orders accepted
by telephone or by mail. A letter written in either
print or braille may be used in place of the standard
order form. $10.00 minimum order.

AMERICAN FOUNDATION FOR THE
BLIND
Customer Service
15 West 16th Street
New York, NY 10011
(212) 862-8838

****

ARCOA INDUSTRIES

Orientation: Physically Challenged
Contents: E-Z Reachers and Accessories; E-Z
Shoe-On; Wheelchair Ash Tray; Wheelchair Cup
Holder; Multi-Purpose Chair (adult and child
sizes); Chair Sling (adult and child sizes).
Comments: Catalog consists of twenty items de-
scribed on three illustrated catalog sheets.

ARCOA INDUSTRIES
A Division of Caliputer, Inc.
888 Rancheros Drive
San Marcos, CA 92069
(800) 621-0852 ext. 165
(619) 489-1170

****

ARJO HOSPITAL EQUIPMENT, INC.

Orientation: Health Care Professionals
Contents: Hydrotherapy Tanks; Extremity
Tank; Therapy Leg Shower; Podiatry Tanks;
Therapy Pool and Pool Lifts; Lifters; Ambulation
Trainers.
Comments: Catalog sheets describing and illus-
trating hydrotherapy, bathing, showering, and lift-
transport equipment for hospitals and nursing
homes.

ARJO HOSPITAL EQUIPMENT, INC.
6380 West Oakton Street
Morton Grove, IL 60053
(800) 323-1245
(312) 967-0360

****

A-T SURGICAL MFG. CO., INC.

Orientation: Health Care Professionals
Contents: Abdominal Binders; Arm Slings; Arm
Supports; Athletic Supporters; Back Supports; Bed
Rail Bumper Pads; Cast Toe Covers; Cervical Col-
lars; Philadelphia Collars; Compression Legging
Garment; Cold or Hot Pack Holder; Elastic Ban-
dages; Finger and Toe Protection; Hand Exerciser;
Knee Braces; Knee Immobilizers; Leg Supports;
Maternity Supports; Rib Belts; Sheeting; Shoulder
Brace and Clavicle Strap; Stockings—Anti-Em-
bolism; Surgical Shields; Sweat Bands; Tens Belts;
Terry Bibs; Thermal Warmers; Trusses; Tube
Holders—Hospital; Badge Holder.
Comments: Catalog offering over forty special-
ized products. Illustrated with black-and-white pho-
tos.

A-T SURGICAL MFG. CO., INC.
115 Park Street
Holyoke, MA 01040-5891
(800) 225-2023
(800) 622-4567 in Massachusetts
(413) 532-4551

✳✳✳✳

BALLERT INTERNATIONAL, INC.

Orientation: Physically Challenged, Health Care Professionals

Contents: Patient Handling Sling; A-F Wire Orthosis; BK (Below Knee) and AK (Above Knee) Training Orthosis; CASH™ Orthosis; Vertetrac™ Ambulatory Traction Unit; Backfriend™ Orthopedically Designed Portable Seat.

Comments: As reported by Donald Perser, President of Ballert International, the BK and AK Training Orthosis has been used in "thousands of hospitals and rehab centers, worldwide to train and evaluate patients."

BALLERT INTERNATIONAL, INC.
3677 Woodhead Drive
Northbrook, IL 60062-1816
(800) 345-3456
(312) 480-0390

✳✳✳✳

CLEO INC.

Orientation: General

Contents: Weights; Hand Exercisers; Elgin Exercise Equipment; Exercise Tables; Treadmills and Rowers; Restorators and Exercise Bikes; Exercise Therapy Equipment; Pulley Systems; Ultrasound Therapy; Biofeedback; Compression Units; Massagers and Vibrators; Gels and Lotions; Diagnostic, Testing Equipment; Traction Equipment and Accessories; Parallel Bars; Walking Belts and Staircases; Balance Training; Rollators and Walkers; Canes, Crutches, and Accessories; Mirrors; Splints; Shoes; Braces; Immobilizers; Collars; Slings; Splinting Materials and Accessories; Positioners; Tumble Forms; Geriatric Chairs; Wheelchair Accessories; Ramps; Protectors and Pads; Pediatric Furniture and Equipment; Play Therapy Aids; Standing Aids; Sports and Games; Craft Supplies; Helmets; Exercise Mats; Bed Rails, Pads and Accessories; Lifters; Baths and Accessories; Heat and Cold Therapy; Storage and Mobile Cabinets and Lamps; Scales; Commodes;

Raised Toilet Seats; Grab Bars and Safety Rails; Bathing and Grooming Aids; Aids for Dressing; Homemaking Aids; Kitchen Aids; Eating and Drinking Aids; Aids for Daily Living; Books, Magnifiers and Writing Aids; Reading, Typing, and Phone Aids; Communication Aids; Driving Aids; Stools; Treatment Tables; Platform and Worktables; Standing Tables; Wheelchair Work Station.

Comments: The main catalog includes over 1800 products illustrated with black-and-white photographs. The supplemental catalog, entitled "The Rehab Shoppe," focuses specifically on products for the physically challenged.

CLEO INC.
3957 Mayfield Road
Cleveland, OH 44121
(800) 321-0595
(216) 382-9700

✳✳✳✳

COLUMBIA MEDICAL MANUFACTURING

Orientation: General

Contents: "Rickshaw" Rehabilitation Exerciser; Car Seat; Toilet and Bath Supports; Bath Chairs; Positioning Seat.

Comments: Catalog is composed of catalog sheets containing photo-illustrated descriptions of twelve products. No minimum order required. All orders shipped within twenty-four hours of receipt.

COLUMBIA MEDICAL MANUFACTURING
P.O. Box 633
Pacific Palisades, CA 90272
(213) 454-6612

✳✳✳✳

CONSUMER CARE™ PRODUCTS INC.

Orientation: General

Contents: Standing Frame; Foot Harnesses; Prone Support Walker; Fasteners; Audio-Light Foot Signal (Communications Aid); Foot- and Hand-powered Tricycles; Hand Positioning Cones and Surface Anchors™; Slant-Board™; Heel Loops; Wheelchair Work Trays; Tablet-Arm Tray for Wheelchairs; Positioning Belt/Belt Materials System; Cushioning; Helmet and Chin Guard; The Care Kids™; Positioning Chair™; Scooter Board.

Comments: No minimum order. All equipment is "ergonomically" designed.

CONSUMER CARE PRODUCTS INC.™
P.O. Box 684
810 N. Water Street
Sheboygan, WI 53082
(414) 459-8368

✳✳✳✳

DANMAR PRODUCTS

Orientation: General
Contents: Head Gear; Swim Aids; Positioning Aids; Participation Products; Specialty Items.
Comments: Company offers over 100 products, fully illustrated and described in Spanish and French, as well as in English. No minimum order.

DANMAR PRODUCTS
2390 Winewood
Ann Arbor, MI 48103
(313) 761-1990

✳✳✳✳

DU-IT CONTROL SYSTEMS GROUP

Orientation: Physically Challenged
Contents: Proportionally Operated Wheelchair Systems; Proportional Control Systems for High-Level Quadriplegics; SCI System Controllers; Recline Control; Computer Access and Simulation; CP Wheelchair Control Systems—Switch Operated; CP Controllers; Control Switches; Environmental Control; Remote Control; "Easicorder" (single switch operated tape recorder); System Accessories; Adapter Cables.
Comments: Du-It designs extensive systems exclusively for very severely disabled people with difficult control problems—high level spinal cord injury (C3-4 to brain stem injured), extensive and severe cerebral palsy, and advanced neuromuscular disease.

DU-IT CONTROL SYSTEMS GROUP
8765 TR 513
Shreve, OH 44676
(216) 567-2906

✳✳✳✳

FLAGHOUSE, INC.

Special Populations
Orientation: Children (body movement, occupational therapy, adapted furniture, toys and games)
Contents: Balance; Adaptive Positioning; Ride-Ons; Movement Education; Athletics/Sports; Water/Swimming; Exercise/Physical Fitness; Therapists Aids/Testing; Manipulatives; Aids For Daily Living; Adapted Toys; Games and Game Tables; Electronic Teaching Aids; Audio-Visual; Adaptive Furniture.
Comments: Catalog has about 3000 items and an almost equal number of photos. No minimum order ($5.00 charge added to orders under $50.00).

FLAGHOUSE, INC.
150 No. MacQuesten Pkwy.
Mt. Vernon, NY 10550
(800) 221-5185
(914) 699-1900 in New York State

✳✳✳✳

FLEETWOOD

Orientation: Health Care Professionals, Educators
Contents: Institutional Furniture (medical and educational facilities, etc.); Wheelchair Accessible Furniture; Adjustable Height Tables, Science Cabinet, Computer Work Stations.
Comments: Catalog includes over 250 products.

FLEETWOOD
P.O. Box 1259
Holland, MI 49422-1259
(800) 257-6390
(616) 396-1142 in Hawaii, Alaska, and Michigan

✳✳✳✳

GUARDIAN—SUNRISE MEDICAL

Orientation: Physically Challenged
Contents: Homecare Patient Lifts (300 lb. capacity); Institutional Patient Lifts (400 & 600 lb. capacities); Slings; Bathing Aids; "Medi-Chair"; Supine Patient Handling System; Portable Scale (attaches to most lifters); Star Ramp™ System; Star Trak™ (portable telescopic ramps); Tub Lifts; Pool Lifts.
Comments: Full color catalog sheets. Products for home and institutional applications.

GUARDIAN PRODUCTS, INC.
12800 Wentworth Street
Box C-4522
Arleta, CA 91331-4522
(800) 255-5022

✳✳✳✳

HAMMATT SENIOR PRODUCTS

Orientation: Health Care Professionals (for Seniors); Recreational Therapy, Physical Therapy, Occupational Therapy

Contents: Games; Sports Equipment; Records and Tapes; Rhythm Band Instruments; Special Fitness Programs (on videotape); Posters; Jumbo Erasable Monthly Calendar.

Comments: Catalog contains over fifty types of recreational products for seniors. Each is fully described, illustrated with black-and-white photos and line art. No minimum order.

HAMMATT SENIOR PRODUCTS
P.O. Box 727
Mount Vernon, WA 98273
(206) 428-5850

****

HAUSMANN INDUSTRIES

Orientation: Health Care Professionals

Contents: Examination and Treatment Tables; Table Accessories; Pediatric Tables; Activity/Therapy Tables; Worktables; Lounges and Couches; Mobile Cabinets and Utility Carts; Cabinets, Desks, Shelves; Stools; Tilt Tables; Mirrors; Pulley Weights; Mat Platforms; Mats and Accessories; Parallel Bars; Exercise Equipment; Staircases; Weights; Convenience Specialties; Self-Help Equipment; Tables, Cabinets and Wardrobes.

Comments: Catalog provides descriptions of over 200 products with medical and rehabilitation applications.

HAUSMANN INDUSTRIES
130 Union Street
Northvale, NJ 07647
(201) 767-0255

****

HOSMER DORRANCE CORPORATION

Orientation: Physically Challenged, Health Care Professionals

Contents: Prosthetic Components; Externally Powered Systems; Orthotics; Tools and Fabrication Supplies.

Comments: Hosmer Dorrance does not sell directly to the end user. Write for more information.

HOSMER DORRANCE CORPORATION
561 Division Street
P.O. Box 37
Campbell, CA 95008
(408) 379-5151

****

HOYLE PRODUCTS INC.

Orientation: Physically Challenged, Low Vision
Contents: Lap Desk; Grippers; Bookstand.

Comments: Information from Hoyle includes catalog sheets and "Health Information Sheets," that describe the products and their applications.

HOYLE PRODUCTS, INC.
302 Orange Grove
P.O. Box 606
Fillmore, CA 93015
(800) 345-1950
(805) 524-1211

****

INDEPENDENT LIVING AIDS, INC. CAN-DO™ PRODUCTS

Orientation: General, Low Vision

Contents: Watches; Clocks and Timers; Magnifiers; Braille Accessories; Canes; Writing Aids; Health Aids; Travel Aids; "Noir" Sunglasses; Communication Aids; Cosmetic and Health Care Ointments and Creams; Incontinence Pants; Daily Living Aids; Positioning Aids; TV and Computer Screen Enlargers; Alarms; Household Aids; Cooking and Feeding Aids; Crafts and Hobbies; Games; Large Print Books; Learning Aids.

Comments: Contains over eighty product categories. Illustrated with photographs and occasionally with line drawings. $20.00 minimum order (for orders under $20.00, 2.00 is added for shipping and handling).

INDEPENDENT LIVING AIDS, INC.
27 East Mall
Plainview, NY 11803
(800) 537-2118
(516) 752-8080

****

J.T. POSEY CO., INC.

Orientation: Health Care Professionals

Contents: Arm Boards; Arm Slings; Bed Accessories; Belts; Catheter Tube Holder Strap; Cervical Collars; Cuffs; Cushions and Pillows; Decubitus Pads; Elbow Splints; Emergency Care Equipment; Eye Protectors; Foot Care Products; Footboards; Foot Elevators; Heel Protectors; "Houdini" Security Suit; I.V. Shields; Incontinent Sheath Holder; Inservice Training Programs; Key and Tab Locks; Leather Restraints; Limb Holders; Locks; Mini Pelvic Holder; Mitts; Operating Room Products; Pads; Patient Lifter; Pediatric Products; Physical Therapy Products; Playboard Line; Poncho/Torso Support; Restraint Net; Safety Bar Kit; Arm Slings; Straight Jacket; Connecting Straps; Traction Equipment; Vests; Vinylflex Cuffs; Weights; Wheelchair Accessories; Wheelchair Belts.

Comments: Catalog contains over 150 products. No minimum order.

J.T. POSEY CO., INC.
5635 Peck Road
Arcadia, CA 91006-0020
(800) 447-6739
(818) 443-3143 in California

****

KAYE PRODUCTS INC.

Orientation: Physically Challenged Children
Contents: Posture Control Walkers; Strollers; Prone Standers and Adjustable Table; Prone Standers with Desk; Bolster Chairs; "Kinder" Chairs; Corner Chairs; Parallel Poles; Adjustable Benches; Posture Inserts; Toilet Trainer; Gymnastik and Therapy Balls; Therapy Mats; Prone Positioner; Therapy Bolsters and Stands; Adjustable Easel; Adapted Tricycle.

Comments: Products in this catalog are described in terms of their uses, features, and specifications. Each is illustrated with a black-and-white photograph. No minimum order.

KAYE PRODUCTS INC.
1010 East Pettigrew Street
Durham, NC 27701-4299
(919) 688-1601

****

KAYE'S KIDS

Orientation: General—Children (Toys and Products)
Contents: Toys to Encourage Looking and Listening; Developing Reaching, Batting, and Swiping; Toys to Develop Grasping, Holding, and Manipulating; Toys to Encourage Two Hands; Coordinating Shoulders, Arms, and Hands; Developing Spatial Concepts, Coordination, and Balance; Products for Daily Care—Feeding, Toileting, and Bathing; Products for Daily Care—Safety and Play; Toys to Develop Grasp and Release; Encouraging Single Finger Movements; Toys to Encourage Size, Shape, Color, and Number Concepts; Developing Labeling, Sorting, and Matching; Coordinating Eyes and Hands; Toys to Develop Grasp with Thumb and Fingers; Toys to Expand Movement Experiences.

Comments: Kaye's Kids is a Division of Kaye Products, Inc. Their catalog contains over 125 products.

KAYE'S KIDS
1010 East Pettigrew Street
Durham, NC 27701-4299
(919) 683-1051

****

LAUREL DESIGNS

Orientation: Physically Challenged, Developmentally Challenged
Contents: "Nancy's Special Workout for the Physically Challenged"; Placket Sweatshirt; A-Line Skirt; Reversible Rain Poncho; Rain Cape; Sport Gloves; Driving Gloves; Pedal Pads; Back Packer; Spare Pocket; Lap Desk; Lok-Tie Shoe Laces; 4-Ingredient Cookbook; Donaldson Clamp; Matey Folding Reacher; Matey Carrying Case; 3-Grip Safety Bar; Telephone Keyboard Enlarger; Telephone Hand Clip; Telephone Amplifier; "Maddatap"; Skidtrol Plus; T-Shirts; "Nancy's Special Workout for the Developmentally Challenged"; Handy Pouch; Fleece Sweatshirt; Fleece Pants; Fleece Skirt; Unisex Pouch Pocket Shirt; Unisex Drawstring Pants.

Comments: Catalog includes illustrated descriptions of thirty-four products. No minimum order.

LAUREL DESIGNS
5 Laurel Avenue, #9
Belvedere, CA 94920
(415) 435-1891

****

LS&S GROUP, INC.

Orientation: Visually Impaired
Contents: Watches; Clocks; Computers; Accessories; Software; Printer; Synthesizers; Computer Keytops; CCTV; Recorders; Radios; Telephones; Answering Machines; Timers; Magnifiers; Monoculars; Binoculars; Special Spectacles; Magnifying Mirrors; Lamps; Mobility Aids; Canes; Cane Accessories; Walkers; Health Aids; Bathroom Aids; Grips; Reachers; Desk, Stands, and Table; Glasses;

Security; Braille; Kitchen Aids; Large Print Books; Large Print Pens; Learning Aids; Recreation; Miscellaneous; Sports Vision Testing/Training.

Comments: Catalog contains over 600 products. Available on cassette for a $3.00 charge, deducted from the first order. No minimum order.

LS&S GROUP, INC.
P.O. Box 673
Northbrook, IL 60065
(800) 468-4789
(312) 498-9777

****

LUMEX

Orientation: General

Contents: Grab Bars and Support Bars; Children's Toilet Seats; Raised Toilet Seats; Commodes; Shower Chairs; Shower Hoses and Accessories; Bath Seats; Canes; Quad Canes; Walkane; Crutches; Walkers and Accessories; Rollators; Ramps; Overbed Tables; Trapezes; Bedrails; Mattress System; Commode Seat Pad; Side Rail Pads; Seating Cushions; Eating and Drinking Aids; Kitchen Aids; Reachers and Turners; Dressing Aids; Accessories to Daily Living.

Comments: Lumex offers over 200 products including the "Swedish Rehab" line, designed and developed in the Scandinavian and Southern European countries.

LUMEX
Division of Lumex, Inc.
100 Spence Street
Bay Shore, NY 11706
(800) 645-5272
(516) 273-2200
(800) 424-2458 in New York

****

MARSHALL MEDICAL

Orientation: Health Care Professionals, Home Health Care

Contents: Sphygmomanometers; Blood Pressure Kits; Disposable Examination Gloves; Stethoscopes; Stethoscope Replacement Parts and Accessories; Blood Pressure Replacement Parts and Accessories; Thermometers; Breast Pump; Food Grinder; Infant Wipes; Canes; Walkers and Forearm Crutches; Crutch, Cane and Walker Parts and Accessories; Infant/Toddler Feeding Accessories; Infant Toddler Orthodontic Products; Emergency

and Paramedical Aids; Surgical Scissors and Instruments; Stainless Steel Utensils; Glass Hypodermic Syringes; Transportation Chair (for children); Infant Stroller.

Comments: Fully illustrated catalog includes over 100 items for professional and home use. Minimum order of $25.00.

MARSHALL MEDICAL
Division of Marshall Electronics, Inc.
Lincolnshire, IL 60069
(800) 323-1482
(312) 634-6300

****

OPTION CENTRAL

Orientation: Visually Impaired

Contents: Canes; Dog Products; Electrical Items; Envelopes; Greeting Cards; Housewares; Medical Supplies; Personal Items; Recreation Products; Talking Products; Tape Cassette Products; Writing Products.

Comments: Catalog contains over sixty items, and is available in braille and cassette formats. Braille catalogs cost $1.00. The tone indexed cassette catalog, containing demonstrations of several products, costs $1.00, or it is free if a blank C60 cassette is supplied. Orders and correspondence may be sent in braille, print, or cassette tape format.

OPTION CENTRAL
Fred Sanderson, Proprietor
1604 Carroll Avenue
Green Bay, WI 54304
(414) 498-9699

****

PCA INDUSTRIES, INC.

Orientation: Educators and Health Care Professionals—Children

Contents: Playground Equipment; Art and Eye /Hand and Primary Balancing Activities and Equipment; Tumbling/Soft Playthings; "Irish Mail," Trikes and Scooters; Sand and Water Play Equipment; Storage Units; Furniture; Wheelchair Swing; Perceptual/Motor Trainers; Block Sets; Fitness Courses; Gymnastic Climbers; Bike Racks; Seating; Gym and Sports Equipment.

Comments: PCA manufactures more than 800 products including Playgrounds™—playgrounds for creative play, PlayLearn™—early years equipment, SportsPlay™—sports and gym equipment, and

TheraPlay™—equipment for special education. Their catalog is printed twice a year, in January and July. $30.00 minimum order.

PCA INDUSTRIES, INC.
5642 Natural Bridge
St. Louis, MO 63120
(800) 325-4794
(314) 389-4140

✶✶✶✶

J.A. PRESTON CORPORATION

Orientation: General

Contents: Therapeutic Instruments; Diagnostic Equipment; Mirrors; Walkers; Crutches and Accessories; Canes; Mobility Accessories; Ambulation Training Aids; Mat Platforms; Exercise Apparatus; Mats; Adaptive Positioning; Perceptual Motor; Protective Helmets; Communications; Reachers; Self Help Aids; Recreation; Special Needs Eating Utensils; Bathing Aids; Intermittent Compression; Electrotherapy; Massage; Pain Control; Heat and Cold Therapy; Hydrotherapy; Lifters; Slings and Orthopedic Splinting Materials; Splints; Lifters; Velcro; Wheelchair Accessories; Pediatric Mobility; Traction; Treatment Furniture.

Comments: Catalog contains over 1500 items.

J.A. PRESTON CORPORATION
60 Page Road
Clifton, NJ 07012
(800) 631-7277
(201) 777-2700 in New Jersey

✶✶✶✶

RADIO SHACK

Selected Products For People With Special Needs
Orientation: General

Contents: Audio Adapters; Audio Amplifier; Batteries; Calculators; CB Equipment; Chess Computer; Clocks; Headphones; Health Care; Lights; Listening Aid System; Microphones; PA Systems; Pager; Personal Protection System; Radios; Remote Control Systems; Room Monitors; Security Equipment; Sound Level Meter; Tape Recorders and Players; Telephones and Telephone Accessories; Indoor/Outdoor Thermometer; Electronic Thermostat; Timers; Tools; Talking Wristwatch.

Comments: Catalog contains over 150 products available at Radio Shack retail stores nationwide. To obtain a copy of the catalog contact your local Radio Shack store.

✶✶✶✶

RAYMO

Orientation: Health Care Professionals

Contents: Medication Cards; Medication Card Racks; Syringe Trays; Bed Record Racks; X-Ray and Chart Holder Wall Racks; Shampoo - Rinse Tray; Walker Caddy's; Wheelchair Trays; Lap Desk; Medication Trays; Thermometer Tray; Reality Orientation Charts; Record and Data Holder Wall Racks; Clip Board-Style Patient Chart Holders; Walker and Caddy Trays.

Comments: Catalog is composed of illustrated catalog sheets describing Raymo's medication equipment, medical record equipment, and health-care equipment.

RAYMO PRODUCTS, INC.
212 South Blake
Olathe, KS 66061
(913) 782-1515

✶✶✶✶

RIFTON

Equipment for the Handicapped
Orientation: Physically Challenged

Contents: Activity Chairs; Adaptive Easel; Adjustable Chairs, Corner Chair; Toddler Chairs; Tables; Standing Frame; Walker; Wedge; Air Chair; Feeding Apron; Arm Chairs; Baby Chairs; Bath Chairs; Foam Blocks; Bolster Chair; Bolster Swing; Therapy Bolsters; Tricycles; Corner Floor Sitters; Foam Cubes; Drop-Off Wedges; Trays; Vestibular Boards; Supine Boards; Foam Ramps; Freedom Standers; Hammock Swing; Mats; Nursery Rocking Boat; Platform Swing; Potty Chairs; Prone-Scooter Boards; Prone Standers; Rainbow Rolls; Reclining Baby Chair; Rocking Balance Board; Therapy Rolls; Scooter Boards; Shower Chairs; Sidelying Boards; Standing Tables.

Comments: Most items in this catalog adjust over a broad range, without special tools. Many of them are built of wood—solid maple and attractive birch plywood. Slides are available, on loan or for purchase, that graphically portray the uses of Rifton Equipment for therapeutic positioning.

RIFTON
Equipment for the Handicapped
Route 213
Rifton, NY 12471
(914) 658-3141/3143

✳✳✳✳

SCIENCE PRODUCTS

Orientation: Visually Impaired

Contents: Talking Health Aids; Talking Instruments and Tools; Talking Calculators; Talking Cash Register; Special Instruments; Measuring Tools; Custom Electronics; Audio Equipment; Audio Accessories; Lighting; Magnifiers; Eyewear; Vision Work Aids; Sensors; Recreation Equipment; Children's Toys, Games, and Books; Book Accessories; Large Print Books; Clocks and Watches; Office Aids.

Comments: Science Products' electronics shop adapts and services electronic equipment for diverse industrial and medical applications. No minimum order.

SCIENCE PRODUCTS
Box 888
Southeastern, PA 19399
(800) 888-7400

✳✳✳✳

SNITZ MANUFACTURING

Orientation: Educators and Recreation Specialists

Contents: Athletic Equipment; Foam Balls; Foam Saucers, Games, and Accessories; Cageballs, Pushballs, Playground Balls, and Mesh Bags; Vinyl Balls; Bite-Proof "Plaeballs;" Miscellaneous Game Balls, Ballbags, and Accessories; Parachutes; Parachute Records; "Edu-Links;" Folding Mats; Early Childhood Equipment; Movement Activities; "Softee" Games; Timers, Scorers, and Watches; Pinnies; Gymnastic Equipment; Game Accessories; Games; Adaptable Gymnastics; Adaptive P.E. Equipment; Playground Equipment; Ropes and Nets; Game Standards; Gym Mats; Display and Bulletin Boards; Trophy Cases; Rhythm Sets and Records; Erasable, Magnetic, and Chalkboards; Achievement Boards and Activity Charts.

Comments: Catalog contains over 2000 products. Minimum order $25.00.

SNITZ MANUFACTURING CO.
2096 South Church Street
East Troy, WI 53120
(800) 642-3991 (for information)
(800) 558-2224 (for orders only)

✳✳✳✳

ST. LOUIS OSTOMY AND MEDICAL SUPPLY

Orientation: General

Contents: Convalescent Products; Diabetic Products; Incontinence Products; Instruments and Blood Pressure Equipment; Urologicals; Breast Pumps and Supplies; Dressing Tapes and Accessories; Feeding Tubes and Sets; Tracheostomy Products; Surgical Stockings; Ostomy Products; Orthopedic Supplies; Skin Care Products.

Comments: St. Louis Ostomy and Medical Supply offers free shipping for orders over $30.00, and a 20% discount for ostomy orders over $50.00. More than 450 types of products are indexed in their catalog. No minimum order.

ST. LOUIS OSTOMY AND MEDICAL SUPPLY
10821 Manchester Road
Kirkwood, MO 63122
(800) 365-3232
(314) 821-7355

✳✳✳✳

TASH, INC.

Orientation: General, Physically Challenged

Contents: Ability Switches; Technical Information; Mounting Hardware; Switch Accessories; Environmental Controls; Computer Aids; Communication and Educational Aids; Mobility Aids.

Comments: Tash is a marketing corporation established in 1978 by the Canadian Rehabilitation Council for the Disabled in conjunction with the National Research Council of Canada. Its purpose is "to make technical aids available which are not readily available from other suppliers." The Rehabilitation Technology Unit of the National Research Council of Canada performs a major role in product engineering as well as ongoing improvements of Tash technical aids. Over 150 products are included in the Tash catalog.

TASH, INC.
70 Gibson Drive, Unit 12
Markham, Ontario L3R 4C2
(416) 475-2212

✳✳✳✳

THERAFIN CORPORATION

Orientation: Physically Challenged, Health Care Professionals

Contents: Wheelchair Trays; Wheelchair Accessories; Control System Components; Transfer

Boards; Wheelchair Hardware; Communication; Dressing Aids; Hygiene Aids; Eating Aids; Clinic/Therapy; Activity/Miscellaneous.

Comments: Therafin is a custom products manufacturer, and can customize products either by adapting any of their existing models or by custom designing and producing an item to suit specific or unique customer requirements. Catalog contains over 130 photo-illustrated product entries.

THERAFIN CORPORATION
3800 S. Union Avenue
Steger, IL 60475
(800) THERAFIN
(312) 755-1535

＊＊＊＊

T.R.S.

Orientation: Physically Challenged
Contents: Prosthesis—GRIPs I, II, and SOFT-TOUCH III; ADEPTs B I, C II, and F III; SUPER SPORTs I, II, III, IV, and Infant; All Terrain Ski Terminal Device (AT-Ski-TD); Amputee Golf Grip; AMP-u-POD (Camera Support); Cable Cleat System; Neo-Axilla Loop Padding; Wrist Units; "Rapid Adjust" Upper-Extremity Prosthetic Harness; Educational Videos—"Training Children with Below-Elbow Prostheses" and "GRIP Training Film."

Comments: Catalog consists of seven illustrated catalog sheets. A video catalog is also available.

T.R.S.
1280 28th Street, Suite 3
Boulder, CO 80303-1797
(303) 444-4720
(800) 621-8385 ext. 150

＊＊＊＊

WHEELCHAIR CARRIER, INC.

Orientation: Physically Challenged
Contents: Scooter and Power Wheelchair Carrier; Tilt 'N Tote® Wheelchair Carrier; Standard Wheelchair Carriers; Budget Non-Folding Carrier; Scooter Carrier; Platform, Ramp, and Chair Carrier; Platform Ready Ramp; Tote A Ramps; Convoluted Foam Pads; Chair Poncho; Lap Desk; Foot Lifter; Handicap Sign; Handicap Stencil; Remedial Weights; Wheelchair Bag; Wheelchair Backpack; Walker Bags; Wheelchair Covers; Carrier Cover; Chair-Bike Carrier for Bumper or Trailer Hitch.

Comments: Illustrated catalog containing over fifty items.

WHEELCHAIR CARRIER, INC.
P.O. Box 79, 726 Farnsworth Road
Waterville, OH 43566-0079
(800) 541-3213

＊＊＊＊

WINCO INCORPORATED

Orientation: Health Care Professionals
Contents: Petite Recliner; Care Cliner; Convalescent Recliner; Golden Years Chair; Relax-A-Cliner; Chart Racks; Shower Chair; Adjustable Commode Chair; Folding Multi-Use Chair; Grab Bars; Assist Rails; Safety Arm Rest; Raised Seats; Footstools; Telescopic Curtain; Folding Screens; Walkers; Compact Travel Chair; Adjust-A-Leg Recliner; Convertible Chair; Treatment Tables; Adjustable Stools; Legrest; Folding Treatment Table; Drop Arm Shower Chair; Ultra Comfort Cliner.

Comments: Over 100 products are described in this catalog.

WINCO INCORPORATED
3062 46th Avenue North
St. Petersburg, FL 33714-3864
(800) 237-3377
(813) 526-2152

BOOKS

Games, Sports, and Exercises for the Physically Handicapped, 4th Edition
 Ronald C. Adams and Jeffrey A. McCubbin

In this fourth edition all chapters have been updated to be consistent with new concepts and changing views of physical education and the therapeutic value of exercise as they relate to handicapped persons. Progress in treatment techniques and methods of evaluating the degree of health impairment have been incorporated, drawing from new research on disabilities, sports, and exercise. Also updated are the survey on prevalent handicapping conditions, elements of treatment, and physical education concepts for various disabilities, including a new section on head trauma. New methods of adapting sports for participation by the disabled are outlined for team sports and sports not previously included—racquet sports, aerobics, and golf.

Ordering information: Lea & Febiger has a telephone recording system. You may telephone any orders or any requests or messages by calling (800) 444-1785. Outside Continental U.S. call (215) 922-1330.

LEA & FEBIGER
600 Washington Square
Philadelphia, PA 19106-4198

****

Locating, Recruiting and Hiring the Disabled
 Rami Rabby

This book offers short and long term strategies for locating qualified job candidates. It assists personnel executives, recruiters, and all other managers and supervisors, and contains over 500 listings including publications directed at the disabled; job banks; private sector training and/or placement projects; information and referral plus other resources for contacting qualified candidates.
 Price: $3.95

Computers—New Opportunities for the Disabled
 Harold Remmes

This sourcebook shows how computer technology can remove barriers to education, employment, and communication for the disabled and also provide an outlet for creative recreation. Special considerations for selecting and using a computer are included as well as supplemental programs and software that facilitate usability and overcome physical handicaps.
 Price: $3.50

PILOT BOOKS
103 Cooper Street
Babylon, NY 11702
(516) 422-2225

****

Multiple Sclerosis Fact Book
 Richard Lechtenberg, M.D.

This concise book explains what multiple sclerosis is understood to be, what is thought to cause it, what types of problems it causes, and what can be done to manage those problems. It will be an invaluable resource for persons with multiple sclerosis and their families, as well as for the professionals who work with them. The spectrum of useful and useless therapies is reviewed concisely, with emphasis on the most valuable treatments currently available. Much of the book considers the management of common problems as well as the implications of these problems. Special coverage is given to the implications of multiple sclerosis in pregnancy, sexual activity, personal hygiene, and employment.
 Price: $14.95

Physical Management for the Quadriplegic Patient, 2nd Edition
 Jack R. Ford and Bridget Duckworth

This popular manual is now available in an expanded second edition. Retaining the step-by-step illustrative format that made the first edition so practical and useful, the book has been updated to include new equipment and techniques. Responding to reviewer requests three new chapters have been added—Sexual Management, Parenthood, and Household Management—and a new appendix including house design plans and functional assessment tools.

Price: $59.00

Other titles include:
Rehabilitation of the Head-Injured Adult, 2nd Edition Edited by Mitchell Rosenthal and Ernest R. Griffith
Lower Limb Amputations: A Guide to Rehabilitation, Gloria T. Sanders and Bell J. May

F.A. DAVIS COMPANY
1915 Arch Street
Philadelphia, PA 19103-9954
(800) 523-4049

****

Mixed Blessings
William and Barbara Christopher
William Christopher played "Father Mulcahy," a sensitive army chaplain, on M*A*S*H, one of the most successful programs in TV history. He and his wife were living a private drama. They were raising an autistic son, Ned. *Mixed Blessings* is the Christophers' unforgettable story of life with this special boy. In a remarkably open and candid way, *Mixed Blessings* invites readers to share in the personal struggles of one of America's most beloved actors and his wife. It is a story filled with hope, persistence, dreams, and love.

Price: $15.95

ABINGDON PRESS
201 Eighth Avenue, South
P.O. Box 801
Nashville, TN 37202
(800) 251-3320
(615) 749-6347

****

Self-Help for the Laryngectomee
Edmund Lauder
This book is written by a laryngectomee who has taught several thousand laryngectomees how to communicate again. Colonel Lauder has a certificate of clinical competence in speech pathology (CCC-SP), from the American Speech and Hearing Association. Sixteen chapters are illustrated and outline important details of interest to laryngectomees, physicians, nurses, speech pathologists, rehabilitation counselors, and others in paramedical professions.

Price: $6.00

EDMUND LAUDER
11115 Whisper Hollow
San Antonio, TX 78230

****

Consumer's Guide to Attendant Care
This book specifically addresses persons with physical disabilities who would like to hire personal care attendants. Functioning as a how-to-manual, a personal checklist, and a general overview, the *Consumer's Guide* discusses the process of recruiting, screening/ inter-viewing, hiring and supervising attendants. In addition to sample ads, applications, and agreements, the *Consumer's Guide* gives important tips concerning emergency back-up care. An invaluable resources for anyone considering attendant care.

Price: $7.50

The Accessible Bathroom
This detailed book was put together by the Design Coalition, Inc., Madison, Wisconsin's community design and planning center. *The Accessible Bathroom* includes many illustrations, with detailed dimensions and construction tips, as well as general discussions about accessible design. Where specific fixtures and accessories are available, the book provides manufacturers' addresses. In addition to pre-made accessories, *The Accessible Bathroom* discusses possible modifications to existing equipment.

Price: $8.50

An Accessible Entrance: Ramps
Another Design Coalition, Inc. book, it is as detailed and comprehensive as *The Accessible Bathroom*.

Price: $7.50
ACCESS TO INDEPENDENCE INC.
1954 East Washington Avenue
Madison, WI 53704
(608) 251-7575 Voice and TTY

****

Handi-Travel: A Resource Book for Disabled and Elderly Travelers

Cinnie Noble

This is a comprehensive travel guide for people with disabilities affecting mobility, hearing, and sight. Cinnie Noble, an expert in travel for the disabled, provides detailed information on transportation by air, rail, bus, and ship—both in North America and overseas. The book contains updated information on:

• how to find a travel agent familiar with the special needs of people with disabilities

• guidelines on acceptable levels of accessibility for wheelchair travelers, and for visually and hearing impaired people

• special tips for travelers with diabetes, epilepsy, respiratory conditions, and those on dialysis

• how to determine whether a disabled traveler's personal attendant would be eligible for a 50% air fare discount

• resources to consult for further information.

Price: $12.95 plus $2.00 postage for Canadian orders.

Orders outside Canada must be prepaid in U.S. funds.

Accentuate the Positive: Expressive Arts for Children with Disabilities

Fran Herman and James C. Smith

"In the foreword to *Accentuate the Positive*, the authors 'hope that the material and suggestions offered will be an aid to therapists, teachers, child care workers and recreationists, programming for a child with disabilities, and for parents who may turn any time of day into a creative period for their child.' Targeted primarily toward children between the ages of three and twelve, the activities suggested in this book will prove, without a doubt, to be an invaluable aid for those working with children with disabilities.

"The book is divided into five parts: 1) Accentuate the Positive, which sets the tone of the book; 2) Finding Out About Ourselves, which examines activities for children from three to six years old; 3) Discovering through Expressive Arts, which concentrates on the child from seven to twelve with chronic disabling conditions ranging from moderate to severe; 4) Large Scale Adventures, which examines the importance of children participating in major activities such as dramatic or musical presentations and; 5) Disabilities, Distress and Remedial Strategies, which focuses on children who are seriously mentally or physically impaired. (Parts two through five are subdivided into themes and sub-units, usually accompanied by an introduction, a set of well-defined objectives, exploration [activities] and possible variations, pictures, and some very touching anecdotes. The book's major strength is that the activities derive from a philosophy which is concerned with the needs of the child first, and then his disability. The authors have identified and developed activities and experiences that all children can enjoy, and have also supplied sufficient information (including a useful appendix) so that the activities can be modified to cater to children with special needs. Because of its unquestionable value for children in general, this book probably surpasses the expectations of its readers.

"There are several areas in which *Accentuate the Positive* could be more "user-friendly." The materials required for the various activities might have been listed under a 'Materials Required' section, so that this information is more readily located. Secondly, as computers are being used in the field of disabilities, a listing of computer software, included in the Appendix section, would be helpful. The authors have clearly shown that by adopting an accentuate the positive attitude, all children can enjoy the rich experiences that creative art and expression have to offer!"

Reviewed by Arron Eisen, a special education teacher with the North York Board of Education.

Price: $18.95 plus $2.00 postage

CANADIAN REHABILITATION COUNCIL FOR THE DISABLED
Suite 2110, One Yonge Street
Toronto, Ontario M5E 1E5
(416) 862-0340

＊＊＊＊

The Human Horizons Series

"It was far sighted to establish this series to provide information for a wide range of individuals on many topics to do with disability."—*The British Medical Journal*

"All the authors are involved with the field they are writing about as parent, patient or worker. This gives their writing a vividness and conviction born of actual experience ... Each book is constructive and informative."—*The Health Services*

The Wheelchair Child

Philippa Russell

Here is a completely revised and updated edition of the highly praised handbook for parents of the child in a wheelchair, covering problems which arise from early childhood to young adulthood. Philippa Russell is Senior Officer to the Voluntary Council for Handicapped Children in the National Children's Bureau in London, and is the mother of a handicapped child.

Things for Children to Make and Do
  Science and Technology Activities
  Alan V. Jones

All children love finding out how and why things work, but too often children who have a physical disability or special educational needs may have been deprived of the opportunity to explore and question.

Produced in a special spiral-bound large format, this book offers a wealth of exciting and imaginative ideas that will enable children of all ages and abilities to enjoy experimenting while absorbing the basic principles of science and technology. The activities use commonplace household odds and ends like spools and dishwashing liquid bottles, and are great fun to do. The simple jargon-free language, combined with clear diagrams, make this a book for any parent or teacher.

Alan V. Jones is Head of the Department of Physical Sciences at Trent Polytechnic. His previous book, *Science for Handicapped Children*, also in the *Human Horizons* series, has proved widely popular.

Other titles include:
Cystic Fibrosis: A Guide for Parents and Sufferers
  Percy Bray

Managing Incontinence
  Edited by Cheryle B. Gartley

Down's Syndrome
  Cliff Cunningham

Multiple Sclerosis
  Alexander Burnfield

Children in Need of Special Care
  Thomas Weihs

Easy to Make Toys for Your Handicapped Child
  Don Caston

Out of Doors with Handicapped People
  Mike Cotton

Computer Help for Disabled People
  Lorna Ridgway & Stuart McKears

Multiply Handicapped Children
  Rosalind Wyman

SOUVENIR PRESS LTD.
43 Great Russell Street
London WC1B 3PA, England

✳✳✳✳

AMERICAN FOUNDATION FOR THE BLIND

The American Foundation for the Blind is a national nonprofit organization that advocates, develops, and provides programs and services to help blind and visually impaired people achieve independence with dignity in all sectors of society. Among programs and resources provided by AFB in partnership with over 1,000 specialized schools, agencies, and organizations nationwide are public education, social and technological research, consumer products, publications, consultation and referrals, government relations, and Talking Books for the Library of Congress. Founded in 1921 and recognized as Helen Keller's cause in the United States, AFB is headquartered in New York City and maintains regional offices in Atlanta, Chicago, Dallas, New York, San Francisco, and Washington, D.C. AFB Toll-Free Hotline Number (800) AFBLIND (232-5463) NY Residents call (212) 620-2147

The hotline supplies information on visual impairment and blindness, and answers queries regarding AFB services, products, publications, technology, the Job Index (a national data and networking resource on the competitive employment of blind and visually impaired persons), and much more.

Foundations of Education for Blind and Visually Handicapped Children and Youth
  Edited by Geraldine T. Scholl

A unique resource of current options in the education of blind and visually handicapped children, from preschool through high school. Twenty-six specialists contributed material to twenty-two chapters. Major sections include Education for the Visually Handicapped: A Social and Educational History; Definitions, Development, and Theory; Components of a Quality Educational Program; and Special Curriculum Considerations.

AFB Directory of Services for Blind and Visually Impaired Persons in the United States, 23rd edition

AFB's resource directory of agencies and other organizations for blind and visually impaired persons. Names, addresses, and services offered by the federal government are listed, with voluntary agencies, schools, and organizations.

Choice Not Chance: A Guide to Computers for Blind and Visually Imparied Persons

This book demystifies the subject by discussing computers in terms of the tasks and functions to be performed and access modalities—synthetic speech, braille, large print. It covers use by blind and visually impaired persons and by professionals to produce materials in alternative media. It includes a comprehensive vendor list, training options, glossary, and illustrations.

How to Thrive, Not Just Survive, A Guide to Developing Independent Life Skills for Visually Impaired Children and Youths

Edited by Kathleen Mary Huebner, Ph.D. and Rose-Marie Wallow, Ed.D.

Designed for parents and others involved in the education of blind and visually impaired children and youths, the book presents guidelines and strategies for helping them develop, acquire, and apply skills necessary for independence in socialization, orientation and mobility, and leisure time and recreational activities.

AMERICAN FOUNDATION FOR THE BLIND
15 West 16th Street
New York, NY 10011
(800) 232-5463
(212) 620-2147 in New York

✶✶✶✶

Peterson's Guide to Colleges with Programs for Learning-Disabled Students

Editors: Charles T. Mangrum II, Ed.D., and Stephen S. Strichart, Ph.D.

For learning-disabled students and their families, this is the most complete and accurate guide to colleges with learning disabilities programs.

This book profiles institutions in two sections so that counselors, parents, and students can distinguish between colleges with full-fledged LD programs and those that offer some services. The first section contains extensive profiles of colleges with fully developed programs, while the second details colleges with support services not designed as comprehensive programs. It now covers two-year colleges as well as four-year colleges. In addition, the editors offer extensive advice and information on:
  • How learning-disabled students are admitted
  • An overview of college services
  • How to select the right college

"Highly informative, concise, geared precisely to the needs of the learning-disabled student considering college."—Dr. Sally E. Shaywitz, Director, Learning Disorders Unit, Yale University School of Medicine

PETERSON'S GUIDES
P.O. Box 2123
Princeton, NJ 08543-2123

✶✶✶✶

Holidays and Travel Abroad 1989: A Guide for Disabled People

An annual guide to accommodation and facilities available abroad for disabled vacationers.

The Directory of Airline Facilities

A guide to the accessibility of air travel for disabled people.

Arts Centres and Creative Opportunities for Disabled People

Information on facilities and special programs at arts centres around the country (England) for disabled people.

Motoring and Mobility for Disabled People

Ann Darnborough and Derek Kinrade

A source of information and guidance on all aspects of mobility, including sections on motoring with a wheelchair, insurance, and assessment centres.

REMAP Yearbook 1989

Describes the many aids, modifications, and adaptations which have been designed, made, and supplied to disabled individuals. Contains a comprehensive list of panel addresses.

Abilities and Disabilities

A booklet aiming to give school children an understanding of the difficulties faced by people with disabilities in the community. Illustrated with drawings and cartoons. Accompanying Teachers' Notes also available.

Working Together Towards Independence

Judith Male and Jean Ward

Directed to non-teaching assistants working with children with physical disabilities.

Employers' Guide to Disabilities

Second edition by Bert Massie and Melvyn Kettle

Aimed at helping employers realize what disabled people can do and to consider their suitability for employment on the strength of their abilities and not their disabilities. Published by Woodhead-Faulkner in association with RADAR.

The Directory for Disabled People

Compiled by Ann Darnborough and Derek Kinrade (5th Edition)

Published by Woodhead-Faulkner in association with RADAR.

THE ROYAL ASSOCIATION FOR
DISABILITY & REHABILITATION
(RADAR)
25 Mortimer Street
London W1N 8AB, England

****

The Children and the Nations
Maggie Black

In *The Children and the Nations*, Maggie Black has told the UNICEF story as it should be told. After many years of writing about development issues, she became editor of publications for the Fund and, with its blessing, undertook the prodigious tasks of research, interviews, and writing that have given us this beautiful book. Above all else, the UNICEF story is a drama about people: the people, mostly children, who need help; the people who have tried to help them; and the people who have molded and expanded an original idea of limited scope into a global doctrine for child survival. Maggie Black knew this and has built her book around the people whose lives and deeds are the UNICEF story.

Readers concerned about disability will find much of interest in *The Children and the Nations*. Among the Fund's earliest projects were those to assist the war torn nations to provide treatment for children crippled and ravaged by the war. Throughout its history most of the programs UNICEF has designed and supported have served to prevent or reduce the impairments consequent to malnutrition, disease, and ignorance. The response to childhood disability has become an integral part of UNICEF's campaign for child survival.

Excerpted from a book review by Norman Acton, *International Rehabilitation Review*, Vol. 39, No. 1, June 1988.

Price: $25.95

UNICEF HISTORY PROJECT
UNICEF House
3 UN Plaza
New York, NY 10017

****

Disabled Policy: America's Programs for the Handicapped

Edward Berkowitz, Director of the Program in History and Public Policy, George Washington University

Interest about disability issues among policy oriented scholars has grown tremendously in recent years, providing a valuable context to the more established literature on rehabilitation and disability. One of the most insightful contributors to this new body of work has been the historian Ed Berkowitz. He has written an important book which is a major contribution to the disability policy literature, as well as to the more general literature on social policy. It provides an informative overview of the five major policy approaches taken by the American government toward disability: workers' compensation, social security disability insurance, vocational rehabilitation, and, more recently, civil rights and independent living programs. Each of the substantive chapters integrates the existing literature while drawing on a wide range of archival materials. Berkowitz succinctly summarizes current policy debates, both within programs and across disability policy as a whole, and concludes with plausible recommendations for reforming and reintegrating American public policies concerning disability. The book also gives a useful conceptual framework for categorizing and evaluating disability programs in relation to each other. Berkowitz suggests a number of specific changes in the various disability benefit programs which would reorient incentives for disabled people and employers to maintain individuals with disabilities in the work force as much as possible. *Disabled Policy* provides a critical overview which should be read by anyone concerned with public policy and disability. It is an excellent book which will be of great use to scholars, practitioners, activists, and students concerned with disability, or with the nature of social policy in the American welfare state.

Excerpted from a book review by Richard K. Scotch, Assistant Professor of Sociology and Political Economy at the University of Texas at Dallas, *International Rehabilitation Review*, Vol. 39, No. 1, June 1988.

Price: $24.95

CAMBRIDGE UNIVERSITY PRESS
32 E. 57th Street
New York, NY 10022

****

Aging and Developmental Disabilities: Issues and Approaches
Edited by Matthew P. Janicki and Henryk M. Wisniewski
Price: $35.95

PAUL H. BROOKES PUBLISHING COMPANY
P.O. Box 10624
Baltimore, MD 21285-0624

****

Open Care for the Elderly in Seven European Countries
Edited by Anton Amann
Price: $52.00

PERGAMON PRESS INC.
Maxwell House
Fairview Park
Elmsford, NY 10523

****

Rehabilitation in the Aging
Edited by T. Franklin Williams, M.D.
Price: $60.00

RAVEN PRESS
1140 Avenue of the Americas
New York, NY 10036

****

The Aging Workforce: Implications for Rehabilitation
Edited by Leonard G. Perlman and Gary F. Austin
Price: $15.00

NATIONAL REHABILITATION ASSOCIATION
633 South Washington Street
Alexandria, VA 22314

To Walk Again!
Carolyn Clawson
"That morning in the fall of 1969 when my husband left for work, I sat in the house a near invalid. That evening . . . I WALKED out to meet him, unaided! He was speechless! I took him into the house and demonstrated the fact that clogs enabled me to walk. We both realized I had possibly stum-bled onto something of great value. How grateful I was for this marvelous gift. I felt I had been given a reprieve, set free from a physical bondage. WHAT A GLORIOUS DAY! Little did I realize . . . I was about to embark on the greatest adventure of my life."

In *To Walk Again!* Carolyn Clawson tells her inspiring story of the chance discovery and subse-quent development of a unique therapeutic aid for persons with walking disabilities, the "Clawson Rocker Shoe."

MOBILITY RESEARCH FOUNDATION
P.O. Box 337
Rexburg, ID 83440

****

There's Lint in Your Bellybutton!
Audrey J. King
There's Lint in Your Bellybutton! presents an honest yet positive and humorous look at the dilemmas of disability. With a minimum of text, this book of cartoons depicts the many barriers that ex-ist in architecture, attitudes, employment, and other areas. The characters face the trials, tribula-tions, and exhilarations that life presents to people with disabilities, and reinforces the fact that people with disabilities are basically the same as anyone else. Well-known cartoonist and writer Audrey King approaches the subject with a keen sense of fun, so that readers of all ages can relax and appre-ciate the genuine amusement that often arises from looking at life literally on a different level.
Price: $4.95 and $2.00 postage

Other titles include:
Connections: Accessibility at Major Transportation Terminals in Canada $5.00

CRCD Rehabilitation Classification Scheme: A Specialized Subject Cataloguing System for Rehabilitation Information $10.00

Rehabilitation Treatment Centres for Physically Disabled Persons in Canada $5.00

Conversations with Non-Speaking People $4.50

Jonathan, Too, Goes to Day Nursery $4.50

Housing and Support Services for Physically Disabled Persons in Canada $5.00

CANADIAN REHABILITATION COUNCIL FOR THE DISABLED
Suite 2110, One Yonge Street
Toronto, Ontario M5E 1E5
(416) 862-0340

****

After the Tears: Parents Talk About Raising a Child With a Disability
Robin Simons

A child born with a disability presents to the parents themselves the danger of being disabled by grief, regret, guilt, anger, and the seemingly unanswerable question,"What are we to do?" Yet the danger must somehow be faced, and it must be overcome, because life will go on after the tears have stopped. In this deeply sensitive book, parents of children with disabilities describe with affecting candor how they first confronted their experience and then recovered to emerge stronger, healthier, abler. They answer here the question that at first seems unanswerable.

Price: $8.00

TASH, INC.
7010 Roosevelt Way N.E.
Seattle, WA 98115
(206) 523-8446

****

Able Scientists—Disabled Persons: Careers in the Sciences
S. Phyllis Stearner, Ph.D.

The scientists with disabilities who share their life experiences in this book are similar to the thousands more who are working each day across our nation. Each one is a story of self-motivation, persistence, patience, ingenuity, assertiveness, and innovation. Truly, each is a profile in achievement, an inspiration to us all.

The disabled persons included have overcome numerous barriers and have demonstrated ability as able scientists and students of science ... They have gained satisfaction in overcoming difficulties and in accomplishing tasks required to function in the larger society, and this satisfaction served as an additional motivating force in their reaching even higher levels of accomplishment.

Each biographical sketch testifies to the importance of encouragement and support of teachers and the educational system as well as that of family and therapists. They illustrate possible career options open to physically disabled students. They are an inspiration to all-disabled and non-disabled. This book is a plea for help for disabled students of science—help in eliminating the barriers that exist in our educational systems, in industry, and in academe. The author, herself an able disabled scientist with a Ph.D. from the University of Chicago, was a research radiobiologist at Argonne National Laboratory for thirty-five years before her recent retirement. This book offers a fascinating glimpse of what is possible and strongly suggests that almost nothing is impossible.

"The fact that these scientists are involved in such diverse fields as geology, meteorology, computers, organic chemistry, clinical psychology, electrical engineering and others is overwhelming evidence that individuals with physical disabilities can succeed in scientific and technical work. Instructors, parents, counselors, and others may find this book the inspiration necessary to encourage students with disabilities to consider a career in science."

Price: $12.95

FOUNDATION FOR SCIENCE AND THE HANDICAPPED, INC.
154 Juliet Court
Clarendon Hills, IL 60514

****

The Sensuous Wheeler: Sexual Adjustment for the Spinal Cord Injured
Barry J. Rabin, Ph.D.

There has long been a need for a book on sexuality and spinal cord injury written to satisfy the needs of the professional and the spinal cord injured alike. Barry J. Rabin, Ph.D. has the background both in academic and clinical settings to appreciate the style necessary to communicate on these two levels. *The Sensuous Wheeler* has recently accomplished this goal; by being widely accepted in academic as well as in rehabilitation institutions, serving the needs of professionals and individuals with spinal cord injury.

The Sensuous Wheeler provides the professional and the spinal cord injured with a broad spectrum of psychological, medical, and practical information to help each one bring optimum sexual adjustment.

Price: $12.95 plus $2.00 postage

BARRY J. RABIN, PH.D.
5595 East 7th Street, Suite 353
Long Beach, CA 90804

****

Gentle Yoga
Lorna Bell, R.N. and Eudora Seyfer

Gentle Yoga is a book especially for people with arthritis, stroke damage, multiple sclerosis, and in wheelchairs, or anyone who needs a gentle, practical guide for improving his health. As competition in the fitness industry increases, emphasis is placed on "perfect" bodies, youth, and traditional beauty. But *Gentle Yoga* is designed for special people with special needs, whether in a wheelchair or just recovering from surgery or illness. This book provides a gentle, practical guide for improving health. It includes easy how-to instructions for yoga exercises with over 135 illustrations. Also included are discussions on nutrition, stress control, breathing, and positive thinking. The book is spiral bound so it lies open as the student of gentle yoga works with it.

Price: $7.95

TEN SPEED PRESS
P.O. Box 7123
Berkeley, CA 94707

****

Volume 1 of the *Breaking New Ground Resource Manual*

In 1979, a severely disabled farmer contacted the Department of Agricultural Engineering requesting information on how he could modify his agricultural equipment to enable him to continue farming. This initial contact eventually led to the establishment of the Breaking New Ground Resource Center (BNG) which has become nationally and internationally recognized as the primary source of rehabilitation technology relating to agricultural worksites.

Since 1979, when Breaking New Ground first initiated research directed at assisting agricultural producers with physical handicaps, it has collected numerous ideas that disabled farmers and ranchers throughout the United States and Canada have developed and are using.

Many of these ideas, along with relevant commercial products, are presented in Volume 1 of the *Breaking New Ground Resource Manual*. This manual contains over 350 pages of ideas and resources currently being used by agricultural producers with physical handicaps, which enable them to remain active in their operations. Each idea contains a description of the concept, method of operation, and brief overview of how the item was constructed. A contact person is also listed for further information. This manual also has a bibliography on rehabilitation technology for agricultural producers with physical handicaps.

Price: $30.00

Other titles include:

Agricultural Tools, Equipment, Machinery & Buildings for Farmers & Ranchers with Physical Handicaps

Price: $30.00

Evaluation of Self-Propelled Agricultural Machines Modified for Operators with Serious Physical Handicaps
T.L. Wilkinson
Price: $25.00

Agricultural Worksite Assessment Tool and User's Guide for Farmers and Ranchers with Physical Disabilities
T. Willkomm and W.E. Field
Price: $10.00

BREAKING NEW GROUND
Department of Agricultural Engineering
Purdue University
West Lafayette, IN 47907

****

Wheelchairs: A Prescription Guide
A. Bennett Wilson, Jr. and Samuel R. McFarland

Wheelchairs: A Prescription Guide is a comprehensive up-to-date handbook written especially for clinicians responsible for development of prescription for wheelchairs.

The contents of the book include:
• The Need for Wheelchairs
• A Brief History of Wheelchairs
• The Basic Wheelchair
• Variations of the Basic Wheelchair
• Accessories
• Seating
• Prescription
• Externally Powered Wheelchairs
• Wheelchairs for Children
• Sports Chairs
• Special Powered Vehicles
• Operation and Maintenance
• Manufacturers of Sports Wheelchairs
Price: $14.95 (shipping and handling free when order is accompanied by payment)

REHABILITATION PRESS
Box 3696
Charlottesville, VA 22903-0696

****

Attendant Care Manual
Maren R. Larson and Daniel Snobl

This manual has been prepared for individuals who provide attendant care to handicapped students attending Southwest State University. The manual provides knowledge about the various types of disabilities and the attendant care which they require on a day-to-day basis.

Price: $7.00 (postage prepaid at library rate)

MAREN LARSON, R.N., C.
Attendant Supervisor
Bellows 158
Southwest State University
Marshall, MN 56258

****

Equipment for the Disabled

Equipment for the Disabled is the NHS-sponsored series of handbooks of disability equipment and other products that can maximize everyone's capabilities. Facts and comments on a wide range of available items are presented along with advice and guidance in the form of points to consider before any purchase is made. Full details of manufacturers or distributors are given and the books are fully illustrated.

Titles in the *Equipment For The Disabled* series include:

Incontinence and Stoma Care; *Outdoor Transport*; *Communication*; *Wheelchairs*; *Walking Aids*; *Hoists and Lifts*; *Home Management*; *Clothing and Dressing for Adults*; *Gardening*; *Housing and Furniture*; *Personal Care*; *Disabled Mother*; and *Disabled Child*.

EQUIPMENT FOR THE DISABLED
Mary Marlborough Lodge
Nuffield Orthopaedic Centre
Headington
Oxford OX3 7LD, England

****

Playing and Coaching Wheelchair Basketball
Edward S. Owen

An indispensable guide for participants in the sport and a necessary reference and text for people in allied health and education fields, this spiral-bound volume covers such aspects of wheelchair basketball as individual and team offense and defense, special drills, coaching philosophy, the organization of teams and leagues, guides to wheelchair maintenance, and national and international rules. Includes 800 action photos and diagrams.

Price: $16.95

Deafness in Childhood
Edited by Freeman McConnell and Paul H. Ward

This highly readable volume is divided into five broad areas: (1) The Problem of Children with Defective Hearing; (2) Diagnosis; (3) Pathology; (4) Medical Treatment and Research; (5) Audiologic Treatment and Research.

"I heartily recommend this book for your library."—Dr. Terrence Cawthorne, British Otologist.

Price: $14.95

UNIVERSITY OF ILLINOIS PRESS
c/o CUP Services
P.O. Box 6525
Ithaca, NY 14851

****

Home Health Aides: How to Manage the People Who Help You
Alfred H. DeGraff

More and more people with physical limitations are using help from home health aides or personal care attendants (PCAs). For these people to be in control of their own lifestyle and schedule, they must first be in control of the PCAs who provide assistance.

Home Health Aides: How to Manage the People Who Help You is the only step-by-step handbook reference which so extensively teaches people who use PCAs how to find, train, manage, and pay these workers while keeping them happy. For over twenty years, the author has recruited, trained, and managed the PCAs whom he has employed. As the spinal-cord injured, quadriplegic user of a motorized wheelchair, he has recruited and managed help in a variety of settings that include college campuses, career offices, urban offices, urban apartments, rural homes, health facilities, and international travel.

Most previous books on "attendant care" have taught nursing methods to those who provide care. This new 352-page handbook is different . . . it teaches the people who use PCAs how to be in control of that help. When this assistance is provided dependably, efficiently, and on a consistent schedule, the recipient of help can lead the lifestyle and daily schedule which he/she chooses. The recipient is in control of his life and lives relatively independently.

In contrast, when assistance is undependable, of poor quality, and provided on a sporadic schedule, the recipient has lost control. In many cases the care provider now controls the recipient's lifestyle and daily schedule, consciously or not.

A recent survey indicates that over 4.9 million adults with physical limitations have a temporary or lifelong need for assistance from personal care aides. Categories of help can include getting dressed, transferring to a wheelchair, grooming, bathing, toileting, cooking and eating, housecleaning, and transportation.

Yet many service recipients lack the skills to manage the people who provide this help. Several studies have concluded that there is one predominant reason for service recipients lacking control of their own lives: their lack of training in attendant management skills.

Over eighty-five topics in this book teach management skills. Topics include reasons PCAs quit/are fired, settings for using help, strategies of a good manager, factors of good work environments, types of needs which do/do not qualify for help, assertive-aggressive-passive ways to request help, making a list of needs, creating a job description, sources and methods for recruiting, interviewing and screening, hiring and training, parting ways by firing and resignation, using agency aides v. personally recruited help, and ten guidelines for maximum independent living.

The book's clear format makes it an easy-to-use reference as well as a well-structured guide for classroom instruction.

Single copies are $18.95 plus $3.00 postage and handling; multiple-copy discounts are available to independent living programs and agencies. A check, money order, or agency purchase order may be sent to:

SARATOGA ACCESS PUBLICATIONS
6 Birch Street
Saratoga Springs, NY 12866-3834
(518) 587-6974

✱✱✱✱

Nursing Home Activities for the Handicapped
M. Laker
A popular book detailing practical activities for the bedridden, visually handicapped as well as stroke victims and those confined to wheelchairs. Eighty activities, including their planning and scheduling.
Price: $18.25

Creative Arts for the Severely Handicapped
C. Sherrill
The reader will learn from twenty-seven major figures in special education. There is mainstreaming, recreation programming, Orff-Schulwerk, inte-grated arts, drama and research plus motor creativity and movement analysis.
Superb photos. Hardbound.
Price: $36.00

Accentuate the Positive—Expressive Arts for Children with Disabilities
F. Herman and J. Smith
Designed to promote an awareness of learning potential in creative abilities for young children who have moderate to severe disabilities. The book includes hundreds of open-ended activities, original songs, clearly stated objectives and goals, case histories showing direct application and much more.
Price: $19.00

Physical Education and Recreation for the Visually Impaired
American Alliance for Health, Physical Education, Recreation and Dance
This guide illustrates programs, trends, and legal issues for visually impaired students and includes information on the nature of visual impairment, practical program suggestions, and instructional methods.
Price: $8.75

Guide to the Selection of Musical Instruments with Respect to Physical Ability and Disability
Kardon Institute and Moss Rehabilitation Center
A resource abounding in unique, well-researched and tested information, this guide is an aid to therapists teaching the disabled to play musical instruments. It fills the gap about the knowledge of what physical abilities are required for playing different instruments. There is a thorough profile of physiology. Also included are photos for each instrument and special charts for instrument selection, skills checklist, student requirements, muscle utilization, and degree of movement. The book is organized by instrument families with a detailed discussion on how they produce and alter sound.
Price: $7.75

MMB MUSIC, INC.
10370 Page Industrial Blvd.
St. Louis, MO 63132

✱✱✱✱

DISABLED LIVING FOUNDATION

The Disabled Living Foundation (DLF), a charitable trust, studies those aspects of daily living which present special problems to disabled people.

It produces publications designed for those who work with disabled people, whether in a voluntary or professional capacity, and for disabled people themselves and their families.

Clothes Sense for Disabled People of All Ages
Peggy Turnbull and Rosemary Ruston
Published by Piel Caru for the DLF

An extensively revised and updated version of the first edition, *Clothes Sense* not only covers all aspects of clothing and dressing for adults, but has been extended to include some of the problems of disabled children. It includes sections on how to select new clothes, adaptations, dressing techniques and aids, and reinforcements and repairs.

Dressing for Disabled People
Rosemary Ruston

Dressing problems can prevent a disabled person from becoming fully independent. The main section of this pioneering book shows pictorially, with full explanation, different ways of getting in and out of clothes, with reference to different types of handicap. Other chapters deal with the processes of dressing and the skills required, suitable clothing, adaptations, the nature of materials, fastenings, and management of clothing when using the lavatory.

Design Data for Wheelchair Children: With Special Reference to Designing Special Schools for Physically Handicapped Children
Brian C. Goldsmith

This book, originally published as a series of papers by the Greater London Council in their architectural bulletin, is intended for architects and all other professionals involved in designing environments planned for the handicapped child. It focuses specifically on the design problems related to children in wheelchairs.

Handicapped at Home
Sydney Foot

This book, with many photographs and line drawings, suggests ways in which a home may be fully shared by able and disabled people, whatever the age or disability. Throughout the book the aim is to encourage the disabled person to live as full and independent a life as possible.

Work Preparation for the Handicapped
David Hutchinson
Published by Croom Helm

The author describes services available to handicapped school leavers. He discusses curriculum development in further education, describes in detail technical aids and teaching/learning resources available, and assesses the role of support agencies.

Kitchen Sense for Disabled People
Edited by Gwen Conacher
Published by Croom Helm for the DLF

This freshly researched and completely revised edition reflects the increasing awareness of the needs and capabilities of disabled people and the wider choice of equipment, appliances, and aids. Problems facing visually handicapped people and those with chronic skin conditions are now included. It contains practical, detailed advice on planning and equipping a kitchen, aids to making life easier for disabled people, short cuts in cooking, and shopping.

Arts and Disabled People
Published by Bedford Square Press

This report of the Committee of Inquiry set up in 1982 and chaired by Sir Richard Attenborough is the first comprehensive review of facilities in the UK which enable disabled people to be involved in the arts.

Coping with Disability
Peggy Jay

Carefully researched and extensively illustrated, this book is a mine of practical information designed to show disabled people how to get help from the health and social services, from voluntary organizations and others. It contains advice on how to make life easier in the home, how to get in and out of the bath and manage independently in the lavatory, how to cope with problems of clothes and dressing, cooking, eating, housework, and laundry. There are sections on mobility, on keeping in touch, on getting out and about, and on pastimes and leisure activities.

Other titles include:

Able to Work
Bernadette Fallon
Published by the Spinal Injuries Association

Early Years—A Book for the Disabled Mother or Father
Morigue Cornwell

Outdoor Pursuits for Disabled People
Norman Croucher
Published by Woodhead Faulkner for the DLF

Directory for the Disabled
Ann Darnborough and Derek Kinrade
Published by Woodhead Faulkner

Handling the Young Cerebral Palsied Child at Home
    Nancie R. Finnie
    Published by William Heinemann Medical Books

Play Helps: Toys and Activities for Handicapped Children
    Roma Lear
    Published by Heinemann Health Books

Toys and Play for the Handicapped Child
    Barbara Riddick
    Published by Croom Helm

Orders for DLF Publications should be sent to:

HAIGH & HOCHLAND LTD.
International University Booksellers
The Precinct Centre
Oxford Road
Manchester M139QA, England

✳✳✳✳

A Bomb in the Brain
    Steve Fishman
    Steve Fishman provides both a medical memoir and a fascinating investigation of the science and surgery that saved his life. His success with surgery and his hope for an uneventful recovery was snatched from him, however, when a year after the operation he began to have seizures. "To be told you have epilepsy is to be welcomed into a world of stigma from the very first moment," he writes. Fishman describes what it is like to be subject to seizures at any moment—in gyms, restaurants, offices. He writes emotionally of confronting his chronic condition, and trying to understand how it changed him forever.

However, epilepsy comprises only a part of this book. The bulk of the book is a story of doctors trying to save Fishman's life after the vein burst in his brain, the medical science which came into play, his stay in the hospital, and his fellow patients.

As a journalist, Fishman was given special access to the intricacies and practice of high powered medicine at one of the country's leading medical institutions. His surgeons became his friends. He watched a videotape of his own operation with his surgeon at his side, and was allowed to observe an operation like his own performed on another patient.

Fishman explores the psychological as well as the physical experience of illness. He portrays life as a patient as a series of impositions on an adult suddenly obligated to accept whatever he is given.

And he discovers that having an illness changes the behavior of healthy people around him. With the help of an epilepsy support group, Fishman eventually came to terms with his epilepsy. "This is not to say that I feel great about epilepsy, that I wouldn't feel blessed if it one day evaporated," he writes. "... but I am able to accept that being subject to seizures is like any limitation, being unemployed, or picked last on the playground ... The attitude I hold to now is this: I'm different, but it's not that big a deal."

From *National Spokesman* January/February 1989

CHARLES SCRIBNER'S SONS
866 Third Avenue
New York, NY 10022

✳✳✳✳

All Things are Possible
    Yvonne Duffy
    The first book on sexuality of Differently Abled women to cover orthopedic characteristics from arthogryposis to the Werdnig-Hoffman syndrome. In their own words, over seventy-five women from Massachusetts to California candidly share their most intimate feelings about themselves, their mates, their children, and their worlds. Celebrate the sometimes glorious, often painful reaffirmation of your own sexual being as you participate in their joys and sorrows, setbacks and solutions, as they struggle to exercise their sexuality as physically challenged women in a changing society.

Chapters on Parental Attitudes, Sex Education, Masturbation, Relationships, Sexual Intercourse, Homosexuality, Birth Control, and Child-rearing contain explicit descriptions and concrete suggestions for overcoming difficulties in these areas and more. Including a bibliography and a glossary of terms, this comprehensive work will be invaluable to Differently Abled women, their partners, family, and friends as well as the doctors, nurses, social workers, and physical, occupational, and recreational therapists who attend them.

Yvonne Duffy became Differently Abled as a result of polio when she was two years old. She was graduated in 1973 from The University of Michigan with a B.A. in English literature. She is a writer, a researcher, a manager, a counselor, a lobbyist, and a public speaker. Most of all, she is a woman with a woman's feelings and sensitivity to other women's needs. It is in response to these needs that this book was written.

Price: $8.95 plus postage and handling.

A.J. GARVIN AND ASSOC.
P.O. Box 7525
Ann Arbor, MI 48107

****

The Nonrestrictive Environment
Steven J. Taylor, Julie Racino, James Knoll, and Zana Lutfiyya

This book outlines some basic principles of community integration, critiques the "continuum concept," describes homes and support services for adults and children with severe disabilities, discusses integrated vocational services, looks at what makes community integration work, and outlines some of the emerging controversies in community integration. Two appendices outline some strategies and resources to aid in day-to-day problem solving and describe forty-one programs which are doing an effective job of integrating people with severe disabilities into the community.
Price: $8.95

Other titles include:
Let Our Children Go
Douglas Biklen, $4.50

Christmas in Purgatory
Blatt & Kaplan, $5.25

Sticks and Stones Book
Elizabeth Pieper, $4.50

Understanding the Law
Edited by Taylor & Biklen, $4.25

Ordinary Moments
Edited by Alan Brightman, $10.95

HUMAN POLICY PRESS
P.O. Box 127
Syracuse, NY 13210

****

Spinal Network
Sam Maddox

Spinal Network provides a starting place for finding answers to the many questions with which a person with a disability must come to terms with. It is also an invaluable resource for the friends and families of injured people, and for the professionals who work in the disability area, in physical medicine, rehabilitation, social work, insurance, and law.

This unique resource functions as a reference almanac, a visually provocative, comprehensive and interesting journal of what might be called the wheelchair lifestyle. It includes the many medical, legal, social and emotional issues readers need to know to exercise control over their lives, supported by a vast compilation of national and local service material.
Price: $24.95

Research on Multiple Sclerosis, 3rd edition
Bryon H. Waksman, M.D., Stephen C. Reingold, Ph.D., and William E. Reynolds, M.D.

Sponsored by the National Multiple Sclerosis Society, this book provides a broad-based overview of current research for those with MS and others interested in this exciting and fast-moving area. Sections discuss the nature of the disease and its diagnosis, promising areas of research, and current approaches to management. This is an invaluable guide for those seeking to understand the underlying rationale for specific therapies directed to retarding the progression of this difficult disease.

Voluntary Health Organizations: A Guide to Patient Services
Labe Scheinberg, M.D. and Diana M. Schneider, Ph.D.

This complete guide to support groups for those with chronic illness was developed to help the newly diagnosed patient reach the appropriate support organization as quickly as possible. For each disorder, a brief description of the condition is followed by listings of major national organizations, including mailing addresses and telephone numbers, the number of members, information concerning local chapters, and contact persons. It explains the services each organization offers, including counseling, publications, equipment loans, support groups, transportation services, educational seminars, and affiliated clinics. Finally, a list of recommended reading is provided. Also included is a listing of more general services for the handicapped and disabled.
Price: $34.95

Other titles include:
Aging with a Disability
Roberta B. Trieschmann, Ph.D., $29.95

Living Well with Epilepsy
Robert Gumnit, M.D., $19.95

The Exercise Program, 2nd edition
Richard Blonsky, M.D., $29.95

A Very Special Child
Joan Hebden, $11.95

Our Aging Parents: A Practical Guide to Eldercare
Colette Browne and Roberta Onzuka-Anderson, $14.95

DEMOS PUBLICATIONS, INC.
156 Fifth Avenue, Suite 1018
New York, NY 10010

✳✳✳✳

Directory for Exceptional Children, 11th edition
Now in its 11th edition, the completely revised Directory is a comprehensive survey of over 3000 schools, facilities, and organizations across the United States serving children and young adults with developmental, organic, and emotional handicaps. Both public and private programs are included, encompassing residential and day treatment facilities, boarding and day schools, outpatient clinics, and summer sessions. Complete statistical data on each facility is given, and the goals, treatment techniques, and special features of each are described in detail. The *Directory* is an invaluable resource for parents and professionals seeking the optimum environment for special needs children. This single-volume reference is a must for all those who need accurate and up-to-date data on special education.
Price: $45.00 clothbound

1987/88 Guide to Summer Camps and Summer Schools, 25th edition
The *1987/88 Guide to Summer Camps and Summer Schools* covers the broad spectrum of recreational and educational summer opportunities. This 25th edition marshals current facts from over 1100 camps and schools to present the definitive guidebook to summer programs. The authoritative *Guide* includes listings of summer camping, travel, pioneering, recreational, and educational programs. The geographic range encompasses the U.S., Canada, Mexico, and abroad. Specialized programs for the physically and mentally handicapped and for those with learning disabilities make the 25th *Guide* an important and helpful reference work for special needs children. For locating, evaluating, and selecting the most appropriate summer opportunity for children and teenagers, the *1987/88 Guide* is the comprehensive and convenient resource.
Price: $26.00 cloth

PORTER SARGENT PUBLISHERS, INC.
11 Beacon Street
Boston, MA 02108

✳✳✳✳

Disabled We Stand
Allen T. Sutherland
"We are not a category, The Disabled, but we do see ourselves as an oppressed minority. Our disabilities are facts with which we must live, but it is the society we live in that disables us."—Allen T. Sutherland

Allen T. Sutherland, who has grand mal epilepsy, refuses to speak of "disabled people." His book, *Disabled We Stand*, is about people with disabilities, addressed both to them and to those who identify themselves as able-bodied, all of whom are members of the same society. In it, he describes many of his own experiences as someone with a disability, as well as those of a group of people he interviewed for the book. He shows how they have acquired new attitudes about their situation, developing a new consciousness that has led them to take a stand and speak for themselves. He challenges the stereotyped passive roles they have inherited from our society; the stigma associated with various forms of disablement, visible or invisible; the fact that people with disabilities seldom have an effective voice in the organizations set up to "help" them; and the reluctance of institutions and individuals to banish even the most basic forms of discrimination—those that could be eliminated by the provision of mobility access, sign language translation, and the simple courtesy of recognizing other people's personal needs. *Disabled We Stand* is impassioned, often angry, but also hopeful and practical. It is imbued throughout with the spirit and energy of people who are determined to take their lives into their own hands, and it ends with a series of suggestions for action that will lead to change.
Price: $17.95 paperback

We Can Speak for Ourselves: Self Advocacy By Mentally Handicapped People
Paul Williams and Bonnie Shoultz
The fundamental right of speaking for oneself has long been denied to people with developmental delays and mental retardation, who have usually had decisions made for them about every detail of their lives. In recent years, however, the Self-Advocacy Movement has been proving that people who can learn dependence can also learn independence. *We Can Speak for Ourselves* offers practical advice and support for parents, group residence workers, and others interested in developing self-advocacy for mentally handicapped people. It includes detailed models of existing projects, lists

teaching materials, and presents personal accounts by participants with mental retardation in self-advocacy projects both in the United States and England.

Price: $17.95 paperback

Other titles include:

Down's Syndrome: An Introduction for Parents
Cliff Cunningham, University of Manchester, England

Disability in Modern Children's Fiction
John Quicke, Ph.D., Sheffield University, $17.95

Using the Creative Arts in Therapy
Bernie Warren, Ph.D., $17.95

No Handicap to Dance
Dina Levete, M.B.E., $17.95

Puppetry for Mentally Handicapped People
Caroline Astell-Burt, $17.95

Yoga for Handicapped People
Barbara Brosnan, M.B., Ch.B., $17.95

BROOKLINE BOOKS
P.O. Box 1046
Cambridge, MA 02238

✱✱✱✱

The Disabled Traveller's International Phrasebook
Compiled & edited by Ian McNeil
The Disabled Traveller's International Phrasebook has been compiled for the physically challenged to help reduce the worry about potential communication problems in foreign countries. Containing a vocabulary of some 200 specialized words and over fifty phrases of particular importance to the disabled, the book is intended as a supplement to ordinary pocket dictionaries and phrasebooks which may be used in conjunction with it. A range of symbols has been designed to assist clarity and speed of reference. By combining different words and phrases and by substitution, a surprisingly wide range of communication becomes possible with *The Disabled Traveller's International Phrasebook*. It is an invaluable help to the elderly as well as the physically handicapped. All profits from the sale of this book and future Disability Press Publications will be devoted to The Multiple Sclerosis Society and The Disabled Driver's Association.

Price: 1.75 pounds including postage and packing.

DISABILITY PRESS LTD.
Applemarket House
17 Union Street
Kingston upon Thames
Surrey, KT1 1RP, England

✱✱✱✱

Accent Buyer's Guide—1988-89 Edition
This guide contains hundreds of new products and sources that can help you do things faster and easier. You can save money by using this guide, which has been completely updated, to compare products and prices.

Price: $10.00 plus .95 shipping.

Traveling Like Everyone Else
This is a practical guide to traveling around the world. The author, who uses a wheelchair, draws on experience during the past twelve years to share what she has learned about "traveling the hard way." Covers toileting and provides what-to-do information if "disaster strikes."

Price: $11.95 plus .95 shipping.

Ideas for Making Your Home Accessible
This book contains over 100 pages (many illustrated) full of tips and ideas to help you remodel or build. It includes many helpful special devices and where to get them.

Price: $6.50 plus .95 shipping.

Wheelchairs and Accessories
This guide offers an idea of what's on the market so you can make the best choice. It includes manual and powered wheelchairs, and their accessories for comfort, safety, and convenience. It also lists makers' names and addresses.

Price: $7.50 plus .95 shipping.

Single-Handed: A Book for Persons with the Use of Only One Hand
This book includes: devices and aids; special techniques; tips on how-to; illustrations; other helpful publications.

Price: $3.50 plus .70 shipping.

Other titles include:

Ideas for Kids on the Go

Recreation & Sports

Bowel Management: A Manual of Ideas and Techniques

Easy Cooking

Going Places in Your Own Vehicle

Laugh with Accent, 2nd edition

A Manual for Below-Knee Amputees

Spinal Network

Home Health Aides

Wheelchair Batteries

Post Polio

Pressure Sores

ACCENT ON LIVING
P.O. Box 700
Bloomington, IL 61702-9956

✳✳✳✳

Beyond Rage: The Emotional Impact of Chronic Physical Illness
JoAnn LeMaistre, Ph.D.

Beyond Rage defines for you the six stages of emotional response to chronic physical illness: crisis, isolation, anger, reconstruction, intermittent depression, and renewal. It illustrates them with vignettes and commentaries. Stage by stage, the book shows how to recognize harmful and unproductive responses and tells how to avoid or eliminate them. Even more, it identifies positive, helpful responses for patient, family, and therapist. Drawing on extensive clinical experience, *Beyond Rage* is direct, informative, positive, and life-affirming. It will show you how to focus on the person rather than the illness, how to find joy in the present when the future seems bleak, and how to build emotional strength when physical strength is ebbing.

The author, Dr. JoAnn LeMaistre, is an inspiring example of the able-heartedness of which she writes. She is a clinical psychologist who counsels the chronically ill and their families. She teaches in the Department of Psychiatry at Stanford Medical Center and is a lecturer, author and consultant to many organizations concerned with chronic illness. A single parent with a daughter, Dr. LeMaistre also has multiple sclerosis. Despite the deep effect MS has had on her sight and muscular capabilities, she has focused her professional experiences and accumulated wisdom to produce a helpful, hopeful message for those similarly afflicted. Dr. LeMaistre's professional capability and personal courage have brought her many honors for achievement and humanity.

"Dr.LeMaistre has written a book for self-help with the emotional impact of chronic conditions. This book is written in plain English, avoiding medical, psychological and sociological jargon ...

This is a highly readable, well written, and psychologically sound book ..."*—Journal of Visual Impairment & Blindness*
Price: $18.95

ALPINE GUILD
P.O. Box 183
Oak Park, IL 60303

✳✳✳✳

Breaking Barriers: How Children and Adults with Severe Handicaps Can Access the World Through Simple Technology
Jackie Levin, M.A., and Lynn Scherfenberg, R.P.T.

Breaking Barriers is a practical resource guide written in response to hundreds of questions from parents and service providers who want to know more about the applications of simple technology. Contents include:
•What are Automated Learning Devices
•Considerations for Using Automated Learning Devices
•Sensory Activities
•Play and Leisure Activities
•In the Kitchen
•Vocational Settings
•Mounting, Repair, and Safety
•Resource Materials
Price: $13.95

Selection and Use of Simple Technology in Home, School, Work, and Community Settings
Jackie Levin, M.A. and Lynn Scherfenberg, R.P.T.

In case study format this book answers many questions raised by parents and professionals involved in the technology decision-making process.

Case Studies of Functional Applications of Simple Technology in Recreation/Leisure, Domestic, Vocational, and Community Settings. A Functional Approach: Where Do I Begin?
Price: $17.95

ABLENET ACCESSABILITY, INC.
360 Hoover Street N.E.
Minneapolis, MN 55413

✳✳✳✳

A Handbook for the Laryngectomee, 3rd edition
Robert L. Keith
In this new edition, the author has again

provided a valuable booklet that addresses questions and doubts faced by the family when a patient returns home, including advice and information on the latest medical instruments, esophageal voice, and financial assistance. It will help to educate the patient and family, as well as to rehabilitate the post-laryngectomee who is beginning a new way of life.

Price: $3.95

International Directory of Services for the Deaf, 1980

Deaf people, the world over, have created their own social and cultural organizations. Theater societies, national associations of the deaf, and local deaf clubs exist in many countries. For many deaf people, cultural activities are built around athletic competition. There are publications either related to deafness or published by organizations of deaf people in many nations. There are also international organizations that influence the welfare of deaf people throughout the world. Lists of these organizations are provided in this edition, which is published by Gallaudet College in an effort to facilitate the interaction of professionals involved in educational programs for deaf people throughout the world.

Price: $5.95

Speaking for Ourselves: Self-Portraits of the Speech or Hearing Handicapped
Edited by Lon L. Emerick

Millions of words have been written about persons with communication disorders. There are only limited and scattered accounts of what a speech, language, or hearing disorder means from a client's point of view. In this slim volume, the speech or hearing handicapped (or their parents in the case of severe childhood disorders) tell their own stories. The reader will find despair, courage, determination, and, perhaps most important of all, hope.

Price: $7.95.

Other titles include:

Dysphagia (Swallowing Disorders): A Manual for Use by Families Under the Direction of a Speech-Language Pathologist
Grant W. Jones, M.C. Feldmann, Jerry V. Ireland, Rae Reinhart and Anastasia Yozwiak

Improving Communication in Parkinson's Disease
Richard Katz, Marsha Davidoff, and Gary Wolfe

Communication for the Laryngectomized
Ralph C. Bralley and Theresa F. Ormond

Basic Sign Language for Special Children
Judy A. Thompson

The Head-Injured Patient: A Family Guide to Assisting in Rehabilitation
Roselyn M. Cera, Nova N. Vulanich, William A. Brady, and Consulting Editor Jean Blosser

THE INTERSTATE PRINTERS & PUBLISHERS, INC.
P.O. Box 50
19 North Jackson Street
Danville, IL 61834-0050
(800) 843-4774
(217) 446-0500 in Illinois

✱✱✱✱

CHAPTER TWELVE

ORGANIZATIONS

52 ASSOCIATION FOR THE HANDICAPPED, INC.

The 52 Association for the Handicapped, Inc., provides free confidence-building sports and post-therapeutic rehabilitation nationwide to physically disabled veterans and civilian handicapped, adults and children.

The 52 Association was founded more than forty years ago to keep a promise made by fifty-two business and civic leaders to returning veterans that "The Wounded Shall Never Be Forgotten."

Over the years the "52" has fulfilled that promise in many different ways: hospital visits by famous entertainers, trips to theaters and restaurants, and coast to coast in-hospital computer training programs. The "52" expanded its efforts with the development of its unique 41-acre Sports & Recreation Center in Ossining, New York.

The Center is visited by more than 8,000 amputees, paraplegics, blind veterans, and civilian disabled each summer. They come as individual members with their families, or they come in groups by bus from VA hospitals in the Metropolitan New York/New Jersey/Connecticut areas. 52 Association Volunteers greet the buses and provide the veterans with breakfast, barbeque lunch, and dinner.

Besides a tranquil setting of quiet beauty, the Center offers a five acre lake with special paddle and sailboats for the disabled, a large swimming pool with wheelchair ramps, basketball and volleyball courts, baseball batting cages, bicycle paths with tandem bikes for use by the blind, and facilities for track and field. There are barbeque pits, wide lawns, and apple orchards; the lake is well stocked with fish.

While Ossining remains open on winter weekends, the "52's" confidence-building programs go nationwide with a series of free, four-day Learn-To-Ski Clinics for amputees and the blind. The 52 Association started its first ski program in Pennsylvania more than thirteen years ago, and today the clinics are held in major ski areas across the country and are attended by skiers from all fifty states, Mexico, and Canada. For many it is their first chance to meet other amputees in a non-hospital environment and offers an incomparable opportunity for camaraderie and the sharing of experiences.

"52" is helped by a network of volunteers—skiers who learned the sport through the clinics and now are helping others to discover that "life is not ended after a crippling injury ... it is only altered." The Association is funded through the generous support of contributors throughout the U.S., corporations, and foundations.

52 ASSOCIATION FOR THE
HANDICAPPED, INC.
441 Lexington Avenue
New York, NY 10007
(212) 986-5281

✳✳✳✳

ABLEDATA

Abledata is the largest single source for information on disability-related consumer products, with over 15,000 commercially available products listed from over 1,800 manufacturers. Products are included from fifteen categories of assistive technology, including Personal Care, Communication, Transportation, and Recreation. A custom search of the database helps you to locate and compare similar products for yourself, your family, or your client. Abledata provides information to individuals as well as rehabilitation professionals, special educators, vendors, designers of accessible buildings, and others interested in products to assist people with disabilities. In October 1988 the Adaptive Equipment Center at Newington Children's Hospital was awarded a contract from the National Institute for Disability and Rehabilitation Research of the U.S. Department of Education to maintain and develop Abledata.

For more information about Abledata, or to request an Abledata search, call (800) 344-5405 or (203) 667-5405 (in Connecticut) voice or TDD.

ABLEDATA
Adaptive Equipment Center
Newington Children's Hospital
181 East Cedar Street
Newington, CT 06111

✳✳✳✳

ALS ASSOCIATION

The ALS (Amyotrophic Lateral Sclerosis) Association (ALSA) is the only national health organization dedicated solely to the fight against ALS. From its beginnings in 1972, this nonprofit organization has grown extensively. Through its headquarters in Southern California and a growing network of local volunteer chapters and support groups, ALSA wages its battle against the disease on four important fronts: encouraging, identifying, and funding quality research into the cause, means of prevention, and possible cure of ALS—to date, over $40 million has been awarded to research scientists seeking the cause and possible cure of ALS; helping ALS patients and families through referrals for counseling, training, and support on how to cope with this devastating illness; serving as the ALS information center for the medical profession, patients, and family members; educating the public about the gravity of this problem in order to stimulate public support in the search for a cure.

Its network of local chapters and support groups sustains ALSA's effort on the grass roots level, fund raising and providing referrals and assistance in their immediate areas.

THE ALS ASSOCIATION
21021 Ventura Blvd., Suite 321
Woodland Hills, CA 91364
(818) 340-7500

✳✳✳✳

AMERICAN AMPUTEE FOUNDATION, INC.

AAF is a non-profit organization designed to assist in meeting the information and referral needs of amputees. The organization maintains contacts with self-help groups around the country, distributes publications, and provides peer counseling training manuals and other self-help guides. The AAF feels it is imperative to provide pre- and post-operative counseling to new amputees, because a knowledge of artificial limbs and their capabilities before surgery can help to alleviate some of the trauma related to the loss of a limb. The AAF has amputees across the nation who are on call to local hospitals and rehabilitation centers to help meet the visitation and counseling needs of their fellow amputees.

Other services offered by the AAF include information and referral services which assist in answering inquiries concerning employment capability, rehabilitation, availability of training, modification of the home and work site, cost and life expectancy of prosthetic devices, and other problems faced by the amputee. Resource information includes prosthetic facilities, recreational outlets and organizations, and rehabilitation services, as well as technical and scientific information concerning the state of the art in appliances and environmental control systems. Through AAF's National Resource Directory, articles in magazines such as *Ability*, brochures from professionals, and newsletters from various chapters, AAF helps to keep the amputee population updated. The Foundation also provides direct grants to amputees not able to afford the costs of prosthetic services. Applications for these grants are reviewed quarterly.

AMERICAN AMPUTEE FOUNDATION
P.O.Box 55218, Hillcrest Station
Little Rock, AR 72225
(501) 666-2523

✳✳✳✳

AMERICAN COUNCIL OF THE BLIND

The American Council of the Blind is a national consumer organization whose members are blind, visually impaired, and sighted. ACB has affiliated organizations in every state and region in the United States as well as twenty special interest affiliated organizations including the American Blind Lawyers Association, the National Alliance of Blind Students, the National Association of Blind Teachers, the Braille Revival League, Guide Dog Users, Inc., and ACB Parents.

ACB promotes the effective participation of blind people in all aspects of life and serves as a national clearinghouse providing information and referral; legal assistance; scholarships; leadership training; consumer advocate support; assistance in technological research; speaker referral services; consultative and advisory services to individuals, organizations, and agencies; and program development assistance.

Established in 1961, ACB publishes a bimonthly free national magazine, *The Braille Forum*, available in braille, large print, and on cassette. The organization also produces "ACB Reports", a half-hour monthly news information program aired on nearly 100 radio reading services nationwide.

AMERICAN COUNCIL OF THE BLIND
(ACB)
1010 Vermont Avenue N.W., Suite 1100
Washington, DC 20005
(202) 393-3666
(800) 424-8666
Oral O. Miller, National Representative

****

AMERICAN FOUNDATION FOR THE BLIND, INC.

The American Foundation for the Blind (AFB) is a national organization whose primary mission is to ensure the development, maintenance, and constant improvement of services for blind and visually impaired people in the United States. It works in partnership with over 1,000 specialized schools, agencies, and organizations nationwide to provide consultation and referrals, social research, technological research and development, publications, information services, public education, governmental relations, consumer products, and Talking Books. AFB operates a toll-free hotline (800) 232-5463, except in New York: call (212) 620-2147. AFB also maintains six regional centers in New York (Northeast), Chicago (Midwest), Dallas (Southwest), San Francisco (Western), Atlanta (Southeast), and Washington, DC (Mid-Atlantic).

AMERICAN FOUNDATION FOR THE
BLIND
15 West 16th Street
New York, NY 10011
(212) 620-2000

****

AMERICAN PARALYSIS ASSOCIATION

The American Paralysis Association, a not-for-profit volunteer organization founded in 1982, focuses on the encouragement and support of research to find a cure for paralysis caused by spinal cord injury, head injury, and stroke, but with an emphasis on the spinal cord. APA's role is one that complements organizations providing medical and rehabilitation services.

Local chapters across the country make up the heart of the APA. Through membership dues, fund-raising events, and the solicitation of corporate and foundation grants, they provide the resources with which the organization can seek out and sponsor paralysis cure research.

Specifically, two categories of activities have been funded, the major thrust being the provision of grants to support research focused on neural regeneration and recovery. Second, APA supports a variety of activities designed to enhance communication among scientists and to promote their increased involvement in cure research, such as scientific conferences, grants to encourage scientists to undertake collaborative research, and travel for graduate students to stimulate their interest in entering the field of CNS regeneration and recovery research.

The APA Spinal Cord Injury Hotline is a toll-free information and referral service for the spinal cord injured, their families, and professionals. It facilitates the search for support and resources by referring callers to individuals having personal experience, other spinal cord injury organizations, rehabilitation facilities, and SCI literature. The Hotline is available to help families organize, prioritize, and solve problems ranging from searching for rehabilitation facilities to obtaining ideas for an accessible home, from adjusting psychologically to selecting a wheelchair. The Hotline is located at the Montebello Rehabilitation Hospital in Baltimore. It can be reached by dialing (800) 526-3456 (Nationally) or (800) 638-1733 (in Maryland).

THE AMERICAN PARALYSIS
ASSOCIATION
500 Morris Avenue
Springfield, NJ 07081
(201) 379-2690
(800) 225-0292

****

AMERICAN SPINAL INJURY ASSOCIATION

Civilian centers for the treatment of spinal cord injury and disease began to appear in the United States in the late 1950s and early 1960s. During the 1960s, physicians and other medical professionals sought to align themselves as a group, in an effort to exchange ideas and work together toward the establishment of a model for care of this special patient population.

One of the groups involved in this effort began as the Association of the Western Spinal Injury

Care Systems in 1970. In 1972, the Association gave way to the Melbourne Society, which included physicians from other parts of the country. This group became the American Spinal Injury Association in 1973. Although annual scientific meetings have been the primary focus of the association, ASIA has produced publications on a variety of timely topics, and committees which consider subjects such as functional outcomes, high quadriplegia, long range planning, and prevention have been formed. In addition The American Spinal Injury Foundation (ASIF) was established to address the questions of private sector support for programs focused on current questions in the field of spinal cord injury research and treatment. Membership in the American Spinal Injury Association currently includes 335 physicians. The association is actively seeking to expand its membership, and encourages interested physicians to contact the Central Office in Chicago for membership applications and additional information. Members are accepted annually, at the October Board of Directors' Meeting, following a six month period of examination of applications received in May each year.

> AMERICAN SPINAL INJURY
> ASSOCIATION
> 250 East Superior Street, Room 619
> Chicago, IL 60611
> (312) 908-3425

✳✳✳✳

AMERICAN WHEELCHAIR BOWLING ASSOCIATION

The American Wheelchair Bowling Association is a non-profit organization established to encourage, develop, and regulate wheelchair bowling and wheelchair bowling leagues. AWBA members bowl under ABC (American Bowling Congress) Rules & Regulations in conjunction with AWBA Rules, especially adapted for wheelchair bowlers.

The AWBA holds National Wheelchair Bowling Tournaments annually. Tournament sites are rotated to assure that bowlers throughout the United States have an opportunity to participate at least once every five years. "Any wheelchair bowler may qualify by bowling in an ABC sanctioned winter league (21 game minimum), and hold valid AWBA and ABC memberships."

The AWBA publishes a national wheelchair bowling newsletter as well as a "how to" book that describes special bowling equipment and techniques. For those interested in forming new leagues, they offer a pamphlet entitled "Suggested League Rules," and have prepared a packet of forms and information needed to host a state tournament, entitled "How to Run a Successful Tournament."

Other features of the AWBA include a "Hall of Fame" honoring its outstanding members for achievement and dedication, and the AWBA Auxiliary for the families and friends of wheelchair bowlers.

The cost for AWBA membership is $15.00 a year. A life membership program is also available to both new and existing members.

> AWBA
> Daryl L. Pfister
> Exec. Secretary-Treasurer
> N54 W15858 Larkspur Lane
> Menomonee Falls, WI 53051

✳✳✳✳

AMPUTEES IN MOTION

Amputees in Motion (AIM) is a group, organized in San Diego County, California in 1973, providing amputees and their families with continuing contacts with other interested amputees and through civic, social, and recreational participation, helps amputees reestablish active and satisfying lives.

Offering understanding, encouragement, and guidance, and fostering self-help, AIM provides monthly recreational and social activities for both the amputee and his (or her) family. AIM works with physicians, physical therapists, prosthetists, and others as part of the amputee rehabilitation team, to provide empathetic support when needed, particularly before and after surgery. AIM "visitors" are matched as closely as possible to the patient's own age, sex, type of amputation, and other personal factors.

A Speakers Program is available to business, professional, social, and civic groups to promote a better understanding of the amputee's world and explain the goals of the organization. AIM also provides training for persons interested in teaching sports and arranging recreational events; transportation for amputee groups to attend concerts, games, and other recreational activities; information on driving attachments, home aids, federal and state funding, education and work benefits, and other opportunities; sporting equipment including skis, saddles, and other gear.

Annual membership is $6.00 for individuals and $12.00 for families.

AMPUTEES IN MOTION
P.O. Box 2703
Escondido, CA 92025
(619) 454-9300

****

CALIFORNIA WHEELCHAIR AVIATORS

Although there have been several handicapped flying organizations over the years, as of December 1988 the California Wheelchair Aviators (CWA) is the only active group we're aware of. CWA is a fraternal organization of over 100 with members from the U.S, Canada, Finland, France, Germany, Portugal, and Austria. Most of the participants are leg handicapped, paraplegic, quad, amputees. Many own their own planes. CWA has monthly "fly-ins" at different airports (usually in the western U.S.). The CWA newsletter is published monthly and contains information about the "fly-ins" and other member activities.

CALIFORNIA WHEELCHAIR AVIATORS
Bill Blackwood, Secretary
1117 Rising Hill Way
Escondido, CA 92025
(619) 746-5018

****

CAMP HOPE

Camp Hope is a Christian camp that serves boys and girls, ages six through sixteen, who are physically and/or mentally handicapped. Although the camp can accommodate children having a broad range of disabilities, they are unable to accommodate those who need special diets, have severe cardiac conditions, are severely or profoundly retarded, or have severe emotional problems. Campers are placed according to social abilities and maturity rather than by age. Before considering a child's application for the first time, an interview is required, either at the camp or at the child's school.

For further details, or to make an appointment for an interview, call the camp between 9:30 AM and 4:30 PM, Monday through Friday.

CAMP HOPE
Mrs. Carole Wickliffe, Camp Registrar
Box 670
Carmel, NY 10512-0670
(914) 225-2005

****

CHOICE MAGAZINE LISTENING

Choice Magazine Listening is an audio anthology for a special audience: the blind, the visually impaired, and the physically handicapped. It was created to bring the joy of reading back into the lives of those unable to read regular print—completely free of charge.

CML selects and records memorable writing from print magazines. Every other month, this unique service offers its subscribers eight hours of the best articles, fiction, and poetry, chosen from over 100 contemporary periodicals and read by professional voices onto 8 rpm phonograph records. (CML provides information on how to obtain the necessary 8 rpm-speed record player which is supplied free to eligible individuals by the National Library Service for the Blind and Physically Handicapped of the Library of Congress. The NLS requires that the player be used in conjunction with its program of free talking books and magazines, as well as for playing Choice Magazine Listening.)

CML, a project of the nonprofit Lucerna Fund, welcomes new subscribers on a first come, first served basis. Enjoy unabridged selections from such diverse periodicals as *Smithsonian*, *The Atlantic*, *The New Yorker*, *Ms.*, *Sports Illustrated*, *BBC Listener*, *Country Journal*, *Esquire*, *Audubon*, *The Wall Street Journal*, and *The New York Times Magazine*, along with occasional material from other media sources.

CHOICE MAGAZINE LISTENING
P.O. Box 10
Port Washington, NY 11050

****

CMT INTERNATIONAL

CMT International is an organization for people around the world who have Charcot-Marie-Tooth disease, a progressively debilitating neuromuscular disorder. CMT's bimonthly newsletter serves some 3,000 families in sixteen countries. The organization regularly publishes research updates and also sponsors research regarding CMT. An index of information published during the last four years is available on request.

CMT INTERNATIONAL
34 Bayview Drive
St. Catharines, Ontario L2N 4Y6
Canada

****

DISABILITY SERVICES

Boston University has over 200 handicapped students, staff, and faculty among the 35,000 members of its total community. Disability Services (DS), a full-time department of the Division of Student Affairs, works to ensure that University community members with various impairments get the accommodations they need for a mainstreamed campus life. A full campus life means access not only to the classroom, but to extracurricular activities, to approximately 250 student organizations, to men's and women's sports, to internationally noted guest speakers, to the physical development programs of a modern athletic center, to the specialized facilities of nine campus libraries, and to residence parties, art galleries, concerts, live theater, and the most popular films. Most routine activities are fully accessible.

Anytime a student has a question about whether a class or an event is accessible, or any time that special needs require an accommodation, DS is available.

DISABILITY SERVICES
William "Kip" Opperman, Director
Boston University
Martin Luther King, Jr. Center
19 Deerfield Street
Boston, MA 02215

****

DISABLED LIVING FOUNDATION

Disabled Living Foundation (DLF) works to reduce the handicapping effects of disability by finding non-medical solutions to the daily living problems facing disabled people of all ages. Its main activities are research and information provision.

Research is carried out into areas of unmet need. If a study shows that further action is necessary, the DLF may take the action itself or prepare the ground for another more appropriate body to do so.

Information is held on all aspects of living with a disability. Particular emphasis is laid on problem-solving using equipment and technical aids. Information on services, benefits, design criteria, and legislation is also included. Information on products for disabled people is held in a computerized database available on-line at the DLF. Information is provided free to disabled people and their families and a subscription service is offered to those with a professional interest.

The DLF provides a number of advisory services including The Clothing and Footwear Advisory Service and The Incontinence Advisory Service. The latter provides information through the enquiry service, regular courses, and resource papers. The Music Advisory Service aims to encourage all kinds of musical opportunities, and the Visual Handicap Advisory Service was set up in response to the need for information on the daily living problems facing people with low vision (as opposed to people who have no useful vision).

The Equipment Centre contains a comprehensive range of adaptive equipment for people of all ages for use at home or elsewhere. Professional staff (occupational therapists and physiotherapists) provide practical information and demonstrate the equipment to potential users and to anyone professionally concerned.

The Reference Library contains a specialized collection of publications on the diverse aspects of living with a disability. A large intake of current periodicals ensures up-to-date news and information.

THE DISABLED LIVING FOUNDATION
380-384 Harrow Road
London W9 2HU, England

****

THE EPILEPSY FOUNDATION OF AMERICA

The Epilepsy Foundation of America (EFA) is the only national, charitable, nonprofit voluntary agency in the United States specifically dedicated to the welfare of people with epilepsy. It is governed by an all-volunteer board of directors and its programs are reviewed by a volunteer professional advisory board, of which 60 percent of the members are physicians.

EFA is committed to the prevention and control of epilepsy and to improving the lives of people who have it. It works to achieve these goals through a broad range of programs of information and education, advocacy, support of research, and the delivery of needed services to people with epilepsy and their families.

EFA conducts national programs and also produces program materials that its affiliates can use in providing local services. Major national programs include:

Research. To develop better treatments, new

drugs, and to solve the medical puzzle of epilepsy. Through its fellowship programs EFA encourages young scientists to become interested in a career in epilepsy research and trains new epilepsy specialists.

Information and Education. To improve public understanding of epilepsy through production of mass media campaigns and annual distribution of more than one million pamphlets and other materials.

Advocacy. To fight discrimination and support the process of deinstitutionalization. Government advocacy volunteers and staff also point out ways in which government action can remove inequities and barriers to the participation of people with epilepsy in the mainstream of American life.

Membership. To ease the financial burdens of epilepsy, EFA offers its members the opportunity to purchase anti-epileptic medication at lower than average retail cost. Members also receive a free subscription to a twelve-page monthly newspaper. Membership in EFA is open to all.

Employment Programs. To aid people with epilepsy to find and keep competitive work. The national office offers a Training and Placement Service in thirteen cities.

The National Epilepsy Library and Resource Center provides authoritative information to professionals and the public. The Center has computer access to major collections of medical information.

The state and local affiliates of EFA provide and obtain needed services for people with epilepsy in the community. The number of programs offered depends on the size of the local organization and the support it has been able to secure from the community.

EPILEPSY FOUNDATION OF AMERICA
4351 Garden City Drive
Landover, MD 20785
(301) 459-3700

✳✳✳✳

THE FRIEDREICH'S ATAXIA GROUP IN AMERICA, INC.

The Friedreich's Ataxia Group in America, Inc. was founded in 1969 by people who have Friedreich's Ataxia. The group is concerned about the physical and emotional well being of each individual and their families. It financially supports research into the cause and treatment of FA. This and other information relating to persons with dis-

abilities is made available to the members through a Newsletter. There are no membership dues.

FRIEDREICH'S ATAXIA GROUP IN AMERICA, INC.
P.O. Box 11116
Oakland, CA 94611
(415) 655-0833

✳✳✳✳

GUIDE DOG FOUNDATION FOR THE BLIND, INC.

The Guide Dog Foundation for the Blind, Inc., established in 1946, is a private non-profit, non-sectarian organization, for the primary purpose of blind rehabilitation through the use of guide dogs. A guide dog, all of its equipment, a formal 25-day residential training program, and a comprehensive aftercare service are all given, at no charge, to deserving people who seek the independence, mobility, and companionship that a guide dog provides.

The dogs for the program, purebred Labrador Retrievers and Golden Retrievers, are provided through the Foundation's breeding program. Volunteer families, termed "puppy walkers," raise the pups from the age of seven weeks to one year, when the dogs are returned to the Foundation to begin formal training. Throughout the puppy walker year, the pups' progress is supervised by a staff member who makes periodic home visits. All veterinary expenses are assumed by the Foundation.

Five or six times a year, a class of ten to twelve students comes to the Smithtown Center for the residential training program. Students are taught to work with and care for their dogs, with a comprehensive curriculum encompassing all forms of public transportation (including the New York City subway system), "country" walks with no sidewalks, shopping malls, restaurants, turnstiles, and elevators. When the students leave with their new helpers, they are ready to meet the challenges awaiting them with confidence and enthusiasm. In order to maintain a high level of performance from the graduate units in the field, a comprehensive aftercare service is provided.

Currently, sixty person/dog units are graduated annually, with a gradual increase to a maximum of 100 units anticipated. Public education regarding blindness and guide dogs is carried out by a Speakers Bureau of graduates, who visit schools and organizations. This is an adjunct activity to the training program itself.

The Guideway is the official newsletter of the Guide Dog Foundation for the Blind and is available on cassette. The Foundation would be pleased to have the name and address of anyone who would like to receive a copy.

THE GUIDE DOG FOUNDATION FOR
THE BLIND, INC.
371 E. Jericho Tpke.
Smithtown, NY 11787
(516) 265-2121 ,(800) 548-4337

****

HANDICAPS WELFARE ASSOCIATION

The Handicaps Welfare Association was set up as a self help group among disabled people in Singapore. The association loans technical aids such as wheelchairs, walking sticks, and commodes to needy members and the public without charge. It also organizes activities of a social and recreational nature to provide members with opportunities to integrate with the community.

Sporting activities such as swimming, bowling, basketball, and track and field events are actively promoted among members to assist them to develop a sense of achievement and good health. The association operates a subsidized transport service to ferry disabled members who encounter difficulties in commuting between their homes and work places.

HWA started its driving service in 1985 to teach the disabled how to drive a car which has been specially adapted with a hand controlled gadget. The service is open to all disabled people.

The association conducts classes to equip members with basic language skills or to enable members to acquire knowledge that would enhance their employment prospects. It also offers financial assistance to members who wish to pursue on their own, studies of an academic, creative, or recreational nature.

Handicaps Digest, a magazine published bimonthly by the association, is essentially in English, with about 10 percent of the articles and editorials in the Chinese language. It is distributed without charge to all disabled members, government departments, other social agencies, companies, individuals, and overseas agencies that exchange periodicals.

HANDICAPS WELFARE ASSOCIATION
Whampoa Drive
(Behind Block 102)
Singapore 1232
Tel: 2543006

****

HELEN KELLER NATIONAL CENTER FOR DEAF-BLIND YOUTHS AND ADULTS

The power of touch is the power of communication. It has the strength and the gentleness to heal, to support, to encourage, and to teach. The endless list of creative ways to convey a thought, share an idea, or make your presence known is awesome and inspiring. Although many of us think of language when we think of communication, it is not necessarily a requirement. A smile, a hug, a handshake, or a pat on the shoulder are telling the person you care. There are many deaf/blind people who have had no formal language development, but who do have a strong awareness of other people and situations.

"My hand is to me what your hearing and sight together are to you. All my comings and goings turn on the hand as a pivot. It is the hand that binds me to the world of men and women. The hand is my feeler with which I reach through isolation and darkness and seize every pleasure, every activity that my fingers encounter."—Helen Keller

Established in 1967 by a unanimous act of Congress, the Helen Keller National Center for Deaf-Blind Youths and Adults, a comprehensive rehabilitation, research, and training facility, is operated by Helen Keller Services For The Blind. The Helen Keller National Center is located on a 25-acre campus in Sands Point, Long Island. The buildings that constitute the Center are newly constructed, utilizing all specially designed features that are necessary for accessibility, comfort, convenience, and safety. The Peter J. Salmon Hall, where deaf-blind individuals share air-conditioned twin bedrooms with private baths, is attractively furnished.

HELEN KELLER NATIONAL CENTER
For Deaf-Blind Youths and Adults
111 Middle Neck Road
Sands Point, NY 11050

****

IN TOUCH NETWORKS

In Touch Networks is a "newsstand of the air" which uses the airwaves to bring the current press to thousands of print-impaired individuals across the country. From its small studios on West 48th Street in New York City, every day of the year, twenty-four hours each day, more than 400 volunteer broadcasters read 104 different current magazines, periodicals, and newspapers, including three in Spanish, to those whose limitations, either visual or physical, necessitate that they "hear" the publications which they cannot see, or hold, to read.

In addition, In Touch presents five public service interview shows, one each day of the week. These programs cover a wide range of subjects including consumerism and daily living skills for the handicapped. In Touch also offers a "Job Bank of the Air," a program describing current employment opportunities for the handicapped from files of the organization, "Just One Break," ("JOB"). With the exception of the Executive Director and one other administrator, all personnel, including the broadcast engineers, are blind or have seriously limited sight. In addition to the paid staff, 400 dedicated readers come to the studios at all hours, and in all weather, weekends and holidays included, to perform all of In Touch's broadcasting.

IN TOUCH NETWORKS, INC.
322 West 48th Street
New York, NY 10036
(212) 586-5588

****

INDEPENDENT LIVING RESEARCH UTILIZATION PROGRAM

The Independent Living Research Utilization Program (ILRU) is a national center for information, training, research, and technical assistance in independent living. Its goal is to expand the body of knowledge in independent living and to improve the utilization of results of research programs and demonstration projects in this field. It is a program of The Institute for Rehabilitation and Research, a nationally recognized, free-standing rehabilitation facility for persons with physical disabilities.

Since ILRU was established in 1977, it has developed a variety of strategies for collecting, synthesizing, and disseminating information related to the field of independent living. ILRU staff—a majority of whom are people with disabilities—serve independent living centers, state rehabilitation agencies, federal and regional rehabilitation agencies, consumer organizations, rehabilitation service providers, educational institutions, medical facilities, and other organizations involved in the field, both nationally and internationally. ILRU provides on-site technical assistance to independent living centers in thirty-two states and five foreign countries.

This organization compiled a national directory of programs providing independent living services, which is updated regularly. ILRU's *Directory of Independent Living Programs* is a comprehensive listing of over 330 programs providing independent living services in the U.S. and other countries. The organization also developed and maintains the ILRU National Database on Independent Living Programs, a computerized listing of data on 167 programs.

ILRU annually distributes more than 6140 books, pamphlets, posters, and videotapes related to independent living. It maintains an ongoing agenda of research, publications, and conferences on attendant services, and publishes a current bibliography on attendant-related literature. ILRU is presently developing a method for assessing the adequacy of attendant services and has developed a variety of resource materials on independent living subjects, including a technical report series; directories of independent living programs, people who provide technical assistance, and independent living support materials; a bi-monthly newsletter; handbooks providing background information on the independent living movement and on establishing and operating an independent living center; posters depicting people with disabilities as active and productive members of society; audio-visual products on different versions of independent living programs, on repairing manual wheelchairs, and on rural independent living.

INDEPENDENT LIVING RESEARCH UTILIZATION
3400 Bissonnet, Suite 101
Houston, TX 77005
(713) 666-6244

****

INTERNATIONAL POLIO NETWORK

The International Polio Network (IPN) is the world center of information on polio and the late effects of polio. IPN was formally established in 1985 by Gazette International Networking Institute (G.I.N.I.) to link polio survivors and to coordinate post-polio support groups.

G.I.N.I. was founded in 1958 by Gini Laurie to publish an international journal, *Rehabilitation Gazette*, written by and for persons disabled by polio. Gini never had polio, but the disease killed her two sisters and later, her brother. The *Gazette* began as a sort of mimeograph gossip sheet to keep former patients in touch. The *Rehabilitation Gazette* has always maintained a network of polio survivors. Therefore, in 1979, it was the first to recognize the increasing numbers of polio survivors reporting new symptoms of pain, fatigue, weakness, and breathing difficulties. The *Gazette* has grown from a local newsletter to a renowned international journal reaching 40,000 readers in eighty-seven countries (with translations in Japanese) and evolved to include other physical disabilities and the aging of all disabled persons.

IPN publishes the *Polio Network News*, a quarterly newsletter. It is an international newsletter for polio survivors, support groups, physicians, and resource centers, to exchange information, encourage research, and promote networking among the post-polio community. The subscription/membership cost for polio survivors is $8.00; $15.00 for health professionals.

IPN compiles and publishes the Post-Polio Directory of 250 support groups, 60 clinics, and 100 health professionals. It also organizes support group leaders' workshops and resources 250 support groups and biennial international polio and independent living conferences for polio survivors and health professionals, and publishes proceedings of these conferences.

IPN publishes the *Handbook on the Late Effects of Poliomyelitis for Physicians and Survivors*. (Available from IPN for $6.75.)

G.I.N.I. publishes the International Ventilators Users Network newsletter and a handbook: *Ventilators and Muscular Dystrophy*. The newsletter explores topics such as equipment, breathing techniques, travel, and family life and includes notices of publications, conferences, and workshops. Published biannually, the cost for ventilator users is $5.00; $15.00 for health professionals.

INTERNATIONAL POLIO NETWORK
(IPN)
4502 Maryland Avenue
St. Louis, MO 63108
(314) 361-0475

✳✳✳✳

MOBILITY INTERNATIONAL USA

Mobility International USA (MIUSA) was founded in 1973 in London and has as its purpose to promote and facilitate opportunities for people with disabilities to participate in international educational exchange and travel.

Mobility International has offices in over twenty-five countries throughout the world. MIUSA offers a travel information and referral service, news of international work-camp openings—volunteer with people of all ages and nationalities to work on community projects throughout the world, and help in selecting and applying to international educational exchange programs.

In addition MIUSA publishes a quarterly newsletter that tells about the latest opportunities concerning travel and international exchange programs, and provides information on scholarships, specialized tours, and new publications. It provides details on MIUSA's community service programs and educational tours, and on upcoming international conferences.

MIUSA publishes two resource books entitled: *A World Option: A Guide to International Educational Exchange, Community Service and Travel for Persons with Disabilities* and *A Manual for Integrating Persons with Disabilities into International Educational Exchange Programs*.

MOBILITY INTERNATIONAL USA
P.O. Box 3551
Eugene, OR 97403
(503) 343-1284 (Voice and TDD)

✳✳✳✳

NATIONAL ARTHRITIS AND MUSCULOSKELETAL AND SKIN DISEASES INFORMATION CLEARINGHOUSE

The National Arthritis and Musculoskeletal and Skin Diseases Information Clearinghouse is a national resource center for information about professional, patient, and public education materials; community demonstration programs and federal programs related to rheumatic, musculoskeletal, and skin diseases. The Clearinghouse is a program of the National Institutes of Health.

The Clearinghouse continually updates its database of references to journal articles, books, audiovisual materials, brochures, fact sheets, newsletter articles, manuals, and other education materials. Many of these materials—the so-called fugitive literature—are not listed elsewhere. The database is part of CHID—the Combined Health Information Database—which incorporates the computerized files of nine health information and education programs supported and managed by the federal government.

CHID can also be accessed through BRS

Information Technologies, a national database vendor, (800) 468-0908. Individuals need a telecommunicating computer terminal or a personal computer with a modem. CHID is also accessible through hospital and university libraries, public libraries, and organizations that subscribe to BRS.

NATIONAL ARTHRITIS AND
MUSCULOSKELETAL AND SKIN
DISEASES INFORMATION
CLEARINGHOUSE
Box AMS
Bethesda, MD 20892
(301) 468-3235

✳✳✳✳

NATIONAL ASSOCIATION OF ANOREXIA NERVOSA AND ASSOCIATED DISORDERS, INC.

The National Association of Anorexia Nervosa and Associated Disorders, Inc. (ANAD) has provided counsel and information to thousands of anorexics and bulimics, families and health professionals. ANAD has located more than 2000 therapists, hospitals, and clinics in the U.S. and Canada treating anorexia nervosa and bulimia, and has developed an early detection program to alert parents, teachers, and others to the dangers of these disorders. The organization also distributes information about eating disorders to health professionals and provides staff or resources to facilitate lectures, workshops, and seminars nationwide.

ANAD is assisting in the formation of chapters and self-help groups in order for anorexics and their families to meet others with similar problems. There are now affiliated groups in most states of the nation as well as in Canada and West Germany. ANAD distributes its quarterly newsletter to thousands of anorexics, bulimics, concerned family members, health professionals, and schools, and has undertaken or assisted in the development of several research projects.

All services of this organization are offered without charge.

ANAD
Box 7
Highland Park, IL 60035
(312) 831-3438

✳✳✳✳

NATIONAL ASSOCIATION OF THE PHYSICALLY HANDICAPPED, INC.

The National Association of the Physically Handicapped, Inc. (NAPH) is a working organization of handicapped persons. Its primary purposes are to promote employment, accessible public transportation, the elimination of architectural barriers, and increased public awareness.

NAPH is the only national organization with membership open to all disability groups. NAPH does nothing in rehabilitation; has no professional staff; offers no services. It is a voluntary, independent self-help association supported mainly by membership dues and run by the members themselves.

For an annual fee of $10.00, members receive all NAPH mailings including the NAPH National Newsletter, President's Memos, "Calls" to Meetings and Conventions.

NAPH is always anxious to start new Chapters. To start a NAPH Chapter requires a minumin of five physically handicapped persons (plus interested non-handicapped persons)—of voting age, at least eighteen years old—who are willing to pay National and Local dues, and work for the goals of the NAPH National Organization, and the needs of the physically handicapped persons in your area. Contact the Chairperson of Membership and Organization in NAPH for starting a NAPH Chapter in your area.

NATIONAL ASSOCIATION OF THE
PHYSICALLY HANDICAPPED, INC.
76 Elm Street
London, OH 43140

✳✳✳✳

NATIONAL ODD SHOE EXCHANGE

National Odd Shoe Exchange is one of the most unusual organizations on record. It is a service to help the foot-handicapped all over the country, those whose feet are not the same size, or persons with only one foot. The exchange brings together those persons with similar shoe problems and helps them in exchanging shoes with those of opposite shoe size.

This exchange deals with shoes, and with names of persons of similar ages and tastes in shoe styles. When two persons wearing the exact opposites are found, they are notified and they make their own arrangements for the disposal of shoes they now have or for the purchase of future pairs. In the case of amputees, the same procedure applies, with only one shoe.

Shoe stores all over the United States are sending the Exchange their new single and mismated shoes that they usually throw away. The Exchange is working with shoe manufacturing companies and stores to sell mismated shoes, too.

The National Odd Shoe Exchange was founded in 1943 by Ruth Rubin Feldman, who has since retired and is living in California. Jeanne Sallman, Director, joined the organization in the 50's because of a birth defect causing the need for a 6B on her left foot and a 4B on the right foot. The National Odd Shoe Exchange does not guarantee that everyone will be successful in finding "mismates," however, as the membership grows, the service will become more helpful.

The initial fee to join the National Odd Shoe Exchange is $35.00 of which $25.00 is a lifetime registration and $10.00 the annual dues. Full refund on shoes and services if the Exchange cannot help in one year.

This organization offers free shoes, socks, and gloves to amputees; they just ask for reimbursement of the postage.

NATIONAL ODD SHOE EXCHANGE
P.O. Box 56845
Phoenix, AZ 85079-6845

****

NATIONAL STROKE ASSOCIATION

National Stroke Association (NSA) is dedicated to educating stroke survivors, families, health professionals, and the general public about stroke. It seeks to reduce the incidence and effects of stroke through activities related to prevention, medical care, rehabilitation, and resocialization.

NSA develops and distributes educational materials and a newsletter; operates a national clearinghouse for information and referral; promotes research and disseminates research findings; advocates; develops workshops; provides guidance in developing stroke clubs and stroke support groups.

NSA publications include:

The Road Ahead: A Stroke Recovery Guide, published in 1986, as a daily handbook for stroke survivors, family members, and professionals. (This rehabilitation guide will be adapted for readers in England and Australia.)

"Be Stroke Smart," a packet of twenty-five one-page leaflets on various subjects dealing with stroke and rehabilitation, updated periodically.

NSA also produces a number of other booklets and brochures of interest to stroke survivors, families, other caregivers, and health care professionals. A complete list of titles and prices is available.

Negotiations are underway for translation of NSA pamphlets into Spanish, allowing this literature to be given to Spanish-speaking patients and caregivers, as well as promoted in Latin and South America.

NSA corresponds with stroke survivors, medical personnel, and physicians in over fifteen countries including Japan, France, Germany and the Soviet Union.

NATIONAL STROKE ASSOCIATION
300 East Hampden Avenue, Suite 240
Englewood, CO 80110-2622
(303) 762-9922

****

NATIONAL WHEELCHAIR ATHLETIC ASSOCIATION

"Dedicated to the Guidance and Growth of Wheelchair Sports," the National Wheelchair Athletic Association was founded in 1956 in New York as pioneers in rehabilitation came to recognize that recreational and competitive sports play an invaluable part in the rehabilitative process and daily life for physically disabled individuals. By 1987, the NWAA had grown to represent over 3,000 athletes and had restructured itself into a wheelchair sports federation. Every year, junior and adult athletes across the country participate in local and regional games.

The NWAA, a Group E member of the United States Olympic Committee, is the governing body for six Olympic sports—Air Guns, Archery, Athletics (Track, Field, Long Distance Racing), Swimming, Table Tennis, and Weightlifting. NWAA also represents wheelchair basketball and wheelchair tennis at Olympic levels venues; nationally and internationally.

NWAA programs include: Publications (annual Rulebook, quarterly newsletter), Video Rental, U.S. Olympic Committee Member, Local and Regional Wheelchair Games for Adults and Juniors, Local Wheelchair Sports Development, National Training Camps, Road Race Series, National Wheelchair Games, Junior National Wheelchair Games, International Team Trials, Pan American Wheelchair Games, World Wheelchair Games, Events in U.S. Olympic Festivals, Events in Summer Olympic Games, and National Workshops.

NATIONAL WHEELCHAIR ATHLETIC
ASSOCIATION
3617 Betty Drive, Suite S
Colorado Springs, CO 80917-5993

✳✳✳✳

PROMOTE REAL INDEPENDENCE FOR THE DISABLED AND ELDERLY

Promote Real Independence for the Disabled and Elderly (PRIDE) is a national organization dedicated to solving clothing problems. Evelyn Kennedy is the moving force behind PRIDE Inc., a non-profit charitable foundation that strongly promotes the message "looking right leads to feeling right." In the late 60's, Kennedy had a skiing accident that left her confined in a hip-to-toe cast for more than a year. When the cast finally came off, she had to struggle with a leg brace and crutches for two additional years. "Getting dressed, if I could find something to wear, was an ordeal. The clothes I could manage to get on looked terrible and felt worse. I became more and more depressed." Drawing upon her sewing skills, she developed comfortable, well-fitting garments that distracted attention from the brace. Kennedy also developed a flexible teaching device which later evolved into a training vest. This vest was the prototype for a copyrighted design used at rehabilitation centers and currently available from PRIDE. People with special clothing needs began to contact her for help. Although she offered her services through Sewtique, a full-service sewing center that she owned in 1972, few of the disabled could afford to pay for a custom design. So she began making things for them at night. As the number of requests grew, her husband helped her establish the PRIDE Foundation and he provided the initial financial support. Today, PRIDE is funded solely by contributions and by monies Kennedy raises through speaking engagements on its behalf. One of her favorite projects is a jacket designed for a little boy with multiple impairments. It usually took two people to put his coat on. Kennedy and an intern from the University of Connecticut designed a jacket that slipped on from the front and closed with Velcro across the back. To provide him with tactile pleasure, they chose corduroy and soft fleece, fabrics that would look good and feel good next to his skin. The jacket was the envy of the other children in his special school.

(Reprinted from "Designer Helps the Handicapped Dress with Pride," by Anne Marie Soto, *Sew News*, May 1987; reprinted by permission, copyright © 1987 by PJS Publications Inc., Peoria, IL.)

The main objective of the PRIDE Foundation based in Groton, Connecticut is rehabilitation assistance for the disabled and elderly in the areas of home management and independence in dressing and personal grooming. Consulting services are provided to agencies and organizations dealing with special needs of special persons. PRIDE tries to meet the needs that are not presently met by clothing manufacturers.

These publications are available:

Dressing with Pride
This book is filled with useful sewing information including shopping tips, a wardrobe planning guide, patterns for custom designs, and suggested adaptive devices for dressing and grooming.

Clothing Lesson Plan
A curriculum guide and in-service training manual which is a resource for members of the health care team and educators involved in training and providing service to the disabled and elderly. The plan is designed for hands-on workshop session(s) with emphasis on clothing as an integral part of the rehabilitation process.

"Scoliosis"
This is a ten-page report describing alteration procedures for off-the-rack clothing, as well as suggested changes to commercial patterns.

"Resources and Clothing for Special Needs"
This is a listing of services, catalogs, books, etc., to provide resource suggestions for the disabled, the elderly, and their families, educators, and health-care professionals.

PROMOTE REAL INDEPENDENCE FOR
THE DISABLED AND ELDERLY
71 Plaza Court
Groton, CT 06340

✳✳✳✳

REHABILITATION INTERNATIONAL

Rehabilitation International (RI) is a federation of national, regional, and international organizations working together to promote the prevention of disability, the rehabilitation of disabled people, and the equalization of opportunities within society on behalf of disabled people and their families throughout the world. RI is currently composed of 120 organizations leading disability prevention and rehabilitation service development in eighty nations in all the world's regions.

RI maintains official relations with the United Nations Economic and Social Council, the World Health Organization, the International Labour Office, UNESCO, UNICEF, the Organization of American States, the Commission of European Communities, and the Council of Europe. It provides the secretariat for the International Council on Disability, a coordinating body of thirty-five international non-government organizations working in the fields of disability prevention and rehabilitation.

RI is an open forum for the exchange of experience and information on research and practice; an advocate for policies and legislation recognizing the rights of disabled people and their families; a deliberative body which develops guidelines for the future development of rehabilitation policy and practice; a catalyst for change of public attitudes to encourage the equal participation of disabled people in education, employment, and the cultural and social life of their communities.

Rehabilitation International produces an comprehensive array of periodicals and publications concerning the international aspects of disability issues and rehabilitation.

Supporting members receive subscriptions to five periodicals reporting on issues and developments in disability and rehabilitation worldwide; invitations to RI World Congresses, regional conferences, and other international meetings and events; and a membership card.

REHABILITATION INTERNATIONAL
25 East 21st Street
New York, NY 10010
(212) 420-1500

＊＊＊＊

THE ROYAL ASSOCIATION FOR DISABILITY AND REHABILITATION

The Royal Association for Disability and Rehabilitation (RADAR) is the champion of Britain's 3 million disabled people. RADAR seeks to ensure that wherever possible and appropriate disabled schoolchildren are educated alongside their able-bodied friends. The Association has also conducted research into the difficulties disabled children experience in learning to become physically and emotionally independent.

RADAR is involved in trying to improve "access." It does this by advising designers, local authorities, and others on how buildings and public and private transport, can be designed, adapted, and managed so that disabled people can use them.

The *RADAR Bulletin* is published monthly and gives details of new legislation, housing, holidays, entertainment, mobility aids, and appliances. The quarterly journal *Contact* deals with these subjects in greater depth. RADAR publishes literature on all aspects of disability, and a copy of its Publications List is available free from the Publications Officer.

RADAR acts with local authorities and others to encourage well designed housing, and also provides help and advice for individuals who want to find and adapt their own homes. RADAR's annual publication, *Holidays for the Handicapped* contains a wealth of information on hotels, self-catering, and purpose-built accommodation, activity holidays, transport, and details about traveling abroad. The Association advises holiday organizations, tour operators and individuals on how best to help disabled people and their families enjoy their holidays.

RADAR seeks to encourage employers everywhere to recognize a disabled person's right to work and to realize that their disability is rarely an insurmountable problem. RADAR achieves this by research, by informing and publicizing the advantages of employing disabled people and by responding to enquiries from would-be employers and employees alike.

THE ROYAL ASSOCIATION FOR
DISABILITY AND REHABILITATION
25 Mortimer Street
London W1N 8A, England
Tel: 01-637 5400

＊＊＊＊

SPECIAL OLYMPICS

Special Olympics contributes to the physical, social, and psychological development of people with mental retardation. Through successful experiences in sports, they gain confidence and build a positive self-image which carries over into the classroom, the home, the job, and the community.

The mission of Special Olympics is to provide year-round sports training and athletic competition in a variety of Olympic-type sports for all children and adults with mental retardation, giving them continuing opportunities to develop physical fitness, demonstrate courage, experience joy, and participate in the sharing of gifts, skills, and friendship with their familiies, other Special Olympics athletes, and the community.

The concept of Special Olympics began in the

early 1960's when Eunice Kennedy Shriver started a day camp for people with mental retardation. From that experience it was clear that people with mental retardation were far more capable in sports and physical activities than even many experts believed. In 1968 Mrs. Shriver organized the First International Special Olympic Games at Soldier Field in Chicago, where 1000 athletes from the United States and Canada competed in track and field and swimming.

Since 1968 more than one million children and adults with mental retardation have participated in Special Olympics. Today there are Special Olympics programs in 25,000 U.S. communities, representing 97% of the counties in the U.S., and in more than seventy countries worldwide. Local, state, and national offices administer their respective programs under the guidance of Special Olympics Headquarters in Washington, D.C.

The official Summer Sports are: Aquatics, Athletics, Basketball, Bowling, Equestrian, Gymnastics, Roller Skating, Soccer, Softball, and Volleyball. The official Winter Sports are: Alpine Skiing, Figure Skating, Floor Hockey, Nordic Skiing, Poly Hockey, and Speed Skating. The Demonstration Sports are: Canoeing, Cycling, Table Tennis, Team Handball, Tennis, and Weightlifting.

Special Olympics is run almost entirely by volunteers. Over 500,000 volunteers provide manpower for Special Olympics programs worldwide. The volunteers include high school and college students, members of civic and fraternal groups, amateur and professional athletes, sports officials and coaches, teachers, parents, and retired persons.

Over 15,000 Local Games, Meets, and Tournaments are held in both Summer and Winter sports each year in communities all over the world. Chapter (or state) Games are also held annually, while National programs either hold National Games or join together for Regional Games.

"In Special Olympics, it is not the strongest body or the most dazzling mind that counts. It is the invincible spirit which overcomes all handicaps. For without this spirit, winning medals is empty. But with it there is no defeat."—Eunice Kennedy Shriver

If you want to join an existing Special Olympics program, or start a local or National Program where none exists, please write to:

SPECIAL OLYMPICS INTERNATIONAL
1350 New York Avenue, N.W., Suite 500
Washington, DC 20005
(202) 628-3630

****

TECHNICAL AIDS AND ASSISTANCE FOR THE DISABLED

In 1981 the Committee on Personal Computers and the Handicapped (COPH-2) recognized that many persons with disabilities knew the usefulness of computers but did not know how to access them. COPH-2 began pulling together scattered information about the ways personal computers could be adapted for persons with visual or physical impairments. At COPH-2's monthly meetings children and adults with disabilities were invited to try some computer systems and adaptive aids. But monthly meetings were not enough. What was needed was a permanent site with both staff and volunteers offering expanded services on a day-to-day basis.

To meet this challenge the TAAD Center was launched. The Center provides several opportunities:

• To use and compare personal computers and suitable adaptive devices
• To receive technical assistance
• To network with others to share common concerns and experiences via the national COPH-2 Bulletin Board
• To access a wide range of literature on personal computers and their adaptability for persons with disabilities
• To avail yourself of information gathered via SpecialNet and AppleNet databases
• To arrange for the loan of computers and special adaptive devices
• To join in seminars for the purpose of problem-solving
• To attend product demonstrations
• To participate in advocacy before manufacturers, distributors, service providers, and others.

"Our needs are great, but the rewards are even greater. Here are two examples of what we have accomplished, and what we can continue to achieve.

A ten-year-old boy with quadriplegia who could not speak, needed to expand his use of the computer to include word processing and math, plus use the computer to develop independence and social skills. COPH-2 gave him the opportunity, through demonstration and instruction, to gain experience on multiple setups of computer systems. As a result, he now can type a letter to his mother and has realized the potential that computer technology holds for his life.

A woman in California contacted us about a

recent disability which forced her to remain flat on her back. She had spent a lifetime teaching the harpsichord and wanted to share her knowledge by writing a text on the subject. We were able to put her in touch with another person in a similar physical condition who had years of experience using a special computer system. With this shared knowledge she has begun to write her book."

TECHNICAL AIDS AND ASSISTANCE
FOR THE DISABLED (TAAD)
1950 West Roosevelt Road
Chicago, IL 60608
(800) 346-2939
(312) 421-3373

✳✳✳✳

TELEPHONE PIONEERS OF AMERICA

Telephone Pioneers of America is one of the world's largest volunteer service organizations having a membership of more than 750,000 working and retired members of the telecommunications industry. Located throughout the United States and Canada, Pioneers, wherever they live, are dedicated to answering the call of those in need: the disabled, the disadvantaged, and the lonely.

The Telephone Pioneers of America are the official repair depot for "talking books" equipment (audiotape cassettes and players) that the Library of Congress furnishes for the blind. Pioneers are also the inventors and adaptors of a whole catalog's worth of special equipment designed to raise the quality of life for those who are hearing, visually, or mobility impaired.

TELEPHONE PIONEERS OF AMERICA
22 Cortlandt Street
New York, NY 10007

✳✳✳✳

U.S. ASSOCIATION FOR BLIND ATHLETES

U.S. Association For Blind Athletes (USABA) was created in 1976 and sent a team to the Summer Paralympic Games in Toronto, Canada. Before 1976, no athletic organization existed for blind or visually impaired athletes. USABA is not only an athletic organization, it is also a support group.

USABA works to encourage and promote athletic participation among blind and visually impaired individuals. They organize competition from national to international levels.

USABA is a non-profit organization and is dedicated to expanding opportunities to blind and visually impaired athletes by developing physical and sociological well being through sports programs. Currently there are eleven events for athletes to choose from. These events are: Judo, Alpine Skiing, Cycling, Goal Ball, Gymnastics, Powerlifting, Nordic Skating, Speed Skating, Swimming, Track and Field, and Wrestling.

The newsletter *SportsScoop* can be received free by other associations/groups which provide services for the blind. International Blind Sports Association (IBSA) and United States Organization for Disabled Athletes (USODA) are organizations similar to USABA.

IBSA was founded in Paris, France in April 1981. It came into being because of a great need to begin the task of developing international rules for those sports that are becoming the official events for international world competition.

USODA is a non-profit corporation which was formed to provide a coordinated network of funding and marking support for sports organizations for physically disabled. Also, USODA, at the request of its member organizations, plans and implements competitions and special events. USABA has fifty-five chapters within the United States working locally and regionally to provide opportunities for blind athletes.

UNITED STATES ASSOCIATION FOR
BLIND ATHLETES
33 N. Institute, Brown Hall, Suite 015
Colorado Springs, CO 80903

✳✳✳✳

UNCAP INTERNATIONAL, INC.

Uncap International, Inc. is a Creative Resource Center which bridges the gaps between programs of education, health, charity, sociology, and recreation. Uncap is committed to programs that will meet the ever-changing needs of the disabled. Uncap's activities include scholarships, information and referral services, and financial planning.

One thing which Uncap has given special recognition to, since the very beginning, is the right of the disabled and the aged to enjoy collectibles as a hobby. From this idea the Collectors Research Library (CRL) was born. It includes thousands of hardcover and paperback books and periodicals pertaining to coin and stamp collecting, as well as a variety of hobbies, clubs, and related associations.

The goals of Uncap International, Inc. are many and varied. The disabled are encouraged to become as self-sufficient as possible; to accept and live with their own problems; to maximize the physical abilities they do have; to share learned information with others; and, to uphold and maintain the responsibilities of citizenship. By working toward these goals, Uncap believes that the lives of the people it serves are enhanced.

Uncap welcomes handicapped and non-handicapped volunteers to donate their time to promote Uncap projects.

UNCAP INTERNATIONAL, INC.
2613 Huron Street
Los Angeles, CA 90065
(213) 222-1870
(213) 222-2012

✳✳✳✳

UNTAPPED RESOURCES INC.

Untapped Resources Inc. is a New York City based, nonprofit organization providing free comprehensive legal services for the disabled, including a number of multiple sclerosis patients. Untapped Resources seeks to remove or modify attitudinal and architectural barriers adversely affecting the severely physically handicapped.

The legal services of UR are provided in the following ways:

(1) By assuring that the special and collective difficulties and needs of the physically handicapped are properly brought to the attention of responsible and responsive civic leaders, legislators, government administrators, and the courts.

(2) By providing administrative liaison or, when necessary, legal assistance in obtaining from the government, or from public or private agencies, benefits and services which should be available to the physically handicapped.

(3) By seeking through legal action to establish the rights of the physically handicapped; UR has begun several legal matters, the proper pursuit of which awaits funding.

Mr. Curtis Brewer, a New York attorney who is paralyzed from the neck down, is founder and executive director of Untapped Resources. In 1978 Brewer expanded the operation of Untapped Resources by launching a radio series,"Law and the Disabled," a biweekly New York City program, over In Touch Networks, WKCR-FM, and WFUV-FM. The series, which he hosts, presents legal cases involving people deprived of their rights, including

the views of the involved agencies, and commentaries from experts in the disability fields.

Untapped Resources has a number of projects in the works. One is called GUTS—Greater Utilization of Tools and Services. It is a comprehensive plan to guarantee legally that all disabled persons are able to play an active role in society. Technological advances would help the disabled increase their mobility and dexterity, and various educational, psychological, and health services would contribute to their overall process of adaptation.

UNTAPPED RESOURCES INC.
60 First Avenue
New York, NY 10009
(212) 532-4422

✳✳✳✳

WORLD INSTITUTE ON DISABILITY

World Institute On Disability (WID) focuses on major policy issues from the perspective of the disabled community. It functions as a research center and as a resource for information, training, public education, and technical assistance. Since its inception, WID has taken on personal assistance services as a priority and conducts a broad and extensive program of research, policy analysis, technical assistance, and public education.

WID publishes a quarterly newsletter, *Attendant Services Network*, which focuses on issues and problems faced by persons who need personal assistance services. The newsletter reports on developments at the state and federal level and discusses major policy issues. In addition, WID has received a grant from the National Institute on Disability and Rehabilitation Research to develop four policy bulletins on health insurance and disability issues from a consumer perspective.

WID has established itself as one of the world's foremost research, training, policy analysis, and resource centers representing the disabled community. One of its missions is to share the Independent Living philosophy of self-determination for disabled people with other countries around the world.

WID designs individualized training programs to help people with disabilities from around the world to meet the diverse needs of their own communities. It offers foreign visitors a unique opportunity to visit many innovative programs for the disabled including Independent Living Centers, technical aids centers, an increasingly accessible community environment and public transportation system, and many severely disabled persons living and working in the community. WID arranges both local and national programs, and has hosted and trained visitors from over thirty countries.

WID serves as an international resource center for the sharing and exchange of knowledge about disability issues between people of different countries and cultures. WID's international affairs department responds to requests from other countries for contacts in the disability field, bibliographies, articles, and other information in a large number of areas.

WID has an experienced staff and consultants available for consultation with government agencies, organizations, and individuals in many countries. International conferences, workshops, and training sessions are tailored to specific needs for information about disability policy issues and services, but draw on the fundamental tenets of the independent living philosophy.

WID provides technical assistance to organizations nationwide interested in developing economically self-sufficient small businesses as transitional supported employment programs for people with developmental disabilities.

WORLD INSTITUTE ON DISABILITY
1720 Oregon Street, Suite 4
Berkeley, CA 94703
(415) 486-8314

✳✳✳✳

APPENDIX

INFORMATION CENTERS

ACCENT ON INFORMATION
P.O. Box 700
Bloomington, IL 61701
(309) 378-2961

ACCESS/ABILITIES
P.O. Box 458
Mill Valley, CA 94942
(415)388-3250

AIDS INFORMATION HOTLINE
CENTER FOR DISEASE
CONTROL
1600 Clifton Road
Atlanta, GA 30329
(800) 342-AIDS
(404) 329-1290

APPLECIDER BBS
GREG TROBAUGH
39-44 24th Street, Apt. 3B
Long Island City, NY 11101
(718) 482-0088 (Voice)
(718) 482-0089 (Modem)

ASSISTIVE DEVICE CENTER
CALIFORNIA STATE
UNIVERSITY, SACRAMENTO
6000 J Street
Sacramento, CA 95819
(916) 924-0280

CLEARINGHOUSE ON THE
HANDICAPPED
Office of Special Education & Re-
habilitation Services
Department of Education
Switzer Building,
Room 3119
Washington, DC 20202
(202) 732-1245

COUNCIL FOR EXCEPTIONAL
CHILDREN AND YOUTHS
1920 Association Drive
Reston, VA 22091
(703) 620-3660

CTG SOLUTIONS
CLOSING THE GAP
P.O. Box 68
Henderson, MN 56044
(612) 248-3294

ERIC–EDUCATIONAL
RESOURCES INFORMATION
CENTER
Department of Education
555 New Jersey Avenue, NW
Washington, DC 20208
(202) 357-6287

ERIC CLEARINGHOUSE ON
HANDICAPPED AND GIFTED
CHILDREN
The Council for Exceptional
Children (CEC)
1920 Association Drive
Reston, VA 22091
(703) 620-3660

HANDICAPPED EDUCATION
EXCHANGE
11523 Charlton Drive
Silver Spring, MD 20902
(301) 681-7372

HANDICAPPED LEARNER
MATERIAL DIST. CENTER
Audio-Visual Center, Indiana
University
Bloomington, IN 47405
(812) 377-1511

HEATH RESOURCE CENTER
National Clearinghouse on Post-
Secondary Education for Handi-
capped Individuals
One Dupont Circle, NW, Suite 800
Washington, DC 20036-1193
(202) 939-9320, (800) 54-HEATH

INFORMATION CENTER FOR
INDIVIDUALS WITH
DISABILITIES, INC.
20 Park Plaza
Boston, MA 02116
(617) 727-5540
(800) 462-5015

JOB ACCOMMODATION
NETWORK
P.O. Box 6122
809 Allen Hall
University of West Virginia
Morgantown, WV 26506
(800) JAN-PCEH

MAINSTREAM, INC.
1200 15th Street, NW
Washington, DC 20006
(202) 833-1136
MAINSTREAM INFORMATION
LINE
(202) 833-1162

NATIONAL CLEARINGHOUSE
FOR DRUG ABUSE INFORMA-
TION
P.O. Box 416
Kensington, MD 20795
(301) 443-6500

NATIONAL CLEARINGHOUSE
FOR REHABILITATION
TRAINING MATERIALS
115 Old USDA Building
Oklahoma State University
Stillwater, OK 74078
(405) 624-7650

NATIONAL COUNCIL OF THE
HANDICAPPED
800 Independence Avenue, S.W.,
Suite 814
Washington, DC 20591
(202) 453-3846

NATIONAL INFORMATION
CENTER FOR HANDICAPPED
CHILDREN AND YOUTH
(NICHCY)
P.O. Box 1492
Washington, DC 20013
(703) 522-0870, Ext. 316

NATIONAL RESOURCE
CENTER FOR CONSUMERS OF
LEGAL SERVICES
3254 Jones Court, N.W.
Washington, DC 20007
(703) 536-8700

NATIONAL SPINAL CORD
HOTLINE
National Study Center for
Emergency Medical Systems
22 South Greene Street
Baltimore, MD 21201
(800) 526-3456 –National
(800) 638-1733 –Maryland

NATIONAL REHABILITATION
INFORMATION CENTER
(NARIC)
8455 Colesville Road, Suite 935
Silver Spring, MD 20910-3319
(800) 34-NARIC
(800) 346-2742
(301) 588-9284 (TDD/Voice)

RECAL INFORMATION
SERVICES
National Centre for Training &
Education in Prosthetics &
Orthotics
University of Strathclyde
Curran Building
131 St. James Road
Glasgow, G4 OLS, Scotland
(041) 552-4400

REGIONAL REHABILITATION
NETWORK
1849 Sawtelle Blvd., Suite 102
Los Angeles, CA 90025
(213) 479-3028

REHABILITATION
INTERNATIONAL
25 East 21st Street
New York, NY 10010
(212) 420-1500

REHABILITATION
INTERNATIONAL USA
1123 Broadway, Suite 704
New York, NY 10010
(212) 620-4040

SPECIAL EDUCATION
SOFTWARE CENTER
LINC Resources
Building B, Room S312
333 Ravenswood Avenue
Menlo Park, CA 94025
(800) 327-5892

SPECIALNET
2021 K Street, NW, Suite 315
Washington, DC 20006
(202) 296-1800

TECH-KNOWLEDGE CENTER
FOR REHABILITATION
TECHNOLOGY, INC.
Georgia Institute of Technology
Atlanta, GA 30332
(404) 894-4960

DATABASE VENDORS

BRS
1200 Route 7
Latham, NY 12110
(518) 738-7251
(800) 345-4BRS

IBM INFORMATION NETWORK
3405 West Buffalo Avenue
Tampa, FL 33607
(813) 872-2111

COMPUSERVE
110 MacKenan Drive
Cary, NC 27511
(919) 469-3325

DIMDI
Weisshausstrasse, 27
P.O. Box 420580
D-5000 Koln 41
West Germany
49-221-4727-1

DIALOG
3460 Hillview Avenue
Palo Alto, CA 94304
(415) 858-3785
(800) 3-DIALOG

NATIONAL LIBRARY OF
MEDICINE
(MEDLARS)
U.S. Department of Health and
Human Services
8600 Rockville Pike
Bethesda, MD 20852
(301) 496-6193

STSC, INC.
Division of Contel
2115 East Jefferson Street
Rockville, MD 20894
(301) 984-5000

NATIONAL PLANNING DATA
CORP.
P.O. Box 610
20 Terrace Hill
Ithaca, NY 14851-0610
(607) 273-8208

TELENET MEDICAL
INFORMATION NETWORK
12490 Sunrise Valley Drive
Reston, VA 22096
(703) 689-6000
(800) 835-3638

EXECUTIVE TELECOM
SYSTEM, INC.
9585 Valparaiso Court
Indianapolis, IN 46268
(800) 421-8884

DATA RESOURCES, INC.
1750 K Street, NW, Suite 900
Washington, DC 20006
(202) 663-7600

ORBIT SEARCH SERVICE
PERGAMMON INFOLINE
8000 West Park Drive, Suite 400
McLean, VA 22102
(703) 442-0900

LEGAL RESOURCES

DISABILITY RIGHTS
EDUCATION AND DEFENSE
FUND, INC. (DREDF)
2212 6th Street
Berkeley, CA 94710
(415) 644-2555

Government Affairs
1616 P Street, NW, Suite 100
Washington, DC 20036
(202) 328-5185
DREDF is a non-profit public benefit corporation dedicated to offering education and training programs on disability civil rights issues; legal support and advocacy; research and policy analysis. DREDF also distributes disability rights publications. Callers can be referred to local sources for help.

FUND FOR EQUAL ACCESS TO
SOCIETY
1 Thomas Circle, NW, Suite 350
Washington, DC 20005
(202) 223-0570
The Fund is a nonprofit corporation formed in 1980 as an advocate for full and equal access for individuals precluded from effective participation in society because of handicaps.

THE NATIONAL CENTER FOR
LAW AND THE DEAF
800 Florida Avenue, NE
Washington, DC 20002
(202) 651-5373 (Voice/TDD)
NCLD provides legal education on issues affecting hearing-impaired and deaf people through conferences, workshops, and classes; it also presents educational programs to the hearing community on compliance with state and federal legislation requirements.

PUBLIC INTEREST LAW
CENTER OF PHILADELPHIA
(PILCOP)
125 South 9th Street, Suite 700
Philadelphia, PA 19107
(215) 627-7100
PILCOP is a nonprofit public law firm with a Disabilities Project specializing in class action suits brought by individuals and organizations. The Center's primary interests are in promoting family-scale local services for people with developmental disabilities and in promoting state-of-the-art education for people with handicaps in the public schools. Lack of accessible transportation is another focus.

U.S. DEPARTMENT OF EDUCATION, REGIONAL CIVIL RIGHTS OFFICES

The Office for Civil Rights, U.S. Department of Education, maintains ten regional offices which would be able to answer questions on matters of legal interpretation concerning Section 504 of the Rehabilitation Act of 1973.

Region I: Connecticut, Maine, Massachusetts, New Hampshire, Rhode Island, Vermont
U.S. Department of Education
Office for Civil Rights, Region I
John W. McCormack Post Office and Courthouse Building, Room 222
Boston, MA 02109
(617) 223-9662
(617) 223-9324 (TDD)

Region II: New Jersey, New York, Puerto Rico, Virgin Islands
U.S. Department of Education
Office for Civil Rights, Region II
26 Federal Plaza, 33rd Floor
New York, NY 10278
(212) 264-4633
(212) 264-9464 (TDD)

Region III: Delaware, District of Columbia, Maryland, Pennsylvania, Virginia, West Virginia
U.S. Department of Education
Office for Civil Rights, Region III
3535 Market Street, P.O. Box 13716
Gateway Building, 6th Floor
Philadelphia, PA 19104
(215) 596-6772
(215) 596-6794 (TDD)

Region IV: Alabama, Florida, Georgia, Kentucky, Mississippi, North Carolina, South Carolina, Tennessee
U.S. Department of Education
Office for Civil Rights, Region IV
101 Marietta Tower, NW, 27th Fl.
P.O. Box 1705
Atlanta, GA 30301
(404) 331-2954
(404) 331-2010 (TDD)

Region V: Illinois, Indiana, Michigan, Minnesota, Ohio, Wisconsin
U.S. Department of Education
Office for Civil Rights, Region V
300 South Wacker Drive, 8th Floor
Chicago, IL 60606
(312) 353-2520
(312) 353-2541 (TDD)

Region VI: Arkansas, Louisiana, New Mexico, Oklahoma, Texas
U.S. Department of Education
Office of Civil Rights, Region VI
1200 Main Tower Bldg., Suite 2260
Dallas, TX 75202
(214) 767-3959
(214) 767-4116 (TDD)

Region VII: Iowa, Kansas, Missouri, Nebraska
U.S. Department of Education
Office of Civil Rights, Region VII
10220 N. Executive Hills Blvd., 8th Floor
Kansas City, MO 64153
(816) 891-8026
(816) 374-7607 (TDD)

Region VIII: Colorado, Montana, North Dakota, South Dakota, Utah, Wyoming
U.S. Department of Education
Office of Civil Rights, Region VIII
Federal Office Building
1961 Stout Street, Room 342
Denver, CO 80294
(303) 844-5695
(303) 844-3417 (TDD)

Region IX: Arizona, California, Hawaii, Nevada, Guam, Trust Territory of the Pacific Islands, American Samoa
U.S. Department of Education
Office of Civil Rights, Region IX
221 Main Street, 10th Floor
San Francisco, CA 94105
(415) 227-8040
(415) 227-8124 (TDD)

Region X: Alaska, Idaho, Oregon, Washington
U.S. Department of Education
Office of Civil Rights, Region X
2901 Third Avenue, Room 100
Seattle, WA 98121
(206) 442-1635
(206) 442-4542 (TDD)

PROTECTION AND ADVOCACY

State Protection & Advocacy agencies are mandated to protect and advocate for the rights of persons with Developmental Disabilities primarily in the areas of Education, Habilitation, Housing, Public Benefits, Employment, and Right to Treatment.

They provide information and referral as well as technical assistance to all eligible clients who need it and also will provide direct intervention by way of mediation, negotiation, and legal advocacy in appropriate cases.

PROTECTION & ADVOCACY
FOR THE D.D.
325 E. 3rd Avenue, 2nd Floor
Anchorage, AK 99501
(907) 274-3658

ALABAMA DD ADVOCACY
PROGRAM
THE UNIVERSITY OF
ALABAMA
P.O. Drawer 2847
Tuscaloosa, AL 35487
(205) 348-4928

ADVOCACY SERVICES, INC.
12th and Marshall Street, Suite 311
Little Rock, AR 72202
(501) 371-2171
(800) 482-1174

CLIENT A & P AND ADVOCACY
PROGRAMS
P.O. Box 3407
Pago Pago, AS 96799
10-ATT-011-684-633-2418

ARIZONA CENTER FOR LAW
IN THE PUBLIC INTEREST
112 North Central Avenue, Suite 400
Phoenix, AZ 85004
(602) 252-4904

CALIFORNIA PROTECTION &
ADVOCACY, INC.
2131 Capitol, Suite 100
Sacramento, CA 95816
(916) 447-3324
(800) 952-5746

CATHOLIC SOCIAL SERVICE
Box 745, North Marianas Islands
Saipan, CM 96950
10288-011-670-234-6981

THE LEGAL CENTER
455 Sherman Street, Suite 130
Denver, CO 80203
(303) 722-0300

OFFICE OF P & A FOR
HANDICAPPED AND DD
PERSONS
90 Washington Street, Lower Level
Hartford, CT 06106
(203) 566-7616
(800) 842-7303 in Connecticut

INFORMATION, PROTECTION,
AND ADVOCACY CENTER
300 I Street, NE, Suite 202
Washington, DC 20002
(202) 547-8081

DISABILITIES LAW PROGRAM
144 E. Market Street
Georgetown, DE 19947
(302) 856-0038

GOVERNOR'S
COMM./ADVOCACY FOR
PERSONS WITH DISABILITIES
Office of the Governor, Capitol
Tallahassee, FL 32301
(904) 488-9070

GEORGIA ADVOCACY
OFFICE, INC.
1447 Peachtree Street, NE, Suite 811
Atlanta, GA 30309
(404) 885-1447
(800) 282-4538

THE ADVOCACY OFFICE
P.O. Box 8830
Tamuning, Guam 96911
10288-011-671-646-9026

P & A AGENCY
1580 Makaloa Street, Suite 860
Honolulu, HI 96814
(808) 949-2922

IOWA P & A SERVICES
3015 Merle Hay Road, Suite 6
Des Moines, IA 50310
(515) 278-2502

COALITION OF ADVOCATES
FOR THE DISABLED, INC.
1409 W. Washington
Boise, ID 83702
(208) 336-5353

PROTECTION AND ADVO-
CACY
175 W. Jackson, Suite A-210-3
Chicago, IL 60604
(312) 341-0022

ADVOCACY SERVICES
850 N. Meridian Street, Suite 2-C
Indianapolis, IN 46204
(317) 232-1150
(800) 622-4845

KANSAS A & P SERVICES
513 Leavenworth Street, Suite 2
Manhattan, KS 66502
(913) 776-1541
(800) 432-8276

OFFICE FOR PUBLIC
ADVOCACY DIVISION FOR
P&A
151 Elkhorn Court
Frankfort, KY 40601
(502) 564-2967
(800) 372-2988

ADVOCACY CENTER FOR THE
ELDERLY & DISABLED
1001 Howard Avenue, Suite 300A
New Orleans, LA 70113
(504) 522-2337
(800) 662-7705

DD LAW CENTER
11 Beacon Street, Suite 925
Boston, MA 02108
(617) 723-8455

DISABILITY LAW CENTER
2510 St. Paul Street
Baltimore, MD 21218
(301) 333-7600

ADVOCATES FOR THE DD
2 Mulliken Court/Box 5341
Augusta, ME 04330
(207) 289-5755, (800) 452-1948

MICHIGAN P & A SERVICE
109 W. Michigan, Suite 900
Lansing, MI 48933
(517) 487-1755

LEGAL AID SOCIETY
323 4th Avenue, S.
222 Grain Exchange
Minneapolis, MN 55415
(612) 332-7301

DD P & A SERVICES, INC.
211 B Metro Drive
Jefferson City, MO 65101
(314) 893-3333, (800) 392-8667

P & A SYSTEM FOR DD
4793 B McWillie Drive
Jackson, MS 39206
(601) 981-8207

MONTANA ADVOCACY
PROGRAM
1410 8th Avenue
Helena, MT 59601
(406) 444-3889, (800) 245-4743

ADVOCACY COUNCIL FOR
PERSONS WITH DISABILITIES
1318 Dale Street, Suite 100
Raleigh, NC 27605
(919) 733-9250

P & A PROJECT FOR THE DD
13th Floor, State Capitol
Bismarck, ND 58505
(701) 224-2972, (800) 472-2670

NE ADVOCACY SERV., INC.
522 Lincoln Ctr. Bldg.
215 Centennial
Lincoln, NE 68508
(402) 474-3183

DD ADVOCACY CENTER, INC.
6 White Street, P.O. Box 19
Concord, NH 03301
(603) 228-0432

DEPT. OF PUBLIC ADVOCATE
OFFICE OF ADVOCACY FOR
DD
Hughes Justice Complex CN 850
Trenton, NJ 08625
(609) 292-9742, (800) 792-8600

P & A SYSTEM
2201 San Pedro NE
Building 4, Suite 140
Albuquerque, NM 87110
(505) 888-0111
(800) 432-4682

DD ADVOCATE'S OFFICE
2105 Capurro Way, Suite B
Sparks, NV 89431
(702) 789-0233
(800) 992-5715

NY COMM. ON QUALITY OF
CARE FOR THE MENTALLY
DISABLED
99 Washington Avenue
Albany, NY 12210
(518) 473-4057

LEGAL RIGHTS SERVICE
8 East Long Street, 6th Floor
Columbus, OH 43215
(614) 466-7264
(800) 282-9181

P & A AGENCY FOR DD
9726 E. 42nd
Osage Building 133
Tulsa, OK 74126
(918) 664-5883

OREGON ADVOCACY CENTER
310 SW 4th Avenue, Suite 625
Portland, OR 97204
(503) 243-2081

PENNSYLVANIA P & A INC.
3540 North Progress Avenue
Harrisburg, PA 17110
(717) 657-3320, (800) 692-7443

PLANNING RESEARCH &
SPECIAL
PROJECTS/GOVERNOR'S
OMBUDSMAN
Chardon Avenue, # 916
Hato Rey, PR 00936
(809) 766-2333

RI P & A SYSTEM (RIPAS), INC.
86 Weybosset Street, Suite 508
Providence, RI 02903
(401) 831-3150

SC P & A SYSTEM FOR THE
HANDICAPPED, INC.
2360-A Two Notch Road
Columbia, SC 29204
(803) 254-1600

SD ADVOCACY PROJECT, INC.
221 South Central Avenue
Pierre, SD 57501
(605) 224-8294

EACH, INC.
P.O. Box 121257
Nashville, TN 37212
(615) 298-1080, (800) 342-1660

ADVOCACY, INC.
7700 Chevy Chase Drive, Suite 300
Austin, TX 78752
(512) 454-4816
(800) 252-9108

LEGAL CENTER FOR THE
HANDICAPPED
455 East 400 South, Suite 201
Salt Lake City, UT 84111
(801) 363-1347, (800) 662-9080

RIGHTS FOR THE DISABLED
101 North 14th Street, 17th Floor
Richmond, VA 23219
(804) 225-2042
(800) 552-3962

ADVOCACY FOR THE DD, INC.
Apt. #2, 31A New Street
Fredericksted, St. Croix, VI
(809) 772-1200

VERMONT DD P & A, INC.
12 North Street
Burlington, VT 05401
(802) 863-2881

WASHINGTON P & A SYSTEM
1550 West Armory Way, Suite 204
Seattle, WA 98119
(206) 284-1037

COALITION FOR ADVOCACY,
INC.
16 N. Carroll Street, Suite 400
Madison, WI 53703
(608) 251-9600
(800) 328-1110

ADVOCACY FOR THE DD, INC.
1200 Brooks Med Bldg.
Quarrier Street #27
Charleston, WV 25301
(800) 642-9205

WYOMING P & A SYSTEM, INC.
2424 Pioneer Avenue, #101
Cheyenne, WY 82001
(307) 632-3496
(800) 632-3496

ORGANIZATIONS

ABLEDATA
Adaptive Equipment Center
Newington Children's Hospital
181 East Cedar Street
Newington, CT 06111

ACOUSTIC NEUROMA
ASSOCIATION
c/o 26 Hines Drive
Willowdale, Ontario M2H 2M1

AIDS COMMITTEE OF
TORONTO
Box 55, Station F
Toronto, Ontario M4Y 2L4

ALEXANDER GRAHAM BELL
ASSOC. FOR THE DEAF, INC.
3417 Volta Place, NW
Washington, DC 20007
(703) 836-7114

THE ALS ASSOCIATION
21021 Ventura Blvd., Suite 321
Woodland Hills, CA 91364
(818) 340-7500

ALZHEIMER SOCIETY OF
CANADA
1320 Yonge Street, Suite 302
Toronto, Ontario M4T 1X2

AMERICAN AMPUTEE
FOUNDATION
P.O. Box 55218, Hillcrest Station
Little Rock, AR 72225
(501) 666-2523

AMERICAN BOARD OF
CERTIFICATION IN
ORTHOTICS AND
PROSTHETICS
717 Pendleton Street
Alexandria, VA 22314
(703) 836-7114

AMERICAN COUNCIL OF THE
BLIND
1010 Vermont Ave. NW, Suite 1100
Washington, DC 20005
(202) 393-3666
(800) 424-8666

AMERICAN FOUNDATION
FOR THE BLIND
15 West 16th Street
New York, NY 10011
(212) 620-2000

AMERICAN OCCUPATIONAL
THERAPY ASSOCIATION
1383 Piccard Drive
Rockville, MD 20850

AMERICAN PARALYSIS
ASSOCIATION
500 Morris Avenue
Springfield, NJ 07081
(201) 379-2690, (800) 225-0292

AMERICAN SPINAL INJURY
ASSOCIATION
250 E. Superior Street, Rm. 619
Chicago, IL 60611
(312) 908-3425

AMERICAN WHEELCHAIR
BOWLING ASSOCIATION
N54 W15858 Larkspur Lane
Menomonee Falls, WI 53051

AMPUTEES IN MOTION
P.O. Box 2703
Escondido, CA 92025
(619) 454-9300

AMYOTROPHIC LATERAL
SCLEROSIS SOCIETY OF
CANADA (ALS)
250 Rogers Road
Toronto, Ontario M6E 1R1

ARKANSAS RESEARCH AND
TRAINING CENTER IN
VOCATIONAL
REHABILITATION
Hot Springs Rehabilitation Center
P.O. Box 1358
Hot Springs, AR 71902

ARTHRITIS SOCIETY
250 Bloor Street E., Suite 401
Toronto, Ontario M4W 3P2

ASSOCIATED REHAB.
COUNSELING SPECIALISTS,
INC.
2628 East Cannon Drive
Phoenix, AZ 85028

ASSOCIATION CANADIENNE
DE L'ATAXIE DE FRIEDRICH
5620 C.P. Jobin Road
Saint-Leonard, Quebec H1P 1H8

ASSOCIATION OF THE DEAF
Suite 311, 271 Spadina Road
Toronto, Ontario M5R 2V3

ASSOCIATION OF LEARNING
DISABLED ADULTS
P.O. Box 9722
Friendship Station
Washington, DC 20016
(202) 338-7111

ASSOC. ON HANDICAPPED
STUDENT SERV. PROG. IN
POST-SECONDARY
EDUCATION (AHSSPPE)
P.O. Box 21192
Columbus, OH 43221

BLIND ORGANIZATIONS OF
ONTARIO WITH SELF-HELP
TACTICS (BOOST)
597 Parliament Street, Suite B3
Toronto, Ontario M4X 1W3

CALIFORNIA WHEELCHAIR
AVIATORS
1117 Rising Hill Way
Escondido, CA 92025
(619) 746-5018

CAMP HOPE
Box 670
Carmel, NY 10512-0670
(914) 225-2005

THE CANADIAN CANCER SOC.
77 Bloor Street W.
Toronto, Ontario M5S 3A1

CANINE COMPANIONS FOR
INDEPENDENCE
P.O. Box 446
Santa Rosa, CA 95402

CANADIAN ASSOCIATION OF
INDEPENDENT LIVING
CENTRES (CAILC)
150 Kent Street, Suite 905
Ottawa, Ontario K1P 5P9

CANADIAN ASSOCIATION OF
PRACTICAL AND NURSING
ASSISTANTS
31 Lawson Street
Regina, Saskatchewan S4R 3P6

CANADIAN ASSOCIATION OF
SPEECH-LANGUAGE
PATHOLOGISTS AND
AUDIOLOGISTS
31144 Eglinton Avenue W.
Toronto, Ontario M4R 1A1

CANADIAN CEREBRAL PALSY
ASSOCIATION
40 Dundas Street W., Suite 222,
P.O. Box 110
Toronto, Ontario M5G 2C2

CANADIAN COALITION FOR
THE PREVENTION OF
HANDICAP
c/o Canadian Institute of Child
Health
17 York Street, Suite 105
Ottawa, Ontario K1N 5S7

CANADIAN CYSTIC FIBROSIS
FOUNDATION
2221 Yonge Street, Suite 601
Toronto, Ontario M4S 2B4

CANADIAN FOUNDATION FOR
ILEITIS AND COLITIS
21 St. Clair Avenue East, Suite 2301
Toronto, Ontario M4T 1L9

CANADIAN GERIATRICS
RESEARCH SOCIETY
1235 Bay Street, Suite 603
Toronto, Ontario M5R 3K4

CANADIAN HEARING
SOCIETY
271 Spadina Road
Toronto, Ontario M5R 2V3

CANADIAN LIVER
FOUNDATION
1320 Yonge Street, Suite 301
Toronto, Ontario M4X 1X2

CANADIAN LONG TERM CARE
ASSOCIATION
135 York Street, Suite 204
Ottawa, Ontario K1N 5T4

CANADIAN MEDIC ALERT
FOUNDATION INC.
293 Eglinton Avenue E.
Toronto, Ontario M4P 2Z8

CANADIAN NEUROLOGICAL
COALITION
Suite 126,
100 College Street
Toronto, Ontario

CANADIAN OSTEOGENESIS
IMPERFECTA SOCIETY
Box 607 Station O
Toronto, Ontario M8Z 5Y9

CANADIAN OSTEOPATHIC
ASSOCIATION
575 Waterloo Street
London, Ontario N6B 2R2

CANADIAN PHYSIOTHERAPY
ASSOCIATION
890 Yonge Street
Toronto, Ontario M4W 3T4

CANADIAN PSORIASIS
FOUNDATION
P.O. Box 5036 Armdale
Halifax, Nova Scotia B3L 4M6

CANADIAN REHABILITATION
COUNCIL FOR THE DISABLED
One Yonge Street, Suite 2110
Toronto, Ontario M5E 1E5

CANDIDA RESEARCH AND
INFORMATION FOUNDATION
(CANADA)
41 Green Valley Court, Box 583
Kleinburg, Ontario L0J 1C0

CHARCOT-MARIE-TOOTH
DISEASE
One Springbank Drive
St. Catharines, Ontario L2S 2K1

CHOICE MAGAZINE
LISTENING
P.O. Box 10
Port Washington, NY 11050

CMT INTERNATIONAL
34 Bayview Drive
St. Catharines, Ontario L2N 4Y6

COMMISSION ON
ACCREDITATION OF
REHABILITATION FACILITIES
2500 North Pantano Road
Tucson, AZ 85715

CONTINENCE CLINIC
Sunnybrook Hospital,
Room H6969
2075 Bayview Avenue
Toronto, Ontario M4N 3M5

D.I.A.L.: ILLINOIS DISABLED
INDIVIDUAL'S ASSISTANCE
LINE
100 West Randolph Street,
Suite 8-100
Chicago, IL 60601
(800) 233-3425 in Illinois

THE DISABLED LIVING
FOUNDATION
380-384 Harrow Road
London W9 2HU, England

DISABILITY INFORMATION
SERVICES OF CANADA
610, 839-5 Avenue, S.W.
Calgary, Alberta T2P 3C8

DISABILITY SERVICES
Boston University
Martin Luther King, Jr. Center
19 Deerfield Street
Boston, MA 02215

DOLE FOUNDATION FOR
EMPLOYMENT OF PEOPLE
WITH DISABILITIES
1819 H Street, NW, Suite 850
Washington, DC 20006-3603
(202) 457-0318 (Voice/TDD)

DYSTONIA MEDICAL RE-
SEARCH FOUNDATION
175 Humbercrest Blvd.
Toronto, Ontario M6S 4L5

EPILEPSY ASSOCIATION OF
METRO TORONTO
80 Richmond Street W., Suite 804
Toronto, Ontario M5H 2A4

EPILEPSY FOUND. OF AMER.
4351 Garden City Drive
Landover, MD 20785
(301) 459-3700

FAMILIES OF CHILDREN WITH
CANCER
c/o 78 Laburnham Avenue
Etobicoke, Ontario M8W 1S8

FAMILIAL POLYPOSIS
REGISTRY TORONTO
GENERAL HOSPITAL
Miss T. Beck, Eaton Building 10-315
200 Elizabeth Street
Toronto, Ontario M5G 2C4

FIFTY-TWO ASSOCIATION FOR
THE HANDICAPPED, INC.
441 Lexington Avenue
New York, NY 10007
(212) 986-5281

FRIEDREICH'S ATAXIA
GROUP IN AMERICA, INC.
P.O. Box 11116
Oakland, CA 94611
(415) 655-0833

GAZETTE INTERNATIONAL
NETWORKING INSTITUTE
4502 Maryland Avenue
St. Louis, MO 63108
(314) 361-0475

GUIDE DOG FOUNDATION
FOR THE BLIND, INC.
371 E. Jericho Tpke.
Smithtown, NY 11787
(800) 548-4337
(516) 265-2121 in New York

HANDICAPS WELFARE
ASSOCIATION
Whampoa Drive
(Behind Block 102)
Singapore 1232

HEART AND STROKE
FOUNDATION OF ONTARIO
576 Church Street
Toronto, Ontario M4Y 2S1

HEAD INJURY ASSOCIATION
OF TORONTO
c/o Richview Public School,
Clement Rd.
Etobicoke, Ontario M9W 1Y5

HELEN KELLER NATIONAL
CENTER
For Deaf-Blind Youths and Adults
111 Middle Neck Road
Sands Point, NY 11050

HELP FOR INCONTINENT
PEOPLE, INC.
P.O. Box 544
Union, SC 29379
(803) 585-8789

HUNTINGTON DISEASE
RESOURCE CENTRE
c/o North Western Health Centre
2175 Keele Street
Toronto, Ontario M6M 3Z4

HYPOGLYCEMIA
ASSOCIATION INC.
18008 New Hampshire Avenue
Ashton, MD 20861

IMPOTENCE SUPPORT GROUP
Sunnybrook Medical Centre, University of Toronto Urology Clinic
2075 Bayview Avenue
Toronto, Ontario M4N 3M5

INDEPENDENT LIVING
RESEARCH UTILIZATION
3400 Bissonnet, Suite 101
Houston, TX 77005
(713) 666-6244

INTERNATIONAL POLIO
NETWORK (IPN)
4502 Maryland Avenue
St. Louis, MO 63108
(314) 361-0475

IN TOUCH, MENTAL
HANDICAP AND RARE
DISORDERS PARENT
CONTACT SERVICE
10 Norman Road, SALE
Chester, M33 3DF, England

IN TOUCH NETWORKS, INC.
322 W. 48th Street
New York, NY 10036
(212) 586-5588

INSTITUTE FOR
REHABILITATION AND
RESEARCH
Texas Medical Center
P.O. Box 20095
Houston, TX 77225

INTERNATIONAL
ASSOCIATION OF
LARYNGECTOMEES
American Cancer Society
1599 Clifton Road, NE
Atlanta, GA 30329

INTERNATIONAL HEARING
DOG, INC.
5901 E. 89th Avenue
Henderson, CO 80640

INTERNATIONAL SOCIAL
SERVICE CANADA
55 Parkdale Avenue
Ottawa, Ontario K1Y 1E5

THE KIDNEY FOUNDATION
OF CANADA
4060 Ste. Catherine Street W., Suite
555
Montreal, Quebec H3Z 2Z3

LEADER DOGS FOR THE
BLIND
1039 S. Rochester Road
Rochester, MI 48063

LEARNING HOW, INC.
P.O. Box 35481
Charlotte, NC 28235

LOW VISION ASSOCIATION OF
ONTARIO
c/o 1105 Saginaw Cres.
Mississauga, Ontario L5H 3W4

LUPUS ASSOCIATION
(ONTARIO)
250 Bloor Street E., Suite 401
Toronto, Ontario M4W 3P2

MAINSTREAM, INC.
1200 15th Street, NW
Washington, DC 20005
(202) 833-1136

METROPOLITAN
WASHINGTON EAR, INC.
35 University Blvd., E
Silver Spring, MD 20901
(301) 681-6636

MIGRAINE FOUNDATION
390 Brunswick Avenue
Toronto, Ontario M5R 2Z4

MOBILITY INTERNATIONAL
USA
P.O. Box 3551
Eugene, OR 97403
(503) 343-1284 (Voice/TDD)

MULTICULTURAL HEALTH
COALITION
1017 Wilson Avenue, Suite 407
Downsview, Ontario M3K 1Z1

MULTIPLE SCLEROSIS
SOCIETY OF CANADA
250 Bloor Street E., Suite 820
Toronto, Ontario M4W 3P9

MUSCULAR DYSTROPHY
ASSOCIATION, INC.
810 Seventh Avenue
New York, NY 10019
(212) 586-0808

MUSCULAR DYSTROPHY
ASSOCIATION OF CANADA
150 Eglinton Avenue E., Suite 400
Toronto, Ontario M4P 1E8

NATIONAL AMPUTATION
FOUNDATION
1245 150th Street
Whitestone, NY 11357

NATIONAL ARTHRITIS AND
MUSCULOSKELETAL AND
SKIN DISEASES INFORMATION
CLEARINGHOUSE
Box AMS
Bethesda, MD 20892
(301) 468-3235

THE NATIONAL ASSOCIATION
FOR THE COTTAGE
INDUSTRY
P.O. Box 14460
Chicago, IL 60614
(312) 472-8116

NATIONAL ASSOCIATION FOR
VISUALLY HANDICAPPED
22 W. 21 Street
New York, NY 10010
(212) 889-3141

NATIONAL ASSOCIATION OF
ANOREXIA NERVOSA AND
ASSOCIATED DISORDERS, INC.
(ANAD)
Box 7
Highland Park, IL 60035
(312) 831-3438

NATIONAL ASSOCIATION OF
THE DEAF COMMUNICATIVE
SKILLS PROGRAM
814 Thaye Avenue
Silver Spring, MD 20910
(301) 587-1788

NATIONAL ASSOCIATION OF
PHYSICALLY HANDICAPPED,
INC.
76 Elm Street
London, OH 43140

NATIONAL ATAXIA
FOUNDATION
600 Twelve Oaks Center
15500 Wayzata Blvd.
Wayzata, MN 55391
(612) 473-7666

NATIONAL CONGRESS OF
JEWISH DEAF
4960 Sabal Palm Blvd.
Tamarac, FL 33319

NATIONAL EASTER SEAL
SOCIETY
2023 West Ogden Avenue
Chicago, IL 60612
(312) 243-8400

NATIONAL FEDERATION OF
THE BLIND
1800 Johnson Street
Baltimore, MD 21230

NATIONAL HANDICAP
HOUSING INSTITUTE, INC.
4556 Lake Drive
Robbinsdale, MN 55422
(612) 535-9771

NATIONAL HEAD INJURY
FOUNDATION
333 Turnpike Road
Southborough, MA 01772
(617) 485-9950

NATIONAL HOME STUDY
COUNCIL
1601 18th Street, NW
Washington, DC 20009

NATIONAL INFORMATION
CENTER FOR HANDICAPPED
CHILDREN AND YOUTH
P.O. Box 1492
Washington, DC 20013
(703) 522-3332

NATIONAL MULTIPLE
SCLEROSIS SOCIETY
205 East 42nd Street
New York, NY 10017

NATIONAL ODD SHOE
EXCHANGE
P.O. Box 56845
Phoenix, AZ 85079-6845

NATIONAL ORGANIZATION
FOR RARE DISORDERS
(NORD)
P.O. Box 8923
New Fairfield, CT 06812

NATIONAL REHABILITATION
INFORMATION CENTER
(NARIC)
8455 Colesville Road, Suite 935
Silver Spring, MD 20910-3319
(800) 346-2742
(301) 588-9284

NATIONAL STROKE
ASSOCIATION
300 E. Hampden Avenue, Suite 240
Englewood, CO 80110-2622
(303) 762-9922

NATIONAL TUBEROUS-
SCLEROSIS ASSOCIATION
238 Forest Hill Road
Toronto, Ontario

NATIONAL WHEELCHAIR
ATHLETIC ASSOCIATION
3617 Betty Drive, Suite S
Colorado Springs, CO 80917-5993

NEUROFIBROMATOSIS
SOCIETY OF ONTARIO
c/o Dept. of Neurosurgery
38 Shuter Street
Toronto, Ontario M5B 1A6

NORTH AMERICAN CHRONIC
PAIN ASSOC. OF CANADA
6 Handel Court
Bramalea, Ontario L6S 1Y4

ODPHP HEALTH
INFORMATION SERVICE
P.O. Box 1133
Washington, DC 20013-1133

ONTARIO PREVENTATIVE
CLEARINGHOUSE
984 Bay Street, # 603
Toronto, Ontario M5S 2A5

OSTEOPOROSIS SOCIETY OF
CANADA
76 St. Clair Avenue W., Suite 502
Toronto, Ontario M4V 1N2

PARKINSON FOUNDATION OF
CANADA
55 Bloor Street W., Suite 232
Toronto, Ontario M4W 1A6

PATIENTS' RIGHTS
ASSOCIATION
40 Homewood Avenue, #315
Toronto, Ontario M4Y 2K2

PEOPLE UNITED FOR SELF-
HELP IN ONTARIO (PUSH)
Suite 204,
597 Parliament Street
Toronto, Ontario M4X 1W3

PERIPHERAL NERVE INJURY
CLINIC—LIMB
RECONSTRUCTION UNIT
Professor Alan R. Hudson
38 Shuter Street
Toronto, Ontario M5B 1A6

POLIO SURVIVORS
ASSOCIATION
12720 La Reina Avenue
Downey, CA 90242
(213) 862-4508

PROMOTE REAL
INDEPENDENCE FOR THE
DISABLED AND ELDERLY
71 Plaza Court
Groton, CT 06340

RARE HANDICAP GROUPS
SUPPORT PROJECT
30 Westwood Drive,
Little Chalfont
Buckinghamshire, HP6 6RJ,
England

RECORDING FOR THE BLIND,
INC.
The Anne T. Macdonald Center
20 Roszel Road
Princeton, NJ 08540
(609) 452-0606

REGIONAL REHABILITATION
RESEARCH INSTITUTE ON
ATTITUDINAL, LEGAL, AND
LEISURE BARRIERS (RRRI-
ALLB)
George Washington University
Academic Center, T-605
Washington, DC 20052

REHABILITATION
INTERNATIONAL
25 East 21st Street
New York, NY 10010
(212) 420-1500

RETINITIS PIGMENTOSA EYE
RESEARCH FOUNDATION
411-185 Spadina Avenue
Toronto, Ontario M5T 2C6

RETINITIS PIGMENTOSA SELF-
HELP GROUP
c/o Hospital for Sick Children
555 University Avenue
Toronto, Ontario M5G 1X8

THE ROYAL ASSOCIATION
FOR DISABILITY AND
REHABILITATION
25 Mortimer Street
London W1N 8A, England

SELF-HELP CLEARINGHOUSE
OF METROPOLITAN
TORONTO
40 Orchard View Blvd., Suite 215
Toronto, Ontario M4R 1B9

SELF HELP FOR HARD OF
HEARING PEOPLE, INC.
7800 Wisconsin Avenue
Bethesda, MD 20814
(301) 657-2248

SENSORY AIDS FOUNDATION
399 Sherman Ave., Suite 12
Palo Alto, CA 94306
(415) 329-0430

SHARE-A-CARE NATIONAL
REGISTER FOR RARE
DISEASES
8 Cornmarket, Faringdon
Oxfordshire, England

SPECIAL OLYMPICS
INTERNATIONAL
1350 New York Avenue, NW, Suite
500
Washington, DC 20005
(202) 628-3630

SPEECH FOUNDATION OF
AMERICA (STUTTERERS)
5139 Klingle Street, NW
Washington, DC 20016

SPINA BIFIDA AND
HYDROCEPHALUS
ASSOCIATION OF CANADA
Toronto Chapter
c/o 61 Stonedene Blvd.
Willowdale, Ontario M2R 3C8

SPINA BIFIDA ASSOCIATION
OF AMERICA
1700 Rockville Pike,
Suite 540
Rockville, MD 20852
(800) 621-3141

SPINA BIFIDA ASSOCIATION
OF CANADA
633 Wellington Cresent
Winnipeg, Manitoba R3M 0A8

ST. CLARE'S-RIVERSIDE
MEDICAL CENTRE SELF-HELP
CLEARING HOUSE
Pocono Road
Denville, New Jersey 07834

STROKE RECOVERY
ASSOCIATION
170 The Donway W.,
Suite 122
Don Mills, Ontario M3C 2G3

TECHNICAL AIDS AND
ASSISTANCE FOR THE
DISABLED (TAAD)
1950 West Roosevelt Rd.
Chicago, IL 60608
(800) 346-2939
(312) 421-3373

TELEPHONE PIONEERS OF
AMERICA
22 Cortlandt Street
New York, NY 10007

TRACHEO-ESOPHAGEAL
FISTULA FAMILY SUPPORT
GROUP
101 Parkside Drive
Toronto, Ontario M6R 2V8

UNCAP INTERNATIONAL, INC.
2613 Huron Street
Los Angeles, CA 90065
(213) 222-1870
(213) 222-2012

UNITED CEREBRAL PALSY
ASSOCIATIONS, INC.
66 E. 34th Street
New York, NY 10016

UNITED OSTOMY
ASSOCIATION, INC.
36 Executive Park, Suite 120
Irvine, CA 92714
(714) 660-8624

UNITED STATES
ARCHITECTURAL AND
TRANSPORTATION BARRIERS
COMPLIANCE BOARD
1111 18th Street, NW, Suite 501
Washington, DC 20036-3894

UNITED STATES ASSOCIATION
FOR BLIND ATHLETES
33 N. Institute, Brown Hall, Suite
015
Colorado Springs, CO 80903

UNTAPPED RESOURCES, INC.
60 First Avenue
New York, NY 10009
(212) 532-4422

U.S.–CANADA
ENDOMETRIOSIS
ASSOCIATION
P.O. Box 92187
Milwaukee, WI 53202

VOICE FOR HEARING
IMPAIRED CHILDREN
271 Spadina Road
Toronto, Ontario M5R 2V3

THE WASHINGTON AREA
GROUP FOR THE HARD OF
HEARING
P.O. Box 6283
Silver Spring, MD 20906
(301) 942-7612 (Voice/TDD)

THE WASHINGTON EAR, INC.
35 University Blvd., E
Silver Spring, MD 20901
(301) 681-6636

WORLD INSTITUTE ON
DISABILITY
1720 Oregon Street, Suite 4
Berkeley, CA 94703
(415) 486-8314

AMPUTEE SUPPORT GROUPS

Arkansas

AMERICAN AMPUTEE FD.
NATIONAL HEADQUARTERS
P.O. Box 55218
Little Rock, AR 72225

California

AMPUTEES ARE ABLE
1632 Garden
8088 Palm Lane (meetings)
San Bernardino, CA 92404

AMPUTEES CARING
TOGETHER
197 Arneill Road
Camarillo, CA 90310

AMPUTEES IN MOTION,
INTERNATIONAL
475 Marview Drive
Solana Beach, CA 92075

DIRECT LINK
P.O. Box 6762
Santa Barbara, CA 93160

DIRECT LINK
22422 W. Alamota
Saugus, CA 91350

MUTUAL AMPUTEE AID
FOUNDATION
P.O. Box 1200
Lomita, CA 90717

SHRINERS HOSPITAL FOR
CRIPPLED CHILDREN
3160 Geneva Street
Los Angeles, CA 90020-1199
    Totally free services for children
including: Orthopaedic Surgery and
Child Amputee Prosthetics Program

Canada

AMPUTEE VISITOR PROGRAM
P.O. Box 8662
Ottawa K1G 3J1

CANADIAN AMPUTEE SPORTS
ASSOCIATION
5417-39 Avenue
Edmonton, Alberta
T1G 1P3

WAR AMPUTATIONS OF
CANADA
2827 Riverside Drive
Ottawa K1V 0C4

Colorado

Gil Gillespie
Plaza Wood Creek/Box 5159
Mt. Crested Butte, CO 81225

District of Columbia

Mary Lilla Browne
P.O. Box 18259
Washington, DC 20036

NATIONAL ORGANIZATION
ON DISABILITY
910 16th Street, N.W.
Washington, D.C. 20006

Florida

Dr. John Bowker
630 Solana Prodo
Coral Gables, FL 33156

AMPUTEE DISCUSSION
GROUP
Baptist Hospital
8900 N. Kendall Drive
Miami, FL 33137

FLORIDA AMPUTEE HOTLINE
P.O. Box 370788
Miami, FL 33137

AMPUTEE SUPPORT GROUP
Bon Secours Hospital
1050 N.E. 125th
North Miami, FL

CENTRAL FLORIDA AMPUTEE
SERVICE GROUP
P.O. Box 561142
Orlando, FL 32856-1142

A.F.T.E.R. INC.—AMPUTEES
FOR TRAINING, EDUCATION,
AND REHAB
8408 W. McNab Road
Tamarac, FL 33321
    A.F.T.E.R. is in the process of
establishing a national network
program for children born missing
limbs. If your child fits into

this category, please contact them
and help get this important program
started.

C.A.L.D.—CHILDREN
AFFLICTED WITH LIMB
DEFICIENCIES
9127 New Orleans Drive
Orlando, FL 32818

PEN-PARENT EDUCATION
NETWORK OF FLORIDA
2215 East Henry Avenue
Tampa, FL 33610

Iowa

Robin Smith
408 S. Dodge
Iowa City, IA 52240

(or 1801 W. 5th
Indianola, IA 50125)

Illinois

Donna Boddy
8826 Butterfield Lane
Orland Park, IL 60462

AMPUTEE SERVICE
ASSOCIATION
P.O. Box A 3819
Chicago, IL 60690

FAMILIES AND AMPUTEES IN
MOTION
10046 S. Western Avenue,
Suite 10
Chicago, IL 60643

Indiana

MICHIANA AMPUTEE
SUPPORT GROUP
3449 S. High
South Bend, IN 46614

Kansas

L.E.A.P.S. ACROSS THE
HEARTLAND (LOWER EX-
TREMITY AMPUTEES
PROVIDING SUPPORT)
P.O. Box 7906
Shawnee Mission, KS 66207

Louisiana

Trisha Cook
10105 Idlewood Place
River Ridge, LA 70123

Massachusetts

COMMONWEALTH OF
MASSACHUSETTS
2513 8th Street
Charlestown, MA 02129

HELPING HANDS
P.O. Box 2348
Farmington, MA 01701
    Support group for families with
children with hand or arm ab-
normalities.

Maryland

AMPUTEE ASSOCIATION OF
MARYLAND
c/o Kernan Hospital
2200 Forest Park Avenue
Baltimore, MD 21207

Michigan

A.L.A.R.M.—AMPUTEE OF
LEGS OR ARMS RESOURCE
MEETINGS
1301 North Main Street
Adrian, MI 49221

AMPUTEE SUPPORT AND
SERVICE GROUP
31917 Wayburn Drive
Farmington Hills, MI 48018

MICHIGAN AMPUTEE FD., INC.
6849 S. Division Avenue
Grand Rapids, MI 49508

Mississippi

MISSISSIPPI AMPUTEE
SUPPORT GROUP
4901 McWillie Circle
Jackson, MS 39206

Missouri

Suzanne King & Dave Farris
c/o St. Joe YMCA
315 S. 6th Street
St. Joseph, MO 64501

AMPUTEES IN MOTION
P.O. Box 335
Columbia, MO 65205

Maureen Raffensperger, R.P.T.
Heartland Centre
Physical Therapy Dept.
701 Faraon Street
St. Joseph, MO 64501

North Carolina

PHYSICALLY CHALLENGED,
INC. OF WESTERN NORTH
CAROLINA
P.O. Box 888
Sylva, NC 28779

Nebraska

HOTLINE FOR THE
HANDICAPPED
P.O. Box 94987
301 Centennial Mall S.
Lincoln, NE 68509

New Jersey

Elaine Naismith
7 Barberry Way
Essex Fells, NJ 07021

PACT—PARENTS OF AMPUTEE
CHILDREN TOGETHER
c/o Kessler Institute for
Rehabilitation
Pleasant Valley Way
West Orange, NJ 07052

IN-STEP
300 Winston Drive, #1212
Cliffside Park, NJ 07010

IN-STEP
Englewood Hospital
350 Engle Street
Englewood, NJ 07631

S.H.A.G. SELF-HELP AMPUTEE
GROUP
c/o Kessler Institute
Pleasant Valley Way
West Orange, NJ 07052

Nevada

NORTHERN NEVADA AM-
PUTEE SUPPORT GROUP
710 Marion Way
Sparks, NV 89431

New York

Thelma W. Ryan
19 Pine Tree Lane
Levittown, NY 11756

Michael Madden
242 Bloomingrove Drive
Troy, NY 12180

AMPUTEE SUPPORT
NETWORK
Box 2501
Liverpool, NY 13090

FEDERATION OF THE
HANDICAPPED
211 W. 14th Street
New York, NY 10011

52 ASSOCIATION
441 Lexington Avenue, Suite 502
New York, NY 10017

NATIONAL AMPUTEE
FOUNDATION
1245 150th Street
Whitestone, NY 11357

STATEN ISLAND AMPUTEE
CLUB
475 Seaview Avenue
Staten Island, NY 10305

Ohio

AMPUTEE SUPPORT GROUP
222 Pleasanthill Court
Centerville, OH 45459

CENTRAL OHIO AMPUTEE
SUPPORT GROUP
P.O. Box 1701
Columbus, Ohio 43216

I CAN
2380 Overlook Road
Cleveland Heights, OH 44118

Oklahoma

Preston Cross
3384 Del Aire Place
Del City, OK 73115

Oregon

Jan Morrissey
4135 North Court Avenue
Portland, OR 97217

Pennsylvania

AMP-PEER
Magee Rehab Hospital
1600 Arch Street
Philadelphia, PA 19102

AMPUTEE SUPPORT GROUP
Harmarville Rehab Ctr.
P.O. Box 11460,
Guys Run Road
Pittsburgh, PA 15238

AMPUTEE SUPPORT GROUP
OF ALTOONA
c/o Mercy Hospital
2500 7th Avenue
Altoona, PA 16603

AMPUTEE SUPPORT GROUP
Rehab Hospital of York
1850 Normandie Drive
York, PA 17404

AMPUTEES & NON-
FUNCTIONAL LIMBS SUPPORT
GROUP
c/o Altoona Rehab Hospital
2005 Valley View Blvd.
Altoona, PA 16602

COMMUNITY AMPUTEE
SUPPORT TEAM
P.O. Box 400, R.D. 6
Coatsville, PA 19320

COMMUNITY AMPUTEE
SUPPORT TEAM
Bryn Mawr Rehab Hospital
414 Paoli Pike
Malvern, PA 19355

COMMUNITY AMPUTEE
SUPPORT TEAM
503 N. Water Street
Lititz, PA 17543

Tennessee

Barbara Lear
447 E. Market Street
Kingsport, TN 37660
Sheryl Jackson, R.N., C.N.S.
D-2120, M.C.N.
Nashville, TN 37232

Texas

EAST TEXAS AMPUTEE
FOUNDATION
915 Old Hickory Road
Tyler, TX 75703

HILL COUNTRY AMPUTEE
FOUNDATION
P.O. Box 706
Kerrville, TX 78028

NORTH TEXAS AMPUTEE
SUPPORT GROUP
5427 Redfield
Dallas, TX 75235

PILOT PARENTS TRAINING
PROGRAM
1704 Seamist, Suite 450
Houston, TX 77008

S.O.A.R., INC.–STEPPING OUT
AND REACHING
3050 Post Oak Blvd.
Houston, TX 77056

TEXAMO HEALTH CARE
CENTER
120 S. Crockett
Sherman, TX 75090

WEST TEXAS AMPUTEE
ASSOCIATION
3521 A. 34th Street
Lubbock, TX 79404

Virginia

Bill Haneke
P.O. Box 11192
Richmond, VA 23230

INDEPENDENT LIVING CENTERS

ACCESS ALASKA
3550 Airport Way #3
Fairbanks, AK 99709
(907) 451-6370

ALASKA DIV. OF VOC. REHAB.
Pouch F, M/S 0581
Juneau, AK 99811
(907) 465-1814

HOPE COTTAGES, INC.
2805 Bering Street
Anchorage, AK 99503
(907) 561-5335

INDEPENDENT LIVING
CENTER
3421 Fifth Avenue, South
Birmingham, AL 35222
(205) 251-2223

I.L. SERVICES CENTER
5800 Asher Avenue
Little Rock, AR 72204
(501) 568-7588

OUR WAY, INC.
10434 W. 36th Street, Rm. 314
Little Rock, AR 72204
(501) 225-5030

SAMOA CENTER FOR I.L.
P.O. Box 3492
Pago Pago, AS 96799
(684) 633-2337

ARIZONA BRIDGE ILC
1229 East Washington
Phoenix, AZ 85034
(602) 256-2245

COMMUNITY OUTREACH
PROGRAM
268 West Adams Street
Tucson, AZ 85705
(602) 792-1906

DISABILITY RESOURCE
CENTER
1023 North Tyndall Avenue
Tucson, AZ 85719
(602) 624-6452

SERVICES TO ADVANCE I.L.
1700 First Avenue,
Suite 114
Yuma, AZ 85364
(602) 783-3177

ADULT INDEPENDENCE
DEVELOPMENT
1190 Benton Street
Santa Clara, CA 95050
(408) 985-1243

BRENTWOOD SOCIAL
PROGRAM
11301 Wilshire Blvd.
Los Angeles, CA 90073
(213) 824-3277

C.A.P.H.-I.L.C.
1617 East Saginaw Way #109
Fresno, CA 93704
(209) 222-2274

C.I.L. SAN GABRIEL VALLEY
114 East Italia Street
Covina, CA 91723
(818) 967-0635

CENTER FOR I.L.
2539 Telegraph Avenue
Berkeley, CA 94704
(415) 841-4776

CENTER FOR I.L.
2231 East Garvey Avenue
West Covina, CA 91791
(818) 339-1278

COMM. REHAB SERVICES – ILC
4716 Brooklyn Avenue
Bldg. B, # 15
Los Angeles, CA 90022
(213) 266-0453

COMMUNITY RESOURCES
576 B Street, Suite 1
Santa Rosa, CA 95401
(707) 528-2745

COMMUNITY
RESOURCES – ILC
439 A Street
Hayward, CA 94541
(415) 881-5743

COMMUNITY
RESOURCES – ILC
340 Soquel Avenue, Suite 115
Santa Cruz, CA 95062
(408) 688-0364

COMMUNITY SERVICE CTR.
2864 University Avenue
San Diego, CA 92104
(619) 293-3500

DARRELL McDANIEL I.L.C.
18 South Chester
Bakersfield, CA 93304
(805) 325-1065

DARREL McDANIEL I.L.C.
44815 Fig Ave., Suite B
Lancaster, CA 93534
(805) 945-6602

DARRELL McDANIEL I.L.C.
14354 Haynes Street
Van Nuys, CA 92401
(818) 785-6934

DAYLE MCINTOSH CENTER
150 W. Cerritos, Bldg. 4
Anaheim, CA 92805
(714) 772-8285

DISABLED RESOURCES CTR.
1045 Pine Avenue
Long Beach, CA 90813
(213) 437-3543

F.R.E.E.D.
154 Hughes Road #1
Grass Valley, CA 95945
(916) 272-1732

GOOD SHEPHERD CENTER
4323 Leimert Blvd.
Los Angeles, CA 90008
(213) 295-5439

HUMBOLDT ACCESS PROJECT
712 Fourth Street
Eureka, CA 95501
(707) 445-8404

I.L.C. OF SAN FRANCISCO
4429 Cabrillo Street
San Francisco, CA 94121
(415) 751-8765

I.L. RESOURCE CENTER
423 West Victoria
Santa Barbara, CA 93101
(805) 963-1359

I.L. SKILLS PROGRAM
875 O'Neill Avenue
Belmont, CA 94002
(415) 595-0783

MARIN C.I.L.
710 4th Street
San Rafael, CA 94901
(415) 595-0783

NORTHERN CALIFORNIA I.L.C.
555 Rio Lindo Avenue, Suite B
Chico, CA 95926
(916) 893-8527

RESOURCES FOR I.L.
1211 H Street #B
Sacramento, CA 95814
(916) 446-3074

ROLLING START, INC.
443 West 4th Street
San Bernardino, CA 92401
(714) 884-2129

SOUTHEAST C.I.L.
12458 Rives Avenue
Downey, CA 90242
(213) 862-6531

U.C.P. ADULT ACTIVITY
CENTER
347 East Poplar
Stockton, CA 95203
(209) 464-4817

WESTSIDE C.I.L.
1516 Cravens Avenue
Torrance, CA 90501
(213) 320-8920

WESTSIDE CENTER I.L.C.
12901 Venice Blvd.
Los Angeles, CA 90066
(213) 390-3611

WINNERS REHAB & I.L.C.
15738 California Avenue
Paramount, CA 90723
(213) 634-4491

ATLANTIS COMMUNITY, INC.
2937 East Galley Road
Colorado Springs, CO 80909
(303) 591-5550

ATLANTIS COMMUNITY, INC.
4536 East Colfax
Denver, CO 80220

ATLANTIS COMMUNITY, INC.
2710 West Alameda Avenue
Denver, CO 80219
(303) 936-1110

CENTER FOR I.L.
1245 East Colfax Avenue, Suite 219
Denver, CO 80218

CENTER FOR PEOPLE WITH
DISABILITIES
1450 15th Street
Boulder, CO 80302
(303) 442-8662

COLORADO SPRINGS I.L.C.
122 South 16th Street
Colorado Springs, CO 80904

GREELEY RESOURCES
P.O. Box 5045
Greeley, CO 80631
(303) 330-6630

GREELEY CENTER
1734 8th Avenue
Greeley, CO 80631
(303) 352-8484

HANDICAPPED INFO. OFFICE
424 Pine, Suite 101
Fort Collins, CO 80524
(303) 482-2700

HELEN CAMPBELL, I.L.C.
835 Colorado Avenue
Grand Junction, CO 81501
(303) 241-0315

I.L. IN HOME TEACHING
524 Social Services Bldg.
1575 Sherman
Denver, CO 80203
(303) 839-2285

PUEBLO GOODWILL CENTER
410 North Main
Pueblo, CO 81003
(303) 543-4483

SAN LUIS VALLEY CENTER
Box 990
Alamosa, CO 81101
(303) 589-5708

C.I.L. OF SOUTHWESTERN
959 Main Street
Stratford, CT 06497
(203) 378-6977

CHAPLE HAVEN, INC.
1040 Walley Avenue
New Haven, CT 06515
(203) 397-1714

INDEPENDENCE UNLIMITED
410 Asylum Street
Hartford, CT 06103
(203) 549-1330

NEW HORIZONS, INC.
410 Asylum Street
Hartford, CT 06103
(203) 249-6275

D.C. CENTER FOR I.L.
1400 Florida Avenue, N.E., #3
Washington, DC 20002
(202) 388-0033

I.L. FOR THE HANDICAPPED
1301 Belmont Street, N.W.
Washington, DC 20009
(202) 797-9803

EASTER SEAL CENTER
240 North James Street, Suite 100
Wilmington, DE 19804
(302) 998-8090

INDEPENDENT LIVING, INC.
159 Willis Road, #D
Dover, DE 19901
(302) 734-9991

INDEPENDENT LIVING, INC.
818 South Broom Street
Wilmington, DE 19805
(302) 628-2253

C.I.L. IN CENTRAL FLORIDA
720 North Denning Drive
Winter Park, FL 32789
(305) 628-2253

C.I.L. OF NORTH FLORIDA,
INC.
1380 Ocala Road, #H-4
Tallahassee, FL 32304
(904) 575-9621

C.I.L. OF NORTHWEST FL.
3789 Nobles Street
Pensacola, FL 32514
(904) 477-8200

CATHEDRAL C.I.L.
3599 University Blvd., S.
Jacksonville, FL 32216
(904) 354-3378

CENTER FOR SURVIVAL
1335 N.W. 14th Street
Miami, FL 33125
(305) 547-5444

FLORIDA INSTITUTE
307 East Seventh Street
Tallahassee, FL 32303
(904) 681-6835

SELF-RELIANCE, INC.
12310 North Nebraska Avenue #5
Tampa, FL 33612
(813) 977-6368

SPACE COAST ASSOCIATION
1127 South Patrick Drive #6
Satellite Beach, FL 32937
(305) 777-2964

SPACE COAST ASSOCIATION
725 DeLeon Avenue, Suite 134
Titusville, FL 32780
(305) 269-7273

ATLANTIC CENTER
1201 Glenwood Avenue, S.E
Atlanta, GA 30316
(404) 656-2952

I.L.C. ROOSEVELT WARM
SPRINGS
P.O. Box 1000
Warm Springs, GA 31830
(404) 655-3321

INDEPENDENT LIVING
PROGRAM
212 West Oglethorpe
Albany, GA 31702

INDEPENDENT LIVING
PROGRAM
707 Pine Street
Macon, GA 31208
(912) 744-6270

INDEPENDENT LIVING
PROGRAM
420 Mall Blvd.
Savannah, GA 31416

INDEPENDENT LIVING
PROJECT
47 Trinity Avenue
Atlanta, Ga 30334
(404) 656-2639

BIG ISLAND C.I.L.
205 Kinoole Street
Hilo, HI 96720
(808) 935-3777

HAWAII C.I.L.
677 Ala Moana Blvd. #615
Honolulu, HI 96813
(808) 537-1941

KAUAI C.I.L.
P.O. Box 3529
Lihue, HI 96766
(808) 245-4034

MAUI C.I.L.
1446-D Lower Main Street, Room
105
Wailuku, HI 96793
(808) 242-4966

CENTER FOR I.L. REHAB
SERVICES
524 4th Street
Des Moines, IA 50309
(515) 281-7999

HOPE HAVEN
1800 19th Street
Rock Valley, IA 51247
(712) 476-2737

INDEPENDENT LIVING INC.
26 East Market
Iowa City, IA 52240
(319) 338-3870

CENTER OF RESOURCES
707 North 7th, Suite A
P.O. Box 4185
Pocatello, ID 83201
(208) 232-2747

DAWN ENTERPRISES, INC.
P.O. Box 388
Blackfoot, ID 83221
(208) 785-5890

HOUSING SOUTHWEST #2
1102-4 West Finch Drive
Nampa, ID 83651
(208) 467-7461

IDAHO I.L. SERVICES
650 West State
Boise, ID 83702
(208) 334-3390

STEPPING STONES, INC.
124 East Third Street
Moscow, ID 83843
(208) 883-0523

ACCESS LIVING METRO
CHICAGO
815 W. Van Buren Street, Suite 525
Chicago, IL 60607
(312) 226-5900

ALMA
1642 North Winchester Avenue,
Suite 100
Chicago, IL 60622
(312) 276-3176

CENTER FOR
COMPREHENSIVE SERVICES
P.O. Box 2825
Carbondale, IL 62901
(618) 529-3060

CENTER FOR DISABLED
STUDENTS
30 East Lake Street, Room 1045
Chicago, IL 60601
(312) 984-2872

CENTRAL ILLINOIS CENTER
FOR INDEPENDENT LIVING
222 North Western Avenue
Peoria, IL 61604
(309) 676-0192

FOX RIVER VALLEY CENTER
730-B West Chicago Street
Elgin, IL 60123
(312) 695-5818

IL DEPARTMENT OF REHAB
SERVICES
623 East Adams Street
Springfield, IL 62705
(217) 785-0218

ILLINOIS I.L.C.
710 East Odgen, Suite 207
Naperville, IL 60540
(312) 357-0077

IMPACT C.I.L.
P.O. Box 338
Alton, IL 62002
(618) 462-1411

LIVING INDEPENDENCE FOR
EVERYONE
1544 East College Avenue
Normal, IL 61761
(309) 452-5433

NORTHWESTERN ILLINOIS
C.I.L.
205 2nd Avenue
Sterling, IL 61081
(815) 625-7860

P.A.C.E. INC.
102 East Main Street, Suite 302
Urbana, IL 61801
(217) 344-5433

R.A.M.P.
104 Chestnut Street
Rockford, IL 61101
(815) 968-7467

SOUTHERN ILLNOIS C.I.L.
780 East Grand Avenue
Carbondale, IL 62901
(618) 457-3318

SPRINGFIELD CENTER
426 West Jefferson
Springfield, IL 62702
(217) 523-2587

WEST COOK C.I.L.
711 South 5th Avenue
Maywood, IL 60153
(312) 450-3810

CENTER FOR I.L.
5800 Fairfield,
Suite 210
Fort Wayne, IN 46807
(219) 745-5491

DAMAR HONES, INC.
6324 Kentucky Avenue
P.O. Box 41
Camby, IN 46113
(317) 856-5201

CENTER FOR THE
HANDICAPPED
1119 West 10th, Suite 2
Topeka, KS 66604
(913) 233-6323

COWLEY CITY, DEVELOP-
MENTAL SERVICES
P.O. Box 133
Arkansas City, KS 67005
(316) 442-3575

INDEPENDENT LIVING OF
SOUTHWESTERN KANSAS
4808 West 9th
Wichita, KS 67212
(316) 942-8079

INDEPENDENCE INC.
1910 Haskell
Lawrence, KS 66046
(913) 841-0333

INDEPENDENT CONNECTION
1710 West Schilling Road
Salina, KS 67401
(913) 827-9383

INDEP. LIVING PROGRAM
2200 Gage Blvd.
VA Med Center
Topeka, KS 66622
(913) 272-3111

LINK, INC.
P.O. Box 1016
Hays, KS 67601
(913) 625-5678

NETWORK FOR THE
DISABLED
313 A Broadway
P.O. Box 35
Valley Falls, KS 66088
(913) 945-6623

RESOURCE CENTER FOR I.L.
107 Barclay
Osage City, KS 66523
(913) 528-3240

THREE RIVERS I.L.C.
810 4th Street
Wamego, KS 66547
(913) 456-9915

C.I.L. OF LOUISVILLE
P.O. Box 35260
Louisville, KY 40232

CENTER FOR ACCESSIBLE
LIVING
835 West Jefferson, Suite 105
Louisville, KY 40202
(502) 589-6620

CENTER FOR I.L.
1900 Brownsboro Road
Louisville, KY 40206
(502) 897-6439

CONTACT, INC.
212 West Broadway
Frankfort, KY 40601
(502) 875-5777

WEST END AWARENESS
402 South 38th Street, #2C
Louisville, KY 40212
(502) 778-6770

INDEPENDENT LIVING
CENTER
320 North Carrolton Avenue, Suite
2C
New Orleans, LA 70119
(504) 484-6400

NEW HORIZONS, INC.
4030 Wallace Avenue
Shreveport, LA 71108
(318) 635-3652

SOUTHWEST LOUISIANA I.L.C.
3104 Enterprise Blvd.
Lake Charles, LA 70601
(318) 478-4748

VOLUNTEERS OF AMERICA,
I.L.C.
3131 1-10 Service Road N.
#100
Metairie, LA 70002
(504) 834-7015

AD-LIB
442 North Street
Pittsfield, MA 01201
(413) 442-7047

ARC-I.L. PROGRAM
38 Hiramar Road
Hyannis, MA 02601
(617) 771-6595

BOSTON CENTER-ILC
50 New Edgerly Road
Boston, MA 02115
(617) 536-2187

CENTER FOR LIVING AND
WORKING, INC.
600 Lincoln Street
Worcester, MA 01605
(617) 853-1068

D.E.A.F., INC.
215 Brighton Avenue
Allston, MA 02134
(617) 254-4041

HIGHLAND HEIGHTS
APARTMENTS
P.O. Box 989
Fall River, MA 02722
(617) 675-3500

INDEPENDENT ASSOCIATES
693 Bedford Street
P.O. Box 146
Elmwood, MA 02337
(617) 559-9091

NORTHEAST I.L. PROGRAM
190 Hampshire Street,
Suite 101 B
Lawrence, MA 01840
(617) 687-4288

RENAISSANCE PROGRAM
21 Branch Street
Lowell, MA 01851
(617) 454-7944

STAVROS, INC.
691 South East Street
Amherst, MA 01002
(413) 256-0473

STUDENT I.L. EXPERIENCE
3 Randolph Street
Canton, MA 02021
(617) 828-2440

VISION FOUNDATION, INC.
818 Mt. Auburn Street
Watertown, MA 02172
(617) 926-4232

MARYLAND CITIZENS FOR
HOUSING
6305-A Sherwood Road
Baltimore, MD 21239
(301) 377-5900

ALPHA I—MAINE I.L.
PROGRAM
169 Ocean
South Portland, ME 04106
(207) 767-2189

ALPHA I—OUTREACH OFFICE
41 Acme Road
Brewer, ME 04412
(207) 989-6016

ALPHA I—OUTREACH OFFICE
71 State Street
Augusta, ME 04330
(207) 623-1115

ALPHA I—OUTREACH OFFICE
373 Main Street-Rear
Presque Isle, ME 04769
(207) 764-6466

INDEPENDENT LIVING CTR.
Bell Dorm, Husson College
Bangor, ME 04401

MAINE I.L. CENTER
74 Winthrop Street
Augusta, ME 04330
(207) 622-5434

MOTIVATIONAL SERVICES, INC.
114 State Street
Augusta, ME 04330
(207) 622-6273

SHALOM HOUSE, INC.
90 High Street
Portland, ME 04101
(207) 874-1080

THE TOGETHER PLACE
150 Union Street
Bangor, ME 04401
(207) 947-6125

ANN ARBOR CENTER FOR I.L.
2568 Packard, Georgetown Mall
Ann Arbor, MI 48104
(313) 971-0277

ARC/OTTOWA COUNTY
1001 East Wesley
Musk, MI 49442
(616) 777-2006

C.I.L. OF NORTHEASTERN MN
2310 First Avenue
Hibbing, MN 55746
(218) 262-6675

CENTER FOR HANDICAPPED AFFAIRS
918 Southland Street
Lansing, MI 48910
(517) 393-0305

CENTER FOR I.L.
2845 Crooks Road
Rochester, MI 48063
(313) 853-0376

CENTER FOR I.L.
6044 Rochester Road
Troy, MI 48098
(313) 828-3500

COMMUNITY LIVING CENTER
935 Barlow
Traverse City, MI 49684
(616) 941-7150

CRISTO REY HISPANIC CTR.
1314 Ballard Street
Lansing, MI 48906
(517) 372-4700

FAMILY RESOURCE CENTER
51 West Hancock
Detroit, MI 48201
(313) 831-0202

GRAND RAPIDS C.I.L.
3375 South Division
Grand Rapids, MI 49508
(616) 243-0846

INDEPENDENT LIVING
246 South River
Holland, MI 49423
(616) 396-1201

KALAMAZOO C.I.L.
833 West South
Kalamazoo, MI 49007
(616) 345-1516

LIFE SKILLS CENTER
1608 Lake Street
Kalamazoo, MI 49001
(616) 344-0202

MIDLAND I.L. PROGRAM
810 East Ashman
Midland, MI 48640
(517) 835-4041

OPPORTUNITIES UNLIMITED
111 South 9th Street,
Suite 211
Columbia, MO 65201
(314) 874-1646

OPTIONS, INTERSTATE RESOURCE CIL
211 Demers Avenue,
Holiday Mall
East Grand Forks, MN 56721
(218) 773-6100

ACCESSIBLE SPACE, INC.
2550 University Avenue,
W. 301 N
St. Paul, MN 55114
(612) 645-7271

HOMEOWNER ACCESSIBILITY LOAN PROGRAM
400 Sibley #300
St. Paul, MN 55101
(612) 296-7613

R.E.A.L.
317 West Main Street
Marshall, MN 2221
(507) 532-2221

VINLAND NATIONAL CENTER
P.O. Box 308
Loretto, MN 55357
(612) 479-3555

ROCHESTER CIL
1306 7th Street NW
Rochester, MN 55901
(507) 285-1815

ALPHA HOME
P.O. Box 30
Hazlehurst, MS 39083
(601) 894-1771

INDEPENDENT LIVING CENTER
300 Capers Avenue
Jackson, MS 39203
(601) 961-4140

OPPORTUNITIES UNLIMITED
111 South 9th Street,
Suite 211
Columbia, MO 65201
(314) 874-1646

THE WHOLE PERSON, INC.
6301 Rockhill Road,
Suite 30 E
Kansas City, MO 64131
(816) 361-0304

REHABILITATION INSTITUTE
3011 Baltimore
Kansas City, MO 64108
(816) 361-0304

INDEPENDENCE CENTER
4380 West Pine Blvd.
St. Louis, MO 63108
(314) 533-6511

PLACES FOR PEOPLE, INC.
4120 Lindell Blvd.
St. Louis, MO 63108
(314) 535-5600

LIFE SKILL FOUNDATION
609 North & South
St. Louis, MO 63130
(314) 863-3913

DISABLED CITIZENS ALLIANCE
Box 675
Viburnum, MO 65566
(314) 244-3315

MONTANA INDEPENDENT LIVING
1301 11th Avenue
Helena, MT 59601
(406) 442-5755

SUMMITT ILC
1280 South Third Street, West
Missoula, MT 59801
(406) 729-1630

HANDICAP REACH OUT, INC.
Box 948,
345 W. Third Street
Chadron, NE 69337
(308) 432-3560

LEAGUE OF HUMAN DIGNITY
1423 O Street
Lincoln, NE 68508
(402) 471-7871

ASSOCIATION FOR THE
HANDICAPPED
P.O. Box 28458
Las Vegas, NV 89126
(702) 870-7050

INDEPENDENT LIVING
PROJECT
6200 West Oakey
Las Vegas, NV 89102
(702) 870-7050

SUCCESS THROUGH IL
EXPERIENCES
1501 Park Avenue
Asbury Park, NJ 07712
(201) 774-4737

IL RESOURCE CENTER
98 James Street,
Suite 205
Edison, NJ 08820
(201) 632-1590

HANDICAPPED IL PROGRAM
44 Armory Street
Englewood, NJ 07631
(201) 568-0817

NEW VISTAS ILC
500 Don Gaspar
Santa Fe, NM 87501
(505) 984-8171

OPTIONS FOR INDEPENDENCE
55 Market Street
Auburn, NY 13021
(315) 255-3447

GLENS FALLS ILC
P.O. Box 453
Glens Falls, NY 12801
(518) 792-3537

MIDDLETOWN CIL
208 Wickham Avenue
Middletown, NY 10940
(914) 344-4055

DIRECTIONS IN IL
2636 West State Street, Suite A & B
Olean, NY 14760
(716) 373-4602

TACONIC RESOURCES FOR
INDEPENDENCE
89 Market Street
Poughkeepsie, NY 12601
(914) 452-3913

ROCKLAND ILC
235 North Main
Spring Valley, NY 10977
(914) 426-0707

TROY RESOURCE CIL
Troy Atrium, 4th & Broadway
Troy, NY 12180
(518) 274-0701

WATERTOWN ILC
Suite 500, Woolworth Bldg.
Watertown, NY 13601
(315) 785-8703

CAPITAL DISTRICT CIL
22 Colvin Avenue
Albany, NY 12206
(518) 459-6422

MODEL APPROACHES FOR
ILPs
Human Resources Center
IU Willets Road
Albertson, NY 11507
(516) 747-5400

IL FOR THE HANDICAPPED,
INC.
408 Jay Street, Room 401
Brooklyn, NY 11201
(718) 625-7500

BUFFALO IL PROGRAM
3108 Main Street
Buffalo, NY 14214
(716) 836-0822

SUFFOLK CITY/HANDICAPPED
SERVICES
65 Jetson Lane
Central Islip, NY 11722
(516) 348-5340

WESTERN NY IL PROGRAM
2015 Transit
Elma, NY 14059
(716) 838-6904

LONG ISLAND CIL/SUNY
Administration Bldg., #115
Farmingdale, NY 11735
(516) 420-2000

RESOURCE CENTER FOR
ACCESSIBLE LIVING, INC.
602 Albany Avenue
Kingston, NY 12401
(914) 331-0541

SERVICES FOR THE
PHYSICALLY HANDICAPPED
240 Old Country Road, #610
Mineola, NY 11501

VISIONS
817 Broadway, 11th Floor
New York, NY 10003
(212) 477-3800

CENTER FOR INDEPENDENCE
OF THE DISABLED IN NEW
YORK
853 Broadway, #611
New York, NY 10003
(212) 674-2300

ROCHESTER CIL
464 South Clinton Avenue
Rochester, NY 14620
(716) 546-6990

INDEPENDENT LIVING IN THE
CAPITAL DISTRICT
2660 Albany Street
Schenectady, NY 12304
(518) 393-2412

ARISE CIL
501 East Fayette Street
Syracuse, NY 13202
(315) 472-3171

RESOURCE CIL
401 Columbia Street
Utica, NY 13502
(315) 797-4642

WESTCHESTER COUNTY ILC
297 Knollwood Road
White Plains, NY 10607
(914) 682-3926

YONKERS ILC
984 North Broadway
Yonkers, NY 10701
(914) 968-4717

METROLINA ILC
1012 S. Kings Drive
Doctor's Building G-2
Charlotte, NC 28283
(704) 375-3977

FRASER HALL
711 South University Drive
Fargo, ND 59103
(701) 232-3301

HOUSING INDUSTRY
TRAINING CIL
1007 NW 18th
Mandan, ND 58554
(701) 663-0376

TOTAL LIVING CONCEPTS
7710 Reading Road, Suite 001
Cincinnati, OH 45237
(513) 761-3399

SERVICES FOR IL
25100 Euclid Avenue, Suite 105
Euclid, OH 44117
(216) 731-1529

GREEN COUNTRY IL
RESOURCE CENTER
P.O. Box 2295
Bartlesville, OK 74005
(918) 336-0700

TOTAL INDEPENDENT LIVING
TODAY
601 North Porter
Norman, OK 73071

ABILITY RESOURCES
1724 East 8th Street
Tulsa, OK 74104
(918) 592-1235

LAUREL HILL CENTER ILP
2621 Augusta Street
Eugene, OR 97403
(503) 485-6340

COLUMBIA GORGE REHAB
CENTER
1306 Taylor Street
Hood River, OR 97031
(503) 386-2544

RESIDENTIAL TRAINING &
CARE FACILITIES
P.O. Box 1072
Medford, OR 97501
(503) 772-1503

ACCESS OREGON
8213 SE 17th Avenue
Portland, OR 97202
(503) 230-1225

RESOURCES FOR ILC
4721 Pine Street
Philadelphia, PA 19143
(215) 471-2265

ALLIED SERVICES FOR THE
HANDICAPPED
475 Morgan Hwy.
Scranton, PA 18505
(717) 348-2221

PARI INDEPENDENT LIVING
CENTER
Independence Square
500 Prospect Street
Pawtucket, RI 02860
(401) 725-1966

INSIGHT INDEPENDENT
LIVING
43 Jefferson Blvd.
Warwick, RI 02888
(401) 941-3322

SC VR ILP
1400 Boston Avenue
West Columbia, SC 29169

PRAIRIE FREEDOM CENTER
FOR DISABLED
INDEPENDENCE
800 West Avenue North
Sioux Falls, SD 57104
(605) 339-6558

MEMPHIS CIL
163 North Angelus
Memphis, TN 38104
(901) 726-6404

EDUCATIONAL SUPPORT
SERVICES
P.O. Box 19028
U.T. at Arlington
Arlington, TX 76019

TEXAS REHAB COMM IL
SERVICES
118 E. Riverside Drive
Austin, TX 78704
(512) 445-8000

DALLAS CENTER FOR IL
8625 King George Drive, Suite 210
Dallas, TX 75235
(214) 631-6900

DISABLED ABILITY RE-
SOURCE ENVIRONMENT
8929 Viscount, Suite 101
El Paso, TX 79925
(915) 591-0800

HOUSTON CENTER FOR IL
3233 Wesleyan, Suite 102
Houston, TX 77027
(713) 621-3703

INDEPENDENT LIFE STYLES
P.O. Box 742485
Houston, TX 77274
(713) 988-7655

OPTIONS FOR IL
47 North 200 East
Logan, UT 84321
(801) 750-2168

VERMONT CIL
174 River Street
Montpelier, VT 05602
(802) 229-0501

ENDEPENDENCE CENTER OF
NORTHERN VIRGINIA
2111 Wilson Blvd., Suite 400
Arlington, VA 22201
(703) 525-3268

CROSSROADS CENTER, INC.
215 North Main Street
Bridgewater, VA 22812
(703) 828-6073

INDEPENDENCE RESOURCE
CENTER
201 West Main Street # 8
Charlottesville, VA 22901
(804) 971-9629

WOODROW WILSON CIL
Box 37, WWRC
Fishersville, VA 22939
(703) 332-7103

INSIGHT ENTERPRISES
11832 Canon Blvd., Suite E
Newport News, VA 23606
(804) 873-0817

ENDEPENDENCE CENTER,
INC.
100 W. Plume, Suite 224
Norfolk, VA 23510
(804) 625-3555

CENTRAL VIRGINIA ILC, INC.
2900 West Broad Street
Richmond, VA 23230
(804) 353-6503

IL PROGRAM VAMC
RICHMOND
1201 Broad Rock Road
VAMC
Richmond, VA 23249
(804) 230-0001

SHENANDOAH VALLEY ILC
21 South Kent Street
Winchester, VA 22601
(703) 662-4452

VISION AND IL SERVICES
119 N. Commercial, Suite 320
Bellingham, WA 98225

KITSAP COMMUNITY ACTION
PROGRAM
1200 Elizabeth Avenue
Bremerton, WA 98310

INDEPENDENT LIFESTYLE
SERVICE
115 West Third
Ellensburg, WA 98926
(509) 925-1448

EVERETT COALITION OF
PEOPLE WITH DISABILITIES
1301 Hewett
Everett, WA 98201
(206) 252-6456

DIVISION OF VOC REHAB IL
SERVICES
P.O. Box 1788 M/A 21-C
Olympia, WA 98504
(206) 753-2756

CENTER FOR INDEPENDENCE
407 14th Avenue, SE
Puyallup, WA 98371
(206) 848-6661 ext. 1118

DISABILITIES LAW PROJECT
1524 Queen Anne North
Seattle, WA 98109
(206) 284-9733

EPILEPSY ASSOCIATION OF
WEST WA
1715 E. Cherry
Seattle, WA 98122
(206) 323-8174

ILP COMMUNITY HOME
HEALTH CARE
100 W. Harrison
South Tower
Seattle, WA 98119-4113
(206) 282-5048

RESOURCE CENTER FOR THE
HANDICAPPED
20150 45th Avenue, NE
Seattle, WA 98155
(206) 362-2273

VISION SERVICES
1401 Madison Street,
Rm 284
Seattle, WA 98104

WASHINGTON COALITION OF
CITIZENS WITH DISABILITIES
3530 Stoneway N.
Seattle, WA 98103
(206) 545-8306

ILC FOR TRANSITIONING
STUDENTS
N. 721 Jefferson,
Suite 403
Spokane, WA 99260
(509) 326-6355

ADVENTURES–INDEPEN-
DENCE DEVELOPMENT
819 S. Hatch
Spokane, WA 98202
(509) 535-9696

SPOKANE COALITION OF
PEOPLE WITH DISABILITIES
107 W. Queen Avenue
Spokane, WA 99205
(509) 328-6446

DISABILITIES LAW PROJECT
949 Market Street,
Suite 416
Tacoma, WA 98402
(206) 383-1848

COALITION OF HANDICAPPED
ORGANIZATIONS
6503-G East Mill Plain Blvd.
Vancouver, WA 98661
(206) 693-8819

APPALACHIAN CIL
1427 Lee St., E.
Charleston, WV 25301
(304) 342-6328

HUNTINGTON CIL, INC.
914-1/2 Fifth Avenue
Huntington, WV 25701
(304) 525-3324

N. CENTRAL WV CIL
1000 Elmer W. Prince Drive
Morgantown, WV 26505
(304) 599-3636

CURATIVE WORKSHOP, INC.
1506 South Oneida Street
St. Elizabeth Hospital
Appleton, WI 54915
(414) 738-2644

ILP CURATIVE REHAB CTR.
2900 Curry Lane, Box 8027
Green Bay, WI 54308
(414) 468-1161

ACCESS TO INDEPENDENCE
1954 East Washington Avenue
Madison, WI 53704
(608) 251-7575

CIL
University of Wisconsin
Menomonie, WI 54751
(715) 232-2150

SOUTHEASTERN WISCONSIN
CIL
1545 S. Layton Blvd.
Milwaukee, WI 53215
(414) 643-0910

IL SERVICES
5000 W. National Avenue
Milwaukee, WI 53295
(414) 384-2000 ext. 2361

SOCIETY'S ASSETS
720 High Street
Racine, WI 53402
(414) 637-9128

CHRISTIAN LEAGUE FOR THE
HANDICAPPED
P.O. Box 948
Walworth, WI 53184
(414) 275-5924

WYOMING IL REHAB
350 North Bighorn
Casper, WY 82601
(307) 266-6956

REHAB ENTERPRISES OF
NORTHEASTERN WYOMING
245 Broadway
Sheridan, WY 82801
(307) 672-7481

DC CIL
1400 Florida Avenue, NE, #3
Washington, DC 20002
(202) 388-0033

IL FOR THE HANDICAPPED,
INC.
1301 Belmont Street NW
Washington, DC 20009
(202) 797-9803

SAMOA CIL
P.O. Box 3492
Pago Pago, AS 96799
(684) 633-2337

CENTRO DE VIDA
INDEPENDIENTE
Apartado 1681
Hato Rey, PR 00919
(809) 758-0424

VIRGIN ISLANDS
ASSOCIATION FOR IL
P.O. Box 3305
Charlotte Amalie
St. Thomas, VI 00801
(809) 775-9740

SIBLING GROUPS

Linda Griffith
Septer
218 Front Street
Juneau, AK 99801
    Grades 6-12, varying handicaps

Lynn Donald
115 Suttle Drive
Springdale, AR 72764
    Grades 1-6, varying handicaps

Paul Whitmore-LNEC
6145 Decena Drive
San Diego, CA 92120
    Severe handicaps and behavior disorders

Claudia Paliaga
Humboldt Child Care Council
805 7th Street
Eureka, CA 95501

Sharon Mitchell & Marion Karian
ARC Children's Center
420 N. Broadway
Fresno, CA 93701
    Ages 5-17, DD and all handicapping conditions

Christine Cone, M.E.
ARC Children's Center
420 N. Broadway
Fresno, CA 93701
    Ages 5-18, all handicapping conditions

Pat Green
5328 Silver Strand Way
Sacramento, CA 95841

Linda Schneider
1216 Ferhside Street
Redwood City, CA 94061

Marita J. Repole
44 Washington Avenue
Danbury, CT 06810
    Ages up to 18, sibling loss

Judy S. Itzkowitz
Willington Ridge
Baxter Road
Bldg. 1, Unit F
West Wellington, CT 06279
    All ages, all disabilities

Evelyn S. Shapiro
22 Parsons Drive
West Hartford, CT 06117
    Varying handicaps

CANDLELIGHTERS
CHILDHOOD CANCER
FOUNDATION
1901 Pennslyvania Avenue, NW,
Suite 1001
Washington, DC 20006
    Ages up to 21, cancer

Nan Williamson
1409 W. Park
Urbana, FL 61801

Jadene Ransvell
Parent to Parent
1998 Sun Tree Blvd.
Clearwater, FL 34623

Sally Linton Burton
111 A Education Bldg.
University of Idaho
Moscow, ID 83843
    Ages 9-12, varying handicaps

Ms. Murry Bruce
Little Friends School
140 N. Wright Street
Naperville, IL 60540
    Varying ages, DD

Linda Bleschke
Children's Med Center
1775 Dempster Street
Park Ridge, IL 60068
    School age, Pediatric Oncology

Judy Feigon Schiffman
838 Michigan Avenue, Apt 4B
Evanston, IL 60202

Anne Martin
6017 Sawmill Woods Drive
Fort Wayne, IN 46835

Bob Carpenter
ARC Polk County
300 E. Locust
Des Moines, IA 50309

Greg Clancy
738 Hawkeye Drive
Iowa City, IA 52204
    Ages 4-18, varying handicaps

Janet Mapel
Div. of Dev. Disabilities
University Hospital School
University of Iowa
Iowa City, IA 52242
    School age to early adolescent, varying handicaps

Marilyn Neel
UCP Kids Center
982 Eastern Parkway, Box 6
Louisville, KY 40217
    Varying ages, varying handicaps

CHILD EVALUATION CENTER
University of Louisville
Dept. of Pediatrics
334 E. Broadway
Louisville, KY 40202
    Ages 12-17, all DD

April Kerr
Council for Ret. Citizens
1146 S. Third Street
Louisville, KY 40203
    Adolescents & school age, mental retardation, DD

Melba Stevens
Access
200 W. 2nd Street, Suite 101
Lexington, KY 40507
    Pre-elementary, elementary, adolescents, all handicapping conditions

DOWN SYNDROME PROJECT
3365 Dalrymple Drive
Baton Rouge, LA 70802
    All ages, Down Syndrome

Ruth Shook
United Cerebral Palsy of
Northeastern Maine, Inc.
103 Texas Avenue
Bangor, ME 04401
    Ages 8-14, DD and others except emotionally disturbed

Connie Korda
Maine Medical Center
Pediatric Clinic
22 Bramhall Street
Portland, ME 04102
    Varying handicaps

Barbara Fairfield
Pediatrics Genetics
Dept. CMSC 1004
Johns Hopkins Hospital
601 N. Broadway
Baltimore, MD 21205
    Genetics

Patricia Timm
Maryland School for the Deaf
P.O. Box 894
Columbia, MD 21044
    Ages 6-13, mainly deafness,
multihandicapped

Flora Smith
Hampton Elem. School
1115 Charmuth
Lutherville, MD 21093
    Elementary, varying handicaps

Cindy Politch
GBARC
1249 Boylston Street
Boston, MA 02215
    All ages, adults −M.R., younger
groups−all disabilities

Brina Neustat
Concord Family Services
Community Agencies Bldg.
Concord, MA 01742
    Elementary, varying handicaps

Terri Wolak
Pilot Parents of Central Minnesota
14 7th Avenue, N., Suite 032
St. Cloud, MN 56301
    All ages, varying handicaps

Meagan Dunhamn & Jennifer Funk
BASIS
15 Silver Doe Lane
Merrimack, NH 03054
    Ages 10-14, varying handicaps

Laurie Savage
Special Families United
P.O. Box 1141
Concord Bldg.
Concord, NH 03302

Rob Fernley
Elm Street School
Elm Street
Laconia, NH 03246

All ages, speech, language, and
all handicapping conditions

Gerard Costa
ARC
365-381 Clendenny Avenue
Jersey City, NJ 07304
    Ages up to 11, varying handicaps

Susan P. Levine
Family Resource Association
35 Haddon Avenue
Shrewsbury, NJ 07702
    Ages 4-9, 10-teen, varying
handicaps

ALTA MIRA SPECIALIZED
Family Services
3501 Campus NE
Albuquerque, NM 87106
    Ages 4-6, 7-9, 10-13, varying
handicaps

Ed Haddad, PH.D.
23 W. 95th Street
New York, NY 10025
    Children & adults, mental re-
tardation and DD

Dr. Jack Gorelick
New York City Association for the
Help of Retarded Children
200 Park Avenue, S.
New York, NY 10003
    Children & adults, mental re-
tardation and DD

Anna Mariana
The Shield Institute
144-61 Roosevelt Avenue
Flushing, NY 11354
    Ages 8-16, varying handicaps

Grace Snowdon
B.O.C.E.S.
Putnam/North Westchester
Yorktown Heights, NY 10598
    Ages 8-11 (residents of West-
chester county), MR & varying
handicaps

THREE VILLAGE C.Y.S., INC.
P.O. Box 593
Stony Brook, NY 11790

Fredda Stimeli
Association for Children with
Down's Syndrome, Inc.
2616 Martin Avenue
Bellmore, NY 11710
    Age 5 & older, Down Syndrome

Tom Fish
OSU Nisonger Center
1581 Dodd Drive
Columbus, OH 43210
    Ages 6-13, varying handicaps

Wendy L. Busch, M.S.
Dept. of Medical Genetics
2801 N. Gantenbein
Portland, OR 97227
    Ages 6-12, varying handicaps

Grace Peters
D.T. Watson Rehabilitation
Hospital and Education Center
Camp Meeting Road
Sewickley, PA 15143
    Any age, DD

Carol Frangicetto, M.ED
PATH (People Acting To Help)
8220 Castor Avenue
Philadelphia, PA 19152
    Ages 7-10, MR

Cathy A. Lucas
MH-MR Program
RD #1, Box 179-A
Towanda, PA 18848
    Ages 5-10, MR

Elizabeth Francis
Richardson Developmental Center
Box 835066
Richardson, TX 75083-5066
    All ages, varying handicaps

Lenore Locastro
P.E.I.D.
357 Butler Road
Falmouth, VA 22405
    Ages birth to 2 years, C.P., Down
Syndrome, Spina Bifida, DD

James May
Merrywood School
16120 NE 8th
Bellevue, WA 98008
    Ages 8-12, 13-17, varying handi-
caps

SPORTS AND RECREATION

Air Guns

CANADIAN WHEELCHAIR
SPORTS ASSOCIATION
333 River Road
Ottawa, Ontario K1L 8H9
Canada

NATIONAL WHEELCHAIR
SHOOTING FEDERATION
3617 Betty Drive,
Suite S
Colorado Springs, CO 80917

Aquatics

ADVISORY PANEL ON WATER
SPORTS FOR THE DISABLED
The Sports Council
70 Brompton Road
London SW3 1EX, England

AMERICAN RED CROSS
Adapted Aquatics
17th and D Streets
Washington, DC 20006

AMPUTEE SPORTS
ASSOCIATION
c/o George Beckmann, Jr.
11705 Mercy Blvd.
Savannah, GA 31419

BEACH WHEELS, INC.
1555 Shadowlawn Drive
Naples, FL 33942

BRITISH DISABLED WATER
SKI ASSOCIATION
Warren Wood, The Warren
Ahstead, Surrey KT 212 SN,
England

CANADIAN WHEELCHAIR
SPORTS ASSOCIATION
See Air Guns

NATIONAL ASSOCIATION OF
DISABLED SWIMMERS
c/o Jim Rice
1555 Shadowlawn Drive
Naples, FL 33942

NATIONAL ASSOCIATION OF
SWIMMING CLUBS FOR THE
HANDICAPPED
63 Dunnegan Road
Eltham, London SE9, England

NATIONAL HANDICAPPED
SPORTS AND RECREATION
ASSOCIATION (NHSRA)
c/o Jack Benedick
P.O. Box 18664
Capitol Hill Station
Denver, CO 80218

NATIONAL WHEELCHAIR
ATHLETIC ASSOCIATION
3617 Betty Drive, Suite S
Colorado Springs, CO 80917

OLYMPIA SPORTS
745 State Circle
P.O. Box 1941
Ann Arbor, MI 48106

PHYSICALLY CHALLENGED
SWIMMERS OF AMERICA
3617 Betty Drive, Suite S
Colorado Springs, CO 80917

Archery & Crossbow

ARCHERY DEVELOPMENT
PROGRAM COURAGE CENTER
3915 Golden Valley Road
Golden Valley, MN 55422

WHEELCHAIR ARCHERY
SPORTS SECTION
3617 Betty Drive,
Suite S
Colorado Springs, CO 80917

Arts

ASSOCIATION OF
HANDICAPPED ARTISTS, INC.
503 Brisbane Bldg.
Buffalo, NY 14203

BARRIER FREE THEATER
3325 Platt Road
Ann Arbor, MI 48104

DISABLED ARTISTS NETWORK
P.O. Box 20781
New York, NY 10025

HAPPI—HANDICAPPED
ARTISTS, PERFORMERS, AND
PARTNERS INC.
P.O. Box 24225
Los Angeles, CA 90024

INSTITUTE OF ARTS AND
DISABILITIES
2839 Ashby Avenue
Berkeley, CA 94705

MASSACHUSETTS
ASSOCIATION OF DISABLED
ARTISTS
114 Floral Street
Newton Highlands, MA 02161

NATIONAL COMMITTEE/ARTS
FOR THE HANDICAPPED
1825 Connecticut Ave. NW, Ste. 417
Washington, DC 20009

NATIONAL THEATRE
WORKSHOP OF THE
HANDICAPPED
106 W. 56th Street
New York, NY 10019

PROJECT MAJIC
c/o Daniel Freeman
Memorial Hospital
P.O. Box 100
Inglewood, CA 90306

PATH (PERFORMING ARTS
THEATRE OF THE
HANDICAPPED)
P.O. Box 9050
Carlsbad, CA 92208

VERY SPECIAL ARTS
JFK Center for the Performing Arts
Washington, DC 20566

Aviation

AMERICAN WHEELCHAIR
PILOTS ASSOCIATION
c/o Dave Graham
1621 East 2nd Avenue
Mesa, AZ 85204

CALIFORNIA WHEELCHAIR
AVIATORS
Bill Blackwood
1117 Rising Hill Way
Escondido, CA 92025

CANADIAN PARAPLEGIC
ASSOCIATION
Kirby Rowe
520 Sutherland Drive
Toronto, Ontario M4O 3V9

UNIVERSITY OF TENNESSEE
REHAB ENGINEERING
c/o Douglas Hobson, Technical
Director
682 Court Avenue
Memphis, TN 38163

WHEELCHAIR PILOTS
ASSOCIATION
11018 102nd Avenue, North
Largo, FL 33540

Baseball

AMERICAN SPECIAL
RECREATION ASSOCIATION
University of Iowa
Iowa City, IA 52240

Basketball

CANADIAN WHEELCHAIR
SPORTS ASSOCIATION
See Air Guns

NATIONAL WHEELCHAIR
ATHLETIC ASSOCIATION
See Aquatics

NATIONAL WHEELCHAIR
BASKETBALL ASSOCIATION
110 Seaton Bldg.
University of Kentucky
Lexington, KY 40506

ROLLINGS WARHAWK
WHEELCHAIR BASKETBALL
CAMP & COACHING CLINIC
Summer Camp Office
Roseman Bldg. 1004
University of Wisconsin
Whitewater, WI 53190

WRIGHT STATE UNIVERSITY
Dept. of Adapted Athletics and In-
tramural
009 Physical Education Bldg.
Dayton, OH 45435
    Has National Inter-collegiate
Wheelchair Basketball Tournament
and Adapted Athletics Program

Boating/Sailing

CANADIAN RECREATIONAL
CANOEING ASSOCIATION
P.O. Box 500
Hyde Park, Ontario, N0M 1Z0
Canada

COMMITTEE FOR
HANDICAPPED SAILING
Baerum Seilforening
Standalleen 8
1320 Stabelk
Norway

HANDICAPPED BOATERS
ASSOCIATION
P.O. Box 1134
Ansonia Station, NY 10023

INDEPENDENCE AFLOAT
c/o Variety Village
3701 Danforth Avenue
Scarborough, Ontario M1N 2G2
    Sailing school designed to teach
physically and visually impaired
children and adults to sail

LAKE MERRITT'S ADAPTIVE
BOATING
1520 Lakeside Drive
Oakland, CA 94612

S'PLORE—SPECIAL
POPULATIONS LEARNING
OUTDOOR RECREATION AND
EDUCATION
699 East South Temple, Suite 120
Salt Lake City, UT 84102

TRI-COUNTY WHEELCHAIR
ATHLETIC ASSOCIATION
Rt. 2, Box 589
Moncks Corner, SC 29461

WATER SAFETY & BOATING
PROGRAM FOR THE
DISABLED
Parks & Recreation Office
Sailboat House
1520 Lakeside Drive
Oakland, CA 94612

Body Conditioning

LABORATORY OF APPLIED
PHYSIOLOGY
Dept. of Physiology and Biophysics
054 Biological Sciences Bldg.
Wright State University
Dayton, OH 45435
    Research-oriented fitness train-
ing programs for wheelchair users

NATIONAL WHEELCHAIR
ATHLETIC ASSOCIATION
See Aquatics

RECREATION & ATHLETIC
REHAB EDUCATIONAL
CENTER
c/o Brad Hedrick
University of Illinois
1207 South Oak Street
Champaign, IL 61820

STRIDA—SPORTS TRAINING
RESEARCH INSTITUTE FOR
DISABLED ATHLETES
115 Wittich Hall
U.W.-LaCrosse
LaCrosse, WI 54601

Bowling

AMERICAN WHEELCHAIR
BOWLING ASSOCIATION
2424 N. Federal Hwy., Suite 109
Boynton Beach, FL 33435

WHEELCHAIR BOWLERS OF
SOUTHERN CALIFORNIA
6512 Cadia Circle
Huntington Beach, CA 92647

Camping/Hiking

ADOLESCENT AMPUTEE
CAMP
Physical Therapy Dept.
c/o Gay Gregg
Children's Hospital of Pittsburgh
125 DeSoto Street
Pittsburgh, PA 15213

BOY SCOUTS OF AMERICA
Scouting for the Handicapped
1325 Walnut Hill Lane
Irving, TX 75062-1296

BRECKENRIDGE OUTDOOR
EDUCATION CENTER
c/o Mike Mobley
P.O. Box 697
Breckenridge, CO 80424

C.W. HOG—COOPERATIVE
WILDERNESS HANDICAPPED
OUTDOOR GROUP
Idaho State University
Student Union,
Box 8118
Pocatello, ID 97756

FEDERATION FOR CHILDREN
WITH SPECIAL NEEDS
312 Stuart Street,
2nd Floor
Boston, MA 02116

GIRL SCOUTS OF THE U.S.A.
Scouting for the Disabled
830 Third Avenue
New York, NY 10022

HANDICAPPED UNBOUND
c/o Tom Carr
P.O. Box 1044
Prescott, AZ 86302

INFORMATION CENTER FOR
INDIVIDUALS WITH
DISABILITIES
20 Park Plaza, Room 330
Boston, MA 02116

Guide to Day Camps

NATIONAL WHEELCHAIR
ATHLETICS ASSOCIATION
See Aquatics

WILDERNESS ON WHEELS
FEDERATION
1136 S. Taos Way
Denver, CO 80223

Cycling

ADAPTIVE SPORTS PROGRAM
Kinesiotherapy Clinic
c/o Dr. Leonard Greninger
University of Toledo
2801 West Bancroft Street
Toledo, OH 43606

AMERICAN SPECIAL
RECREATION ASSOCIATION
Rec. Education Program
University of Iowa
Iowa City, IA 52240

FUN CYCLES
966 North Elm Street
Orange, CA 92667-5471

NEW ENGLAND HANDCYCLES
48 Bogle
Weston, MA 02193

ROWCYCLE
3164 North Mrks #120
Fresno, CA 93711

SUN CYCLE
P.O. Box 1285
Tavares, FL 32778

UNICYCLE
CP 276, Station N
Montreal, Quebec H2X 3M4
Hand-operated unicycle for use with
a wheelchair

Dance

AMERICAN ALLIANCE FOR
HEALTH, PHYSICAL
EDUCATION, RECREATION,
AND DANCE
Programs for the Handicapped
c/o Dr. Razor
1900 Association Drive
Reston, VA 22091

AMERICAN DANCE THERAPY
ASSOCIATION
2000 Century Plaza
Columbia, MD 21044

COMMITTEE OF RECREATION
AND LEISURE
President's Committee on
Employment of the Handicapped
c/o Gerald Hitzhuser
Washington, DC 20210

DEJA VU DANCE THEATRE
Barry Martin Dance Theatre
484 West 43rd Street, Suite 110
New York, NY 10036
    Founded by Barry Martin, a
quadriplegic who is the chore-
ographer

Disc Sports

FOSTER ANDERSON
190 Norman Road
Rochester, NY 14623
    "Quad-Bee" modified disc with
two adaptive clips for easier throw-
ing

U.S. DISC SPORTS
462 Main Road
West Hampton, NY 11978

Fishing

ADAPTIVE PHYSICAL
EDUCATION & RECREATION
Alfred I. duPont Institute
P.O. Box 269
Wilmington, DE 19899
    Special fishing gear

MIYA EPOCH COMPANY
1635 Crenshaw Blvd.
Torrance, CA 90501
    Adaptive gear

PHYSICALLY CHALLENGED
OUTDOOR ASSOCIATION
3006 Louisiana Avenue
Cleveland, OH 44109

ROYAL BEE CORP.
703 Kihekah
Pawhuska, OK 74056
    Electric retrievable fishing reel

Football

52 ASSOCIATION FOR THE
HANDICAPPED
441 Lexington Avenue, Suite 502
New York, NY 10017

NATIONAL WHEELCHAIR
ATHLETIC ASSOCIATION
See Aquatics

RECREATION & ATHLETIC
REHAB-ED. CENTER
University of Illinois
1207 South Oak Street
Champaign, IL 61820

Gardening

MILWOOD TRAINING CENTER
5606 Dower House Road
Upper Marlboro, MD 20870

NATIONAL COUNCIL FOR
THERAPY AND REHAB
THROUGH HORTICULTURE
9041 Comprint, Suite 103
Gaithersburg, MD 20877

Golf

AMPUTEE SPORTS
ASSOCIATION
11705 Mercy Blvd.
Savannah, GA 31419

INTERNATIONAL SR.
AMPUTEE GOLF SOCIETY,
INC.
14039 Ellesmere Drive
Tampa, FL 33624

NATIONAL AMPUTEE GOLF
ASSOCIATION
P.O. Box 1128
Amherst, NH 03031

EASTERN AMPUTEE GOLF
ASSOCIATION
10 Amherst Drive
Bethlehem, PA 18015

AKRON AMPUTEE GOLF
ASSOCIATION
1373 Lott Drive
Uniontown, OH 44685

MICHIGAN AMPUTEE GOLF
ASSOCIATION
8041 Ridgeview
Lake City, MI 49651

W.I.S.E. AMPUTEE GOLF
ASSOCIATION
P.O. Box 146
Stoughton, WI 53589

WESTERN AMPUTEE GOLF
ASSOCIATION
3719 Oak Park Court
Concord, CA 94519

SENIORS (50+) AMPUTEE
GOLF ASSOCIATION
504 LaJoffa
Sun City, FL 33570

SOCIETY OF ONE-ARMED
GOLFERS
11 Coldwell Lane
Felling, Tyne Wear
NE10 9EX, England

NATIONAL HANDICAPPED
SPORTS & RECREATION
ASSOCIATION (NHSRA)
P.O. Box 18664
Capitol Hill Station
Denver, CO 80218

PROJECT FORE, GOLF FOR
THE PHYSICALLY DISABLED
Singing Hills Country Club
3007 Dehesa Road
El Cajon, CA 92021

RECREATIONAL CENTER FOR
THE HANDICAPPED
207 Skyline Blvd.
San Francisco, CA 94132

U.S. AMPUTEE ATHLETIC
ASSOCIATION
Rt. 2, County Line Road
Fairview, TN 37062

WAR AMPUTATIONS OF
CANADA
c/o Armand Viau & H.C.
Chadderton
2277 Riverside Drive, Suite 210
Ottawa, Ontario K1H 7X6

Hiking

See Camping

Horseback Riding

BRECKENRIDGE OUTDOOR
EDUCATION CENTER
See Camping/Hiking

NATIONAL FOUNDATION FOR
HORSEMANSHIP FOR THE
HANDICAPPED
c/o Maudie Hunter-Warfel
P.O. Box 462
Malvern, PA 19355

NORTH AMERICAN RIDING
FOR THE HANDICAPPED
ASSOCIATION
111 East Wacker Drive,
Suite 600
Chicago, IL 60601

THERAPEUTIC EQUESTRIANS
c/o Pat Morris
8401 Bella Vista
Alta Loma, CA 91701

THERAPEUTIC
HORSEMANSHIP
3209 18th Avenue South
Minneapolis, MN 55407

WINSLOW RIDING FOR THE
HANDICAPPED
Mr. & Mrs. Wolf
4 Colleen Court
Novato, CA 94947

WINSLOW THERAPEUTIC
RIDING UNLIMITED, INC.
c/o Virginia G. Mazza
3408 South Route 94
Warwich, NY 10990

Hunting

DISABLED SPORTSMEN OF
AMERICA
P.O. Box 26
Vinton, VA 24179

Ice Skating

BRECKENRIDGE OUTDOOR
EDUCATION CENTER
See Camping/Hiking

INTERNATIONAL COUNCIL
ON THERAPEUTIC ICE
SKATING
P.O. Box 13
State College, PA 16801

SKATING ASSOCIATION FOR
BLIND AND HANDICAPPED
c/o Elizabeth O'Donnell
3236 Main Street
Buffalo, NY 14214

Ice Sledding

BRECKENRIDGE OUTDOOR
EDUCATION CENTER
See Camping/Hiking

Kayaking

NANTAHALA OUTDOOR
CENTER
Star Route Box 68
Bryson City, NC 28613

RICK CICCOTTO
Route 2, Box 589
Moncks Corner, SC 29461

Motorcycling

BRITISH WHEELCHAIR
MOTORCYCLING ASSOC.
55 Lochinvar
Birchill, Bracknell
Berks RG12 4LD, England

NATIONAL WHEELCHAIR
ATHLETIC ASSOCIATION
See Aquatics

PARALYZED VETERANS OF
AMERICA
c/o Jack Powell
801 18th Street, NW
Washington, DC 20006

WHEELCHAIR MOTORCYCLE
ASSOCIATION
c/o Dr. Eli Factor
101 Torrey Street
Brockton, MA 02401

Mountain Climbing

BRECKENRIDGE OUTDOOR
EDUCATION CENTER
See Camping/Hiking

NATIONAL HANDICAPPED
SPORTS AND RECREATION
ASSOCIATION
See Aquatics

RICK RILEY
c/o Orthotics & Prosthetics Assoc.
500 Jackson Street
Methuen, MA 01844

S.O.A.R. (SHARED OUTDOOR
ADVENTURE RECREATION)
c/o Linda Besant
P.O. Box 14583
Portland, OR 97214

S'PLORE
See Boating/Sailing

WILDERNESS II
c/o Greg Lais
1313 5th Street, SE, Suite 327A
Minneapolis, MN 55414

Music

NATIONAL ASSOCIATION FOR
MUSIC THERAPY
P.O. Box 610
Lawrence, KS 66044

Racquet Sports

AMERICAN AMATEUR
RACQUETBALL ASSOCIATION
U.S. Wheelchair Racquet Sports
Association
1941 Vienta Veraro Drive
Diamond Bar, CA 91765

NATIONAL WHEELCHAIR
RACQUETBALL ASSOCIATION
c/o AARA, Luke Street Onge
815 North Weber, Suite 203
Colorado Springs, CO 80903

RECREATION & ATHLETIC
REHAB EDUCATION CENTER
See Football

U.S. AMPUTEE ATHLETIC
ASSOCIATION
See Golf

Rugby

U.S. QUAD RUGBY ASSOC.
c/o Brad Mikkelson
811 Northwestern Drive
Grand Forks, ND 58201

Roller Skating

AMPUTEE SPORTS
ASSOCIATION
See Aquatics

CHILDREN'S HOSPITAL
ADOLESCENT & YOUNG
ADULT AMPUTEE PROGRAM
c/o Gay Gregg
P.O. Box 99776
125 DeSoto Street
Pittsburgh, PA 15233

DREW A. HITTENBERGER
Prosthetics Research Study
1102 Columbia
Seattle, WA 98104

U.S. AMATEUR
CONFEDERATION ROLLING
SKATING ASSOCIATION
Special Olympics
c/o Nancy Kirk
P.O. Box 81846
Lincoln, NE 68501

Running

ADAPTIVE SPORTS PROGRAM
Kinesiotherapy Clinic
University of Toledo
c/o Dr. Leonard Greninger
2801 W. Bancroft Street
Toledo, OH 43606

AMERICAN AMPUTEE
RUNNING TEAM
c/o George DuPontis
P.O. Box 370788
Miami, FL 33137

INTRN. RUNNING CTR.
c/o Dick Traum
9 East 89th Street
New York, NY 10128

RECREATION & ATHLETIC
REHAB EDUCATION CENTER
See Football

Sailing

See Boating

Scuba Diving

CANADIAN WHEELCHAIR
SPORTS ASSOCIATION
1875 W. 8th Avenue, #403
Vancouver, British Columbia V6J
1V9

HANDICAPPED SCUBA
ASSOCIATION
1104 El Prado
San Clemente, CA 92672

NATIONAL HANDICAPPED
SPORTS & RECREATION
ASSOCIATION (NHSRA)
See Aquatics

Self Defense

HAKKORYU MARTIAL ARTS
FEDERATION
Dennis Palumbo
12028F E. Mississippi Avenue
Aurora, CO 80012

STANLEY K. GORDON
VA Spinal Cord Injury Clinic
Long Beach, CA 90822

Skateboarding

ADAPTIVE SPORTS PROGRAM
See Running

AMERICAN SPECIAL
RECREATION ASSOCIATION
Rec. Education Program
University of Iowa
Iowa City, IA 52240

U.S. AMPUTEE ATHLETIC
ASSOCIATION
See Golf

Skydiving

BRECKENRIDGE OUTDOOR
EDUCATION CENTER
See Camping/Hiking

UNITED STATES PARACHUTE
ASSOCIATION
c/o Mike Johnston
1440 Duke Street
Alexandria, VA 22314

Snowmobiling

NEW ENGLAND
HANDICAPPED SPORTSMEN'S
ASSOCIATION
c/o Earl Plummer
26 McFarlin Road
Clemsford, MA 01824

SEATTLE HANDICAPPED
SPORTS & REC. ASSOC.
(NHSRA)
c/o Dee Melchow
17017 Tenth Avenue, NE
Seattle, WA 98155

S.O.A.R.
See Mountain Climbing

S'PLORE
See Boating/Sailing

VETERANS ADMINISTRATION
MEDICAL CENTER
Prosthetic Treatment Center
c/o Ellis Hensley
1660 S. Columbian Way
Seattle, WA 98108

WILDERNESS INQUIRY II
c/o Greg Lais
1313 5th Street, SE, Suite 327A
Minneapolis, MN 55414

WINTER PARK SPORTS &
LEARNING CENTER
c/o Hal O'Leary
P.O. Box 36
Winter Park, CO 80482

Snow Skiing

ADAPTED SPORTS
ASSOCIATION
c/o Allen A. Hayes
P.O. Box 299
Miller Place, NY 11764

ALBERTA ASSOCIATION FOR
DISABLED SKIING
Box 875, Station M
Calgary, Alberta T2P 2J6

ALPINE ALTERNATIVES
c/o Marty Decker
1634 West 13th Street
Anchorage, AK 99501

ARROYA CERTIFICATION
GUIDELINES
Rehabilitation R & D 153
V.A. Medical Center
3801 Miranda Avenue
Palo Alto, CA 94304

ASPEN HANDICAPPED SKIERS
Box 5429/0174 Meadows Road
Snowmass Village, CO 81615

BRECKENRIDGE OUTDOOR
EDUCATION CENTER
See Camping/Hiking

CANADIAN ASSOCIATION FOR
DISABLED SKIING
P.O. Box 307
Kimberly, British Columbia, V1A
2Y9

CHILDREN'S HOSPITAL
ADOLESCENT & YOUNG
ADULT AMPUTEE PROGRAM
See Roller Skating

DISABLED SKIERS
ASSOCIATION OF BRITISH
COLUMBIA
1200 Hornby Street
Vancouver, British Columbia, V6Z
2E2

52 ASSOCIATION
See Football

NATIONAL HANDICAPPED
SPORTS & RECREATION
ASSOCIATION (NHSRA)
See Aquatics

NEW ENGLAND
HANDICAPPED SPORTSMAN
ASSOCIATION
See Snowmobiling

ONTARIO HANDICAPPED SKI
ASSOCIATION
1220 Sheppard Avenue, East
Willowdale, Ontario M2K 2X1

OUTDOOR WILDERNESS
PROGRAM
Crotched Mountain Center
Greenfield, NH 03047

RECREATION & ATHLETIC
REHAB EDUCATION CENTER
See Football

RICK RILEY
c/o Orthotics & Prosthetics
500 Jackson Street
Methuen, MA 01844

SKI-FOR-ALL FOUNDATION
c/o Joan C. Steck
4160 86th Street SE
Mercer Island, WA 98040

SNOWBIRD HANDICAPPED
SKIER PROGRAM, INC.
c/o Peter Mandler
2274 Arbor Lane, Apt. 6
Salt Lake City, UT 84117

SNOWMASS SKI SCHOOL (FOR
THE HANDICAPPED)
c/o Edwin H. Lucks
P.O. Box 5429
Snowmass Village, CO 81615

S.O.A.R.
See Mountain Climbing

S'PLORE
See Boating/Sailing

STATE OF COLORADO
DIVISION OF REHAB
c/o Mark Litvin
835 Second Avenue #425
Durango, CO 81301

TAHOE HANDICAPPED SKI
SCHOOL
c/o Larry Young
P.O. Box 1636
Truckee, CA 95734

WILDERNESS INQUIRY II
See Snowmobiling

WINTER PARK SPORTS &
LEARNING CENTER
See Snowmobiling

Soccer

INTERNATIONAL GAMES FOR
THE DISABLED
c/o Michael Mushett
Eisenhower Park
East Meadow, NY 11554

RECREATION & ATHLETIC
REHAB EDUCATION CENTER
See Football

UNITED CEREBRAL PALSY
c/o Jeffrey Jones
7700 Second Avenue
Detroit, MI 48202

Softball

NATIONAL WHEELCHAIR
SOFTBALL ASSOCIATION
P.O. Box 22478
Minneapolis, MN 55422

NATIONAL WHEELCHAIR
SOFTBALL ASSOCIATION
c/o Dave Van Buskirk
P.O. Box 737
Sioux Falls, SD 57101-0737

Tennis

INTERNATIONAL
FOUNDATION OF
WHEELCHAIR TENNIS
1909 Ala Wai Blvd.
#1507
Honolulu, HI 96815

NATIONAL FOUNDATION OF
WHEELCHAIR TENNIS
15441 Red Hill Avenue,
Suite A
Tustin, CA 92680

TENNIS FOUNDATION OF
NORTH AMERICA
Jr. Wheelchair Sports Camp
200 Castlewood Drive
North Palm Beach, FL 33408

U.S. AMPUTEE ATHLETIC
ASSOCIATION
See Golf

U.S. TENNIS ASSOCIATION
Education & Research Center
729 Alexander Road
Princeton, NJ 08540

U.S. WHEELCHAIR TABLE
TENNIS ASSOCIATION
3617 Betty Drive, Suite S
Colorado Springs, CO 80917

Track & Field

NATIONAL WHEELCHAIR
ATHLETIC ASSOCIATION
See Aquatics

PARALYZED VETERANS OF
AMERICA
c/o Jack Powell
801 18th Street, NW
Washington, DC 20006

U.S. AMPUTEE ATHLETIC
ASSOCIATION
See Golf

Triathlon

BACHMAN RECREATION
CENTER
2750 Bachman Drive
Dallas, TX 75220
   Annual Dallas Wheelchair Tri-
athlon

NATIONAL TRIATHLON FOR
THE PHYSICALLY DISABLED
VA Medical Center
3801 Miranda Avenue
Palo Alto, CA 94304
also
De Anza College
P.O. Box 1484
Cupertino, CA 95015

Volleyball

CANADIAN WHEELCHAIR
SPORTS ASSOCIATION
See Air Guns

Wheelchair Racing

CAPITOL CITY MARATHON
ASSOCIATION
c/o Dr. James McDowell
P.O. Box 1681
Olympia, WA 98507

INTERNATIONAL
WHEELCHAIR ROAD RACING
CLUB
c/o George Murray
165 78th Avenue, NE
St. Petersburg, FL 33702

MOSS REHABILITATION
HOSPITAL
c/o Lois S. Levy
12th Street & Tabor Road
Philadelphia, PA 19141

NATIONAL WHEELCHAIR
ATHLETIC ASSOCIATION
See Aquatics

NATIONAL WHEELCHAIR
MARATHON
c/o Bob Hall
15 Marlborough Street
Belmont, MA 02178

NATIONAL WHEELCHAIR
MARATHON COMMITTEE
149 California Street
Newton, MA 02158
Wilderness Activity Programs

BLUE SPRUCE LODGE GUEST
RANCH
451 Martin Creek Road
Trout Creek, MT 59847

BRECKENRIDGE OUTDOOR
EDUCATION CENTER
See Camping/Hiking

COOPERATIVE WILDERNESS
HANDICAPPED OUTDOOR
GROUP
Idaho State University
P.O. Box 8118
Pocatello, ID 83209

WILDERNESS INQUIRY II
See Snowmobiling

ACCESSIBLE TRAVEL

ABILITY TOURS, INC.
719 Delaware Avenue S.W.
Washington, DC 20024

ACCESS TO THE SKIES
R.I.U.S.A.
1123 Broadway
New York, NY 10010
Information concerning all aspects of travel for persons with disabilities, especially airline accessibility features.

ACCESSIBLE ADVENTURES
1050 Brownlee Road
P.O. Box 16137
Memphis, TN 38116

ALL OUTDOORS, INC.
P.O. Box 1100
Redmond, OR 97756
Year-round outdoor challenge trips for the physically challenged.

AMERICAN AUTOMOBILE ASSOCIATION
Traffic Safety Dept.
8111 Gatehouse Road
Falls Church, VA 22047
Or your local AAA Office, "Handicapped Driver's Mobility Guide"

AMIGO TRAVEL
2125 Louisiana NE, Suite 140
Albuquerque, NM
Official agent for U.S. Disabled Team competing in the 1988 Paralympic in Seoul, Korea.

AMTRAK PUBLIC AFFAIRS
955 L'Enfant Plaza SW
Washington, DC 20024
(800) 523-5720
Information on accessibility of trains and stations and assistance for handicapped passengers; also a brochure, "Access Amtrak."

ANYONE CAN TRAVEL
24000 Alicia Parkway,
Suite 16
Mission Viejo, CA 92691

AUSTRALIAN TRAVEL FOR THE DISABLED
105 William Street
Perth, WA 6000 Australia

BOOK PASSAGE
57 Post Street
San Francisco, CA 94104
Books: *Access to the World*; *Access in London, A Guide for the Disabled Traveler.*

BRIDGES FOR PEACE
P.O. Box 33145
Tulsa, OK 74153
Study mission tour series of the Holy Land for the disabled traveler.

BLACKWOOD TRAVEL CENTER, INC.
One Union National Plaza # 100
Little Rock, AR 72201

CANADIAN PARAPLEGIC ASSOCIATION
520 Sutherland Drive
Toronto, Ontario M4G 3V9 Canada
Will provide specialized information on travel through their provincial divisions.

CAN WE TRAVEL
553 Broadway
Massapequa, NY 11758

CATHOLIC TRAVEL OFFICE
4701 Willard Avenue, Suite 226
Chevy Chase, MD 20815
Sponsors worldwide group tours and pilgrimages to Lourdes.

CLUB ACCESS
P.O. Box 502
Manhattan Beach, CA 90266
Non-profit organization serving the disabled community—provides driver and van, a specialized transportation service.

DEANZA COLLEGE (STUDY TOURS)
21250 Stevens Creek Blvd.
Cupertino, CA 95014

ENVIRONMENTAL TRAVELING COMPANIONS
Fort Mason Center
Bldg. C
San Francisco, CA 94123
Non-profit agency provides access to the wilderness and environmental education activities.

EVERGREEN TRAVEL SERVICE
19505 44th Street West
Lynnwood, WA 98036
(800) 435-2288
(800) 562-9298 in Washington

FABER TRAVEL, INC.
540 East Liberty
Ann Arbor, MI 48104

FLYING WHEELS TRAVEL, INC.
143 West Bridge
P.O. Box 382
Owatonna, MN 55060
(800) 533-0363
(800) 722-9351 in Minnesota
Offers tours for accompanied or unaccompanied disabled travelers.

GREYHOUND LINES, INC.
Section S
Greyhound Tower
Phoenix, AZ 85077
Has "Helping Hand" service, where a companion and the disabled person travel on a single ticket, also brochure "Reach for Greyhound's Helping Hand."

HANDICAPPED TRAVEL CLUB
Jim Bley
945 North Pasadena
#49
Mesa, AZ 85201-4312
Mostly people with recreational vehicles.

HANDICAPPED TRAVELER ASSOCIATION
1291 East Hillside Blvd.
Foster City, CA 94404
Helps to arrange airline accommodations.

HAPPY HOLIDAY TRAVEL
2550 N.E. 15th Avenue
Wilton Manor, FL 33305

IAMAT
(INTERNATIONAL
ASSOCIATION FOR MEDICAL
ASSISTANCE TO TRAVELERS)
417 Center Street
Lewiston, NY 14092

INCREDIBLE JOURNEYS
5721 Oso Avenue
Woodland Hills, CA 91367

INTERMEDIC
777 Third Avenue
New York, NY 10017
Directory of physicians around
the world; yearly membership fee.

IRISH TOURIST BOARD
590 Fifth Avenue
New York, NY 10036
Free booklet: "Discover Ireland:
Activities and Facilities for Disabled
Persons."

KEROUL
1415 rue Jarry E
Montreal, Quebec H2E 277
Membership travel organization.

LTD TRAVEL
116 Harbor Seal Court
San Mateo, CA 94404
Also publishes a newsletter for
disabled travelers.

MOBILITY INTERNATIONAL
62 Union Street
London SE1 1TD, England
Non-profit organization encouraging a mix of disabled and able-
bodied persons—offices in twenty-
five countries.

MOBILITY INTERNATIONAL
USA
P.O. Box 3551
Eugene, OR 97403

NATIONAL EASTER SEAL
SOCIETY
2023 West Ogden Avenue
Chicago, IL 60612
Maintains a list of motels which
accommodate wheelchair users.

NATIONAL PARK SERVICE
For information on park facilities, fees, or special programs for
handicapped persons, write to the
regional office serving your area of
interest:

NORTH ATLANTIC REGIONAL
OFFICE
15 State Street
Boston, MA 02109

MID-ATLANTIC REGIONAL
OFFICE
143 South Third Street
Philadelphia, PA 19106

NATIONAL CAPITAL
REGIONAL OFFICE
1100 Ohio Drive SW
Washington, DC 20242

SOUTHEAST REGIONAL
OFFICE
1895 Phoenix Blvd.
Atlanta, GA 30349

MIDWEST REGIONAL OFFICE
1709 Jackson Street
Omaha, NE 68102

ROCKY MOUNTAIN
REGIONAL OFFICE
655 Parfet Street
P.O. Box 25287
Denver, CO 80225

SOUTHWEST REGIONAL
OFFICE
P.O. Box 728
Santa Fe, NM 87501

WESTERN REGIONAL OFFICE
450 Golden Gate Avenue
P.O. Box 36063
San Francisco, CA 94102

PACIFIC NORTHWEST
REGIONAL OFFICE
601 Fourth & Pike Bldg.
Seattle, WA 98101
For a complete listing of all national parks, including a description
of services for handicapped visitors,
send $3.50 for the publication "Ac-
cess National Parks," #024-005-
0069-5 to:

U.S. Government Printing Office,
Washington, DC 20402.

NEW HAVEN TRAVEL
SERVICE
900 Chapel Street, Suite 325
New Haven, CT 06510
(800) 243-1806
European tours for the disabled
traveler accompanied by an able-
bodied companion.

OUTBACK RANCH
OUTFITTERS
Ken Wick
P.O. Box 384
Joseph, OR 97846

PALEX TOURS
59 Ha'atzmouth Road
Haifa 31033 Israel
Special tour package for disabled
travelers.

PARALYZED VETERANS OF
AMERICA
801 18th Street
Washington, DC 20014
PVA has a list of motels with
accessible facilities.

PINETREE TOURS, INC.
3600 Wilshire Blvd., Suite 1712
Los Angeles, CA 90010

POWERS TRAVEL AGENCY
(Dream Spinner Tours)
23901 Michigan Avenue
Dearborn, MI 48124

PROFESSIONAL RESPITE
CARE
6460 East Yale CD 261
Denver, CO 80222
Provides nurses as medical
traveling companions.

RAMBLING TOURS, INC.
P.O. Box 1304
Hallandale, FL 33009

REHABILITATION
INTERNATIONAL, USA, INC.
20 West 40th Street
New York, NY 10018
Publishes "International Dir-
ectory of Access Guides."

RENTAL CARS WITH HAND
CONTROLS:
AVIS: All locations, minimum of
two weeks' notice, call toll-free
(800) 331-1212.
HERTZ: Major cities plus
numerous Florida locations, minimum of ten days' notice, call toll-
free (800) 654-3131.

NATIONAL: In Atlanta, Chicago, Detroit, the District of Columbia, Minneapolis /St. Paul, Houston, Los Angeles, Miami, Phoenix, and San Francisco —minimum of 48 hours notice —available in other cities if requests for reservations are made well in advance, call toll-free (800) 328-4567.

ROYAL ASSOCIATION FOR DISABILITY & REHABILITATION-RADAR
25 Mortimer Street
London WIN 8AB, England
Has access guides on airports, country-side, railway, cities, underground, and public conveniences.

SOCIETY FOR ADVANCEMENT OF TRAVEL FOR THE HANDICAPPED
26 Court Street
Brooklyn, NY 11242
Clearinghouse for information on accessible lodgings. It consists of travel agents, innkeepers, and sightseeing companies with an interest in travelers who have disabilities.

SWEDISH TOURIST BOARD
P.O. Box 7473
S-103 92 Stockholm,
Sweden
Special tours for disabled.

TRAVEL INFORMATION CENTER MOSS REHABILITATION HOSPITAL
12th Street and Tabor Road
Philadelphia, PA 19141
(215) 329-5715
Maintains a travel information center for persons with physical disabilities. Includes an extensive collection of data on topics such as accessible hotels, restaurants, transportation and cultural facilities, airline regulations, and cruises. Request for information can be handled by phone or mail.

TWIN PEAKS PRESS
P.O. Box 8097
Portland, OR 97207
Travel for the Disabled: A Handbook of Travel Resources and 500 Worldwide Access Guides

WALT DISNEY WORLD
Guest Letters Department
P.O. Box 40
Lake Buena Vista, FL 32830

Walt Disney World offers a booklet for disabled guests who are planning to visit the theme park in Orlando, Florida. *Disabled Guests Guidebook* gives information about wheelchair access and answers questions about accommodations for the sight and hearing impaired. A copy may be obtained at guest relations locations in the Magic Kingdom's City Hall or Epcot Center's Earth Station or by writing the address above.

WHEELCHAIR WAGON TOURS
P.O. Box 1270
Kissimmee, FL 32742
Walt Disney World, Epcot Center, Sea World, Cypress Gardens, Kennedy Space Center, Water Mania, and various Dinner Theater Tours for the Disabled.

WHOLE PERSON TOURS
P.O. Box 1084
Bayonne, NJ 07002-1084
Offers accessible tours for travelers with disabilities; also publishes *The Itinerary* (a bi-monthly travel magazine for the disabled traveler).

WINGS ON WHEELS
Evergreen Travel Tours Service
19505L 44th Avenue West
West Lynwood, WA 98036

MAGAZINES AND NEWSLETTERS

ABILITY

A semi-annual (Fall & Summer) full color glossy covering a variety of disabilities, with special emphasis on amputees. Issues are divided into features on living, working, playing, and entertainment.
P.O. Box 370788, Miami, FL 33137
(305) 751-2525

ABLE BODIES

A quarterly tabloid mostly oriented toward member-professionals who work with people with disabilities in physical education, but its coverage of sports, competitive and recreation activities is of interest to consumers, too. AAHPERD also offers an extensive publications service for books, audiovisuals, and periodicals on the topics of adapted PE, dance, fitness, research, etc.
AAHPERD, 1900 Association Drive, Reston, VA 22091
(703) 476-3430

ACCENT ON LIVING MAGAZINE

In the early 1950's Raymond C. Cheever, Publisher, was totally paralyzed from polio and spent some time in an iron lung. When he regained partial use of his muscles, he began looking for assistive devices to help him be more independent. He soon realized he couldn't even find a place to buy a wheelchair. Therefore, in 1956, he and his wife started *Accent on Living Magazine* to provide a means for disabled people to find out about products that were available but hard to find. It has become a place where products are presented and ideas introduced. Information comes from rehabilitation professionals, other experts in the field, advertisers, and professional writers across the country. A unique and important source of information is the readers themselves —the people who understand the problems and have worked out solutions.

Gillun Road and High Drive, P.O. Box 700, Bloomington, IL 61701
(309) 378-2961

ACHIEVEMENT
925 N.W. 122nd, North Miami, FL 33161 (monthly)

ADVOCATE, NEW YORK STATE NEWSLETTER FOR THE DISABLED
Office of Advocate for the Disabled, One Empire State Plaza, Albany, NY 12223-0001

AGEING INTERNATIONAL

A periodical which regularly covers aging with a disability. It is published twice a year in English and Spanish by the International Federation On Ageing.
1909 K. Street N.W., Washington, DC 20049

AMERICAN JOURNAL OF ART THERAPY
6010 Board Branch Road, N.W., Washington, DC 20015

AMERICAN REHABILITATION
Superintendent of Documents, U.S. Government Printing Office Washington, DC 20402 (quarterly)

BE STROKE SMART

Published quarterly by: National Stroke Association (NSA), 300 East Hampden Avenue, Suite 240, Englewood, CO 80110-2622
(303) 762-9922

BREAKING NEW GROUND

A newsletter for farmers with physical disabilities. Department of Agricultural Engineering, Agricultural Engineering Building, Purdue University, West Lafayette, IN 47907

BREAKOUT

A national magazine, features on services and consumer products.
400 E. Randolph, Suite 223, Chicago, IL 60601

BULLETINS ON SCIENCE AND TECHNOLOGY FOR THE HANDICAPPED

American Association for the Advancement of Science, Office of Opportunities in Science, 1776 Massachusetts Avenue N.W., Washington, DC 20036 (No subscription charge; quarterly.)

CAN-DO

A newsletter for the exchange of information on devices and methods to reduce physical limitations.
5427 Redfield, Dallas, TX 75235

CAPITOL NEWS

The purpose is to inform NOD Community partners in 1900 towns, cities, and counties throughout the U.S. about pending and enacting federal legislation.
National Organization on Disability, 910 16th Street, N.W., Suite 600, Washington, DC 20006
(202) 293-5960

CAREERS AND THE HANDICAPPED

Equal Opportunity Publication, Inc., 44 Broadway, Greenlawn, NY 11740

CHALLENGED AMERICAN (formerly MOVING FORWARD)

A colorful bi-monthly national tabloid newspaper for people with disabilities. Includes interviews, new products, legal, business, and entertainment articles.
Box 4310, Sunland, CA 91040
(818) 353-3380

COMPUTER-DISABILITY NEWS

The National Easter Seal Society's quarterly technology publication. C-DN makes computer news exciting and easy to understand, listing numerous key resources and contacts for readers to follow up for more information.
c/o The National Easter Seal Society, 2023 West Ogden Avenue, Chicago, IL 60612
(312) 667-7400

DIALOGUE MAGAZINE

Founded in 1961 by Lion Don O. Nold and originally called "The Talking Lion." It is the only independently published magazine of general interest written and edited for the blind. It is a quarterly magazine produced on 1/2 speed cassette, 8 1/2 rpm disc, in braille, and in large print editions. Every issue contains interviews with successful blind people, reports on recent legislation, new products and services, homemaking and gardening tips, recipes, and information about vocational, recreational, and travel opportunities. Every issue also features stories, articles, and poems by blind authors. *Dialogue Magazine* is read in all fifty states, the District of Columbia, and in over fifty countries around the world.
World Headquarters Building, 3100 South Oak Park Avenue, Berwyn, IL 60402-3095
(312) 749-1908

DISABLED USA

A quarterly published by the President's Committee on Employment of the Handicapped. Emphasis is on work, rehabilitation issues, independent living, politics and civil rights, tools for access, and opportunity. Articles range from job strategies to sex surrogates, to computers to unobvious disabilities. The President's Committee also makes a few complimentary subscriptions available.
1111 20th Street N.W., Washington, DC 20036

FORUM PWI

Multi Resource Centers, Inc., 1900 Chicago Avenue South, Minneapolis, MN 55404.
Published six times a year.

HANDICAP NEWS

3060 East Bridge Street, # 342, Brighton, CO 80601

HANDICAPPED AMERICANS REPORTS

951 Pershing Drive, Silver Spring, MD 20910

HANDICAPPED SPORTS REPORT

National Handicapped Sports and Recreation Association, Farragut Station, P.O. Box 33141, Washington, DC 20033

ILRU INSIGHTS

The National Newsletter for Independent Living
A publication of the ILRU Research and Training Center on Independent Living at The Texas Institute for Rehabilitation and Research (TIRR).
Independent Living Research Utilization, 3400 Bissonnet, Suite 101, Houston, TX 77005
(713) 666-6244

IN-STEP NEWSLETTER

A self-help group for amputees, their families and friends.
350 Engle Street, Englewood, NJ 07631.

IN THE MAINSTREAM, Mainstream Inc.

Counsels consumers, business, government, and school systems on barrier removal, affirmative action, and attitude change.
1200 15th Street N.W., Washington, DC 20005
(202) 833-1139

INCITEMENT

American Disabled for Accessible Public Transportation
2810 Pearl, Austin, TX 78705

ITINERARY

P.O. Box 1084, Bayonne, NJ 07002
(bi-monthly)

IT'S ABOUT TIME

Joseph Bulova School, 4024 62nd Street, P.O. Box 465, Woodside, NY 11377 (quarterly)

JODIE, A Newsletter

JODIE is a newsletter that started because of a need for communication among people with disabilities. The name *JODIE* is an acronym for Join Other Disabled for Information Exchange. The newsletter is made up almost entirely of reader input and pro-vides the means whereby people help each other.
P.O. Box 1045, Mill Valley, CA 94942

JOURNAL OF REHABILITATION

633 S. Washington Street, Alexandria, VA 22314 (bi-monthly)

KALEIDOSCOPE

An international magazine of literature and fine arts for people who have disabilities. The magazine accepts tough-minded, unsentimental, disability-related fiction, poetry, visual art, and cartoons.
326 Locust Street, Akron, OH 44302

MAINSTREAM

A full color glossy national magazine "of the able disabled". Covers the full gamut of topics for people with a variety of disabilities—from civil rights to aerobics to travel to interviewing tips for job hunters. The emphasis is shifting somewhat toward more political activism, with regular columns on disability issues, and on legal rights/disability law.
861 Sixth Avenue, Suite 610, San Diego, CA 92101 (monthly)

MATILDA ZIEGLER MAGAZINE FOR THE BLIND

Published at no cost to its readers since 1907. Named for its founder, Mrs. William Ziegler, who endowed it for free distribution to those unable to read print. *The Ziegler* features topical articles selected from a wide range of periodicals, book excerpts, fiction, poetry, and humor. It includes news of special interest to blind and visually impaired people and has a Reader's Forum, where readers express opinions and exchange ideas. *The Ziegler* is issued ten times a year in two editions: Grade 2 braille and disc (8 rpm, playable only on Library of Congress talking book record player).
20 West 17th Street, New York, NY 10011
(212) 242-0263

MENTAL AND PHYSICAL DISABILITY LAW REPORTER

Published by the American Bar Association's Commission on the Mentally Disabled. A bimonthly journal containing recent court decisions, case updates, legislative and regulatory developments, timely articles, legal analyses, and periodic statutory reviews.
American Bar Association Commission on the Mentally Disabled, 1800 M Street, NW, Washington, DC 20036

MRC RELAY

A newsletter with innovative approaches to human services.
Multi Resource Centers, Inc., 1900 Chicago Avenue, Minneapolis, MN 55404

NCILP NEWSLETTER

Published quarterly by the National Council of Independent Living Programs.
4397 La Clede Avenue, St. Louis, MO 631208

NATIONAL INFORMATION CENTER FOR HANDICAPPED CHILDREN AND YOUTH NEWSLETTER

P.O. Box 1492, Washington, DC 20013 (bi-monthly)

NATIONAL SPOKESMAN

This newsletter reports on new developments in a wide range of fields of interest to people with epilepsy and to those who provide services to them.
The Epilepsy Foundation of America, 4351 Garden City Drive, Landover, MD 20785

PALAESTRA: THE FORUM OF SPORT & PHYSICAL EDUCATION FOR THE DISABLED

P.O. Box 508, Macomb, IL 61455
(309) 833-1902

PARAPLEGIA LIFE

National Spinal Cord Injury Association, 149 California Street, Newton, MA 02158

PARAPLEGIA NEWS

5201 N. 19th Avenue, Suite 111, Phoenix, AZ 85015

POSITIVE APPROACH

CTEC, 1600 Malone Street, Municipal Airport, Millville, NJ 08332
(609) 327-4040

PROGRAMS FOR THE HANDICAPPED—CLEARING-HOUSE ON THE HANDICAPPED

Office of Special Education and Rehabilitation Services, U.S. Dept. of Education, Room 3119, Switzer Bldg., Washington, DC 20202 (bi-monthly)

PROJECT NEWSLETTER

Model For Interagency Coordination Of Technology Resources

The goal of this project is to facilitate access to technology devices for individuals who have disabilities.
Interagency Coordination Project, SUNY/Buffalo, 3435 Main Street, 517 Kimball Tower, Buffalo, NY 14214

REGIONAL MOBILITY LIMITED

Printed for the Colorado and Rocky Mountain Region eleven times a year. Lots of features on a wide range of topics including legal matters, self-defense, research, travel, etc. The publication also follows the stocks of publicly-traded companies in the disability field.
401 Linden Drive, Fort Collins, CO 80524
(303) 484-3800

REHABILITATION DIGEST

Offers news, views, and in-depth articles on physical rehabilitation, for professionals and disabled people. The magazine reaches a unique audience of active and concerned people, both nationally and internationally. It is published by the Canadian Rehabilitation Council for the Disabled, CRCD, an association of over eighty non-profit organizations whose objectives and activities are directed towards ensuring the provision of comprehensive rehabilitation services for physically disabled adults and children.
One Yonge Street, Suite 2110, Toronto, Ontario M5E 1E5

REHABILITATION GAZETTE

Gazette International Networking Institute, 4502 Maryland Avenue, St. Louis, MO 63108 (annual)

REHABILITATION INTERNATIONAL NEWSLETTER

Provides brief items of information on significant events and developments around the world. Published between issues of the *International Rehabilitation Review*, the *Newsletter* reports on meetings, people, awards, and Rehabilitation International activities.

Rehabilitation International, 25 East Street, New York, NY 10010

REHABILITATION TECHNOLOGY REVIEW

A newsletter for the Association for the Advancement of Rehabilitation Technology.
1101 Connecticut Avenue, N.W., Suite 700, Washington, DC 20036

REHABILITATION WORLD

Rehabilitation International USA, 1123 Broadway, New York, NY 10010

RURAL TRANSPORTATION REPORTER

1312 18th Street N.W., Washington, DC 20036

SHHH SELF HELP FOR HARD OF HEARING PEOPLE

This is a bi-monthly journal published specifically for hard of hearing people. An important service offered by SHHH is attention to individual problems. Everyone requesting assistance and advice is answered personally by someone on the staff with a particular area of expertise.
7800 Wisconsin Avenue, Bethesda, MD 20814

THE SOURCE

P.O. Box 7956, Rockford, IL 61126
(815) 397-9638

SIA NEWSLETTER

Spinal Injuries Association, Yeoman House, 76 St. James's Lane, London N10 3DF, England

SPORTS N' SPOKES

News, feature stories, calendar, product reports, profiles, and resource lists.
PVA Publications, 5201 N. 19th Avenue, Phoenix, AZ 85105-9986
(602) 246-9426

TASH NEWSLETTER—THE ASSOCIATION FOR PERSONS WITH SEVERE HANDICAPS

Aims to disseminate information on any/ all aspects of the education of people who have severe/profound handicaps, and to facilitate communication among its readers.
7010 Roosevelt Way N.E., Seattle, WA 98115
(206) 523-8446

TOGETHER
News for the rehabilitation community.
20 Park Plaza, Room 330, Boston, MA 02116

TRAVEL TALK
The publication of Wheelchair Journeys, published four times a year.
Division of Redmond Travel, 16979 Redmond Way, Redmond, WA 98052
(206) 885-2210

VOICE OF THE PHYSICALLY CHALLENGED (formerly PYRAMID)
News features, resources, book reviews, calendar, sports, profiles, etc.

Contact: L.I. Family Publications, 222 Sunrise Highway, Rockville Center, New York, NY 11570
(516) 536-4900

VOICE: THE MAGAZINE FOR HEARING IMPAIRED PEOPLE
A five-year-old national magazine. Hearing impaired consumers, parents, and professionals read this publication which does not distinguish between "deafness" and "hearing impairment." *The Voice* is not affiliated with any organization.
Rt. 1, Box 177, Ingleside, TX 78362
(512) 776-2003

WHOLE ACCESS QUARTERLY
A quarterly report to consumers and caregivers, published by the authors of *The First Whole Rehab Catalog.* Includes reviews of products and services and continuously updated information about funding opportunities. *Whole Access Quarterly* is available by subscription to libraries, educational institutions, rehabilitation agencies, professionals, and physically and/or perceptually challenged consumers.
SR 12479, Box 209, Phoenicia, NY 12464
(914) 688-2091

THE WRITE AGE–FIRST MAGAZINE OF WRITING THERAPY
Popular style by and for mid-age to older general readers, the physically impaired, those in transition, and group facilitators.
P.O. Box 722, Menomonee Falls, WI 53051
(414) 255-7706

✶✶✶✶

INDEX